Nursing Research and Statistics

Nursing Research and Statistics

Anurag Bhai Patidar

MSc (N), PhD Scholar

Lecturer, Bhopal Nursing College

Bhopal Memorial Hospital & Research Centre

Indian Council of Medical Research, Department of Health Research

Ministry of Health & Family Welfare, Union Government of India

Universities Press

UNIVERSITIES PRESS (INDIA) PRIVATE LIMITED
Registered Office
3-6-747/1/A & 3-6-754/1, Himayatnagar, Hyderabad 500 029, Telangana, India
e-mail: info@universitiespress.com: www.universitiespress.com

Distributed by
Orient Blackswan Private Limited

Registered Office
e-mail: info@universitiespress.com; www.universitiespress.com

Other Offices
Bengaluru/ Bhopal/ Chennai/ Ernakulam/ Guwahati/ Hyderabad
Jaipur/ Kolkata/ Lucknow/ Mumbai/ New Delhi/ Noida/ Patna

First published by Universities Press 2016

ISBN: 978-81-7371-979-0

Typeset in Adobe Garamond Pro 12/14 *by*
Bookcraft Publishing Services (I) Pvt Ltd, Chennai

Printed in India at
B.B. Press, Noida

Published by
Universities Press (India) Private Limited
1/24 Asaf Ali Road, New Delhi 110002, India

To my parents,

Shri Sawai Lal
and
Smt Jawala Patidar,

who have been a great source of inspiration and encouragement for me. Without their blessings and unconditional support, this endeavour would not have been possible. I always knew that you believed in me and wanted the best for me.

Preface

Nursing research has evolved rapidly over the last few decades in India. However, the consumers of nursing research – nurse practitioners – are lacking in knowledge about sound research methodology. Indian Nursing Council (INC) set a new milestone in its recent revision of the GNM and BSc Nursing curricula by incorporating the subject of research methodology to ensure that newly qualified nurses are not only the producers but also the consumers of scientific evidence in nursing.

Most Indian books on research methodology lack clarity about basic research and statistical concepts. This has created an aversion among novice nurse researchers to studying research methodology. This book addresses this problem by incorporating basic terminology at the beginning of each chapter to serve as a springboard to grasping and understanding the complexities of research methodology. Tailor-made according to the latest syllabus prescribed by INC, this book includes examples specific to the Indian context, which makes the text more relevant to situations that Indian nursing students will face. The use of many line diagrams helps break down complex concepts to simpler forms and enables better understanding of the research fundamentals. Concrete examples and figures, given throughout the book, will help students easily grasp the sophisticated statistical procedures and also instruct them in how to use software for data analysis. Special attention has been given towards explaining how to select the appropriate sample and research design, which are key areas in research methodology. Statistical tests have been elucidated with the use of examples. The unique feature of this book is the self-evaluation section provided at the end of every chapter.

This book interweaves the basic principles of research into the nursing discipline and is in accordance with the current syllabus prescribed by INC for GNM, BSc (Basic) Nursing, Post-Basic BSc Nursing and MSc Nursing. I hope this book will be welcomed by the Indian nursing fraternity and that readers will find it useful.

Anurag Bhai Patidar

Acknowledgements

Firstly, I must express my deep gratitude to Prof (Dr) Manoj Pandy, Director, BMHRC, Bhopal, for allowing me to undertake this endeavour. He has been a great source of inspiration for me.

It is my proud privilege to express my deepest regards and heartfelt gratitude to my PhD Supervisor, Dr (Mrs) Asha Sharma, Ex-Principal, RAK College of Nursing, New Delhi, for her cutting-edge guidance in advanced research methodology.

I am indebted to Dr Manju Vasta, Principal, College of Nursing, AIIMS, New Delhi; Dr Sandhya Gupta, Lecturer, AIIMS College of Nursing; and Mrs Deepika Khakha, Lecturer, AIIMS College of Nursing, who introduced me to research methodology with a concept-based approach which assisted me greatly while writing this book.

A deep sense of gratitude is due to Dr (Mrs) Jasbir Kaur, Principal, DMCH College of Nursing, Dayanand Medical College and Hospital, Ludhiana, for her visionary guidance and encouragement at the outset of this project.

My special thanks to Mrs Prabhjot Saini, Professor, DMCH College of Nursing, Dayanand Medical College and Hospital, Ludhiana, for her constant encouragement and valuable suggestions to improve the book.

I am grateful to Ms Mamta Choudhary, Lecturer, Sri Guru Teg Bahadur College of Nursing, Ludhiana, for her valuable support in completing this project.

My sincere thanks to Ms Anita Nand, Principal; Mrs Radha K, Vice Principal; Mrs Prabha Agnibhoj, Lecturer, all from Bhopal Nursing College, BMHRC, for providing support and guidance to enable me to accomplish this task successfully.

I am indebted to the staff of Universities Press, especially Mr Ravi Vishwakarma, for his cooperation and careful attention to detail, and Ms Madhavi Sethupathi for her speedy and thorough editing of this text.

A very special thanks to my brother, Mr Chirag Patidar, Scientist, Department of Atomic Energy; and my sister Mrs Reena Patidar, for assisting me in writing the statistical section of this book.

Words cannot express my deep gratitude to my loving wife, Mrs Leela Patidar, for her intense care and concern, which provided mental support to me in accomplishing this task.

Last but not least, credit must go to my sweet daughter, Nischal Patidar, and son, Yash Patidar, for their love and understanding when they had to spend time alone as I was busy writing this book.

Anurag Bhai Patidar

Contents

Preface *vii*
Acknowledgements *viii*

SECTION A: NURSING RESEARCH

Chapter 1: Research and the Research Process **1**
Introduction to Nursing Research 1
Need for Nursing Research 2
Definition of Research and Nursing Research 3
Methods of Acquiring Knowledge: Problem-solving and the Scientific Method 4
Characteristics of Good Research 8
Evolution of Nursing Research in the West—Important Dates 9
Evolution of Nursing Research in India—Important Dates 10
Concept of Evidence-based Nursing Practice 12
Ethics in Nursing Research 14
Research Process: Quantitative Research 19
Research Process: Qualitative Research 25

Chapter 2: Research Problem/Question **32**
Definition of Terms 32
Introduction to Research Problems 34
Identification of the Research Problem 35
Sources of Research Problems 36
Characteristics of a Good Problem Statement 38
Evaluation of the Research Problem 38
Research Question 40
Research Objectives 42
Research Variables 43
Assumptions 46
Limitations and Delimitations 47
Hypothesis 48

Characteristics of a Good Hypothesis 49
Types of Hypotheses 49
Hypothesis Testing 52
Errors in Hypothesis Testing 53

Chapter 3: Review of Literature **60**
Introduction to Review of Literature 60
Definition of Literature Review 60
Purpose of Literature Review 61
Sources of Literature Review 62
Electronic Sources 62
Printed Sources 66
Reviewing Literature 66
Review Format 69

Chapter 4: Research Approaches and Designs **74**
Introduction to Research Approach/Design 74
Definitions of Research Design 74
Factors Influencing Selection of Design 75
Research Approaches 76
Quantitative Research 76
Qualitative Research 76
Mixed Methods Approach/Pragmatic Approach 77
Participatory Approach/Action Research 78
Research Designs 78
Quantitative Research Designs 78
Qualitative Research Designs 96
Other Research Designs 104

Chapter 5: Theoretical/Conceptual Framework **113**
Introduction to Theoretical/Conceptual Framework 113
Definition of Terms 114
Characteristics of Theories 115
Significance of Theory 116
Common Concepts in Nursing Theory 116
Theory, Research and Practice Relationship 117
Classification of Theories 120
Conceptual Model/Framework/Schemes 121
Selecting the Appropriate Conceptual Framework 122
Criteria for Evaluating Conceptual Models/Frameworks 123

Systems Theory as a Framework 124
Criticisms of Nursing Theories 127

Chapter 6: Sampling Techniques **132**
Need for a Sample 132
Characteristics of a Good Sample 132
Definition of Key Terms 133
Factors Influencing the Sampling Process 134
Process of Sampling 135
Types of Sampling Techniques 136
Probability Sampling Techniques 137
Non-probability Sampling Techniques 143
Sampling Errors 151

Chapter 7: Data Collection Tools and Techniques **156**
Introduction to Data Collection 156
Developing the Data Collection Plan 157
Questionnaires 157
Interviews 160
Observations 164
Vignettes 174
Projective Techniques 176
Q Sorts 176
Bio-physiological Methods 177
Pilot Study 184
Data Collection Procedure 184

Chapter 8: Analysis of Data **192**
Introduction to Data Analysis 192
Classification of Data 192
Organisation of Data 193
Tabulation of Data 196
Graphical Presentation of Data 198
Analysis and Interpretation of Data 205

Chapter 9: Communication and Utilisation of Research **213**
Introduction to Communication of Findings 213
How to Communicate Research Findings? 214
Disseminating Research Results at Conferences 215
Presenting a research poster 216
Publishing a Journal Article 217

Research Utilisation 228
Barriers to Research Utilisation 228
Facilitators of Research Utilisation 229
Innovation Diffusion Model 230

Chapter 10: Critiquing Research Articles/Reports 235
Introduction to Critiquing Research Articles 235
Definition of terms 235
Steps in Quantitative Research Critiquing 236
Steps in Qualitative Research Critiquing 243

Chapter 11: Research Proposals 247
Introduction to Research Proposals 247
Types of Proposals 248
Writing a Research Proposal 248
Budget Plan 256
Action Plan 256
Final Proof Reading and Editing 257
Common Reasons for Proposal Rejection 257

SECTION B: STATISTICS

Chapter 12: Introduction to Statistics 262
Introduction 262
Basic Statistical Terminology 263
Types of Statistical Methods 265
Application and Scope of Statistics in Health 266
Vital Health Statistics 267
Types and Levels of Data and their Measurement 270

Chapter 13: Measures of Central Tendency 275
Introduction to Measures of Central Tendency 275
Mean (Arithmetic) 276
Median 280
Mode 282
Selecting the Appropriate Measure of Central Tendency 284
Position of Measures of Central Tendency 284

Chapter 14: Measures of Variability 289
Introduction to Measures of Variability 289
Range 289
Interquartile Range 290

Variance 293
Standard Deviation 295
Choosing the Appropriate Measure of Variability 298

Chapter 15: Measures of Relationship **302**
Correlation: Meaning and Need 302
Scatter Diagram Method 303
Types of Correlation 303
Correlation Statistics 306
Simple Linear Regression 314

Chapter 16: Parametric and Non-parametric Tests **321**
Introduction to Parametric and Non-parametric Tests 321
Parametric Tests 321
t-Test 322
z-Test 326
Analysis of Variance (ANOVA) 327
ANCOVA 331
Non-Parametric Tests 332
Chi-square Test 333
Sign Test 336
Wilcoxon Signed Rank Test 338
Mood's Median Test 341
McNemar's Test 342
Mann–Whitney U Test 343
Fisher's Exact Test 346
Kruskal–Wallis Test 348

Chapter 17: Use of Computers for Data Analysis **357**
Introduction to Computers 357
Use of Computers in Statistics 358
Statistical Packages for Quantitative Research 358
SPSS 358
STATA 359
Microsoft Office Excel 359
Statistical Packages for Qualitative Research 364
Advantages of Statistical Packages 366
Disadvantages of Statistical Packages 366

Annexures *369*
Model Question Papers *391*
Index *399*

INC Syllabus
Nursing Research and Statistics

Placement: Fourth Year Internship | Time: Theory – 45 Hours, Practical – 45 Hours

Course Description: The Course is designed to enable students to develop an understanding of basic concepts of research, research process and statistics. It is further, structured to conduct/participate in need based research studies in various settings and utilize the research findings to provide quality nursing care. The hours for practical will be utilized for conducting individual/group research project.

Unit	Time	Learning Objectives	Content	Training Learning Activities	Assessment Methods
I	4	• Describe the concept of research, terms, need and areas of research in nursing. • Explain the steps of research process	**Research and research process** • Introduction and need for nursing research • Definition of research & nursing research • Steps of scientific method • Characteristics of good research • Steps of research process-overview	• Lecture Discussion • Narrate steps of research process followed from examples of published studies	• Short answer • Objective type
II	3	• Identify and state the research problem and objectives	**Research Problem/Question** • Identification of problem area • Problem statement • Criteria of a good research problem. • Writing objectives	• Lecture Discussion • Exercise on writing statement of problem and objectives	• Short answer • Objective type
III	3	• Review the related literature	**Review of Literature** • Location • Sources • On line search; CINHAL, COCHRANE etc. • Purposes • Method of review	• Lecture Discussion • Exercise on reviewing one research report/ article for a selected research problem • Prepare annotated bibliography	• Short answer • Objective type

Unit	Time	Learning Objectives	Content	Training Learning Activities	Assessment Methods
IV	4	• Describe the research approaches and designs	**Research approaches and designs** • Historical, survey and experimental • Qualitative and quantitative designs	• Lecture Discussion • Explain types of research approaches used from examples of published and unpublished research studies with rationale.	• Short answer • Objective type
V	8	• Explain the sampling process • Describe the methods of data collection	**Sampling and data collection** • Definition of population, sample, sampling criteria, factors influencing sampling process, types of sampling techniques. • Data-why, what, from whom, when and where to collect. • Data collection methods and instruments: ❑ Methods of data collection ❑ Questioning, interviewing ❑ Observations, record analysis and measurement ❑ Pilot study ❑ Data collection procedure	• Lecture Discussion • Reading assignment on examples of data collection tools. • Preparation of sample data collection tool. • Conduct group research project	• Short answer • Objective type
VI	4	• Analyze, interpret and summarize the research data	**Analysis of data:** • Compilation, tabulation, classification, summarization, presentation, interpretation of data	• Lecture Discussion • Preparation of sample tables	• Short answer • Objective type

Unit	Time	Learning Objectives	Content	Training Learning Activities	Assessment Methods
VII	15	• Explain the use of statistics, scales of measurement and graphical presentation of data • Describe the measures of central tendency and variability and methods of correlation	**Introduction to statistics** • Definition use of statistics, scales of measurement. • Frequency distribution and graphical presentation of data. • Mean, median, mode, standard deviation • Normal probability and tests of significance • Co-efficient of correlation • Statistical packages and its application	• Lecture Discussion • Practice on graphical presentations • Practice on computation of measures of central tendency, variability & correlation	• Short answer • Objective type
VIII	4	• Communicate and utilize the research findings	**Communication and Utilization of Research** • Communication of research findings ❑ Verbal report ❑ Writing research report ❑ Writing scientific article/paper – Critical review of published research – Utilization of research findings	• Lecture Discussion • Read/ Presentations of a sample published/ unpublished research report. • Writing group research project	• Short answer • Objective type • Oral presentation • Assessment of group research project.

1 Research and the Research Process

Chapter overview

- Introduction and need for nursing research
- Definition of research and nursing research
- Methods of acquiring knowledge—problem-solving and the scientific method
- Characteristics of good research
- Historical evolution of research in nursing
- Concept of evidence-based practice
- Ethics in research
- Steps of the research process

INTRODUCTION TO NURSING RESEARCH

In any profession, research is necessary to enable the invention of new technology and techniques to make human life more comfortable, as well as to advance the body of knowledge on which the practice of professionals is based. Research in nursing equips nurses with the scientific knowledge required to be a competent nurse practitioner. Nursing as a discipline borrows knowledge from psychology, sociology, medicine, surgery and various other subjects. Thus, the scope for research in nursing is vast. Various paradigms from these related fields were incorporated into nursing by the early nurse researchers. Nursing research in India evolved predominantly when nursing education became a part of higher education and strove to seek its own body of knowledge, different from that of medicine.

Research in nursing is aimed at improving the clinical outcome of the patient and at helping society achieve good health. Since the inception of the profession, by Florence Nightingale, progress in nursing research has acquired exceptional speed. Today, it is considered essential for a competent nurse to have knowledge of nursing research methodology. Nursing practice is sensitive to changes and advances in medical and surgical practices. This has necessitated design-related research studies to improve nursing practice so that advances in medical and surgical practices can be successfully incorporated into nursing care.

NEED FOR NURSING RESEARCH

Is nursing a science or an art?—this is the most debated question among nursing professionals. Needless to say, it is research that provides the status of 'scientific discipline' to any profession. Without the enormous store of scientific evidence generated through systematic enquiry (research), no profession can be considered a science. Therefore, to affirm that nursing is a scientific discipline whose practice is based on scientific evidence generated through rigorous research is essential in nursing.

Research also generates new knowledge for clinical practice, nursing administration and education. It is the only acceptable way through which an objective scientific database of knowledge can be developed for the continuous growth of the profession. The ultimate purpose of nursing practice is to provide high-quality patient care. Clinical practice without research is practice based on tradition, without any scientific basis. Nursing practice based on research evidence replaces traditional nursing practice with scientific or evidence-based nursing practice and ensures the use of scientific reasoning by the nurse practitioner.

Research is also needed to evaluate the effectiveness of nursing treatment modalities, to determine the impact of nursing care on the health of patients and to test nursing theory. Today, with the cost of healthcare skyrocketing and reforms to contain these costs, research confirms the relevance of nursing and the effectiveness of care, not only to the profession but also to consumers (patients). Research findings help nurses eliminate nursing actions that do not achieve the desired results and identify those practices that can change outcomes.

The horizons of nursing education can be broadened by the use of innovative teaching and learning strategies and of evaluation tools developed and tested by research. Research also provides scope for the development and use of innovative management strategies to enhance the nurse's control, discipline, performance appraisal and nursing care approaches. It is also helpful in designing and evaluating effective, high-quality and cost-effective ways to deliver care.

Nursing theories developed by eminent nurse theorists can be tested for clinical use in a variety of healthcare settings through nursing research. Therefore, research is an integral and essential part of any scientific profession, without which that profession cannot be considered as a scientific discipline. It is only through research that nurses can, in a real sense, improve their effectiveness and enhance their professional lives.

Research in nursing will help identify the recent advances and trends in nursing practices, establish standards in writing scientific papers, develop skills in applying sophisticated data analysis and, most importantly, promote qualitative studies in nursing practice. Research has been used to legitimise nursing as a profession; education has been radically reformed to reflect a research base.

Unlike other countries, where clinical trial and research in nursing has advanced greatly, the research base for nursing in India is yet to develop.

From the above discussion, it can be concluded that:

- Research paves the way for the uninterrupted development of a scientific body of knowledge in the nursing sciences.
- Research provides a framework from empirical data which determines the unique role of nursing sciences as a profession.
- Incorporating research evidence in clinical decision-making enhances the professional accountability of nurses.
- The cost of healthcare expenses is on the rise; therefore cost-containment policies have been enforced in many institutions. Research helps avoid the costlier trial-and-error method of knowledge generation as well as nursing interventions that are unsafe.
- Research generates evidence for nursing practice which enables nurses to make more informed decisions about patient care.
- Qualitative research enables nurses to understand and appreciate a phenomenon about which little is known.

DEFINITION OF RESEARCH AND NURSING RESEARCH

According to Wikipedia, the word *research* is derived from the French *recherche* which means *to go about seeking*. In simple words, research is made up of two words: *re* and *search,* which means searching again and again to obtain information or facts to solve a problem.

Research has been defined in numerous ways. Some of the important definitions are given below:

- Scientific research can be defined as a systematic and objective attempt to provide answers to certain questions.
- The Merriam–Webster Online Dictionary defines research in more detail as, "A studious inquiry or investigation or experimentation aimed at the discovery and interpretation of facts, revision of accepted theories or laws in the light of new facts, or practical application of such new or revised theories or laws".
- Research aims to generate new facts or validate the facts generated through previous investigations; solve existing problems in nursing practices; and develop and test theories relevant to the nursing profession. It also purports to validate data collection instruments and intervention; and expand the previous work in the field.
- According to Calmorin et al., "Research is defined as the scientific investigation of phenomena which includes collection, presentation, analysis and interpretation of facts that link an individual's speculation with reality".
- According to Schotfeldt, "Nursing research is defined as the application of scientific inquiry to phenomena of concern to nursing. The systematic investigation of patients and their health experience is the primary concern of nursing".

METHODS OF ACQUIRING KNOWLEDGE: PROBLEM-SOLVING AND THE SCIENTIFIC METHOD

As mentioned earlier, influx of new knowledge is necessary for the continued growth of any profession. New knowledge can be acquired by different methods. These may include intuition, belief, trial and error, problem-solving, life experiences, scientific method, and so on. It must be noted here that most of these methods generate knowledge that is coloured by the personal perceptions and prejudices of the person engaged in knowledge generation. Therefore, this new knowledge may not be acceptable to others. The scientific method and problem-solving are accorded the most respect as they eliminate subjective bias and prejudice during the process of new knowledge generation; therefore, knowledge generated using these methods is widely accepted.

Problem-solving Method

This method is undertaken to solve a problem systematically, thereby generating new knowledge. It is a logical process that follows certain steps to produce an answer or solutions to the problem of interest. It is a means by which an individual uses previously acquired knowledge, skills and understanding to meet the demands of an unfamiliar situation. Problem-solving is among the core skills of a competent nurse. A problem is viewed as a gap between 'what is' and 'what should be'. Traditional problem-solving usually involves the six steps elaborated in Fig. 1.1.

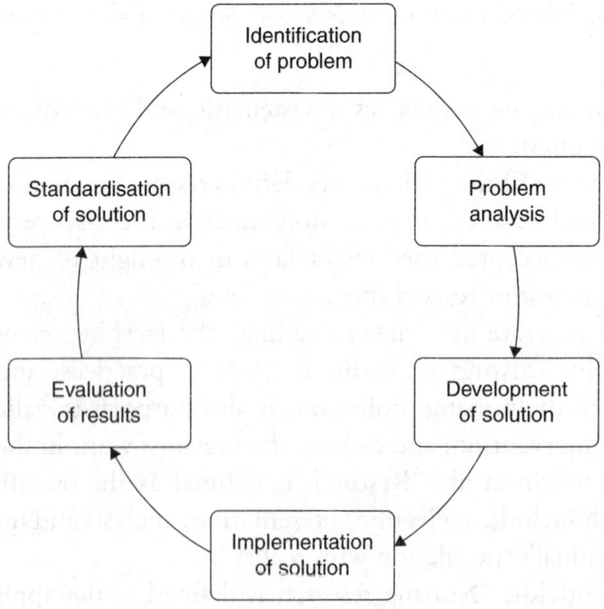

Figure 1.1 Steps in problem-solving

Steps in problem-solving

1. **Identify the problem**: The first step in problem-solving is identification of the problem itself. In this step, the nurse must identify and define the problem clearly so that a precise problem statement is formulated. It is noteworthy that problem identification may be influenced by the information available, and by the values, attitudes, time and experience of the problem solver. Similarly, it is important to differentiate a problem from the manifestation of the problem. By doing so, the most appropriate solution can be identified and implemented.
2. **Analyse the problem**: In this step, data relating to the factors contributing to the problem is gathered to identify the root cause of the problem. The information gathered should be valid, accurate, relevant and timely. Data is further analysed to refine the problem statement and identify problem solutions. Without identifying the root cause of the problem, it is almost impossible to solve the actual problem; otherwise, the problem solver may arrive at a solution for the manifestation of the problem and not for the actual problem. Therefore, it is necessary to carry out a critical analysis of the problem to understand it thoroughly. Collection of additional data may be required to verify the root causes of the problem.
3. **Develop the solution**: After gaining sufficient insight into the problem, potential solutions are generated that address the root cause of the problem. Each possible solution is evaluated in terms of its pros, cons and applicability in the given situation. The solution that fulfils the established criteria is selected and its implementation is planned. The problem-solver should be flexible enough to consider a range of possible solutions. She must set aside preconceived notions and personal ideas as that enables the generation and consideration of a wide range of solutions.
4. **Implement the solution**: After carefully considering each generated solution against the objective criteria, the most suitable one that fulfils the set criteria is implemented on a pilot basis.
5. **Evaluate the results**: Data is gathered from the pilot run of the solution. Thereafter, it is analysed to determine whether the selected solution was appropriate for solving the problem of interest. If the desired results have been achieved by implementing the solution, the problem solver can proceed to the next step; otherwise, she must return to Step 1.
6. **Standardise the solution**: The solution that showed the greatest effectiveness in solving the problem is adopted and applied fully. Training needs and systemic changes are identified for full implementation. This step also focuses on ongoing monitoring of the solution as well as improvement opportunities to continuously refine the solution.

The solution generated through the problem-solving process is applicable for the given situation, setting and individual. The same solution may not be applicable for a similar problem in a different situation and setting and with some other individual. Therefore, the results derived from the problem-solving process have limited generalisability as compared to the scientific method.

Scientific Method

Personal and cultural beliefs influence the perceptions and interpretation of natural phenomena. Therefore, the use of standard procedures and criteria is required to minimise these influences when developing a nursing theory. The scientific method is one of the most respected methods of knowledge generation as it yields objective information which is widely accepted by the professional community.

It is based on empirical and measurable evidence which reduces the chances of bias. Results, data and methodology are reported and archived in scientific literature/journals so they are available for careful scrutiny by other scientists, giving them the opportunity to verify results by attempting to reproduce them.

In summary, the scientific method attempts to minimise the influence of bias or prejudice in the experimenter when testing a hypothesis or theory, thus generating knowledge that is based purely on objective observation/data.

Characteristics

The scientific method has some distinct features that make it superior to other methods of knowledge generation. These features or characteristics are explained in detail.

Order and control: The scientific method proceeds in a systematic and orderly way to solve the problem. To reduce interference, tight control is placed over extraneous factors that can influence the outcome of the process. For example, in a study to explore the relationship between food habits and hypertension, the researcher must take steps to control other possible causes of hypertension like stress, cigarette smoking, as well as age and sex.

Empirical: The scientific method seeks real evidence gathered through observations and verified through our senses—touch, smell, sight, taste and hearing. For example, the colour of mucosa and the odour of wound drainage. Sometimes, our senses may not be able to record what is real. Therefore, extensions of the senses in the form of instruments, equipment and tools (weighing scale, thermometer, questionnaire or other instruments) that aid the senses are used to collect empirical evidence.

Generalisation: An important aspect of the scientific method is generalisation of the findings. The generalisability of research findings is an important criterion for evaluating the quality of the research.

Theory development: Theories are an important requirement for any scientific profession. Scientific methods use qualitative as well as quantitative research to enhance theory development within the professional boundary to improve nursing practice. (Quantitative research deals with data collected in the form of quanta or numbers, whereas qualitative research aims to collect data in the form of descriptions).

Steps of the scientific method

Being a systematic, orderly process, the scientific method follows certain steps, described in Fig. 1.2.

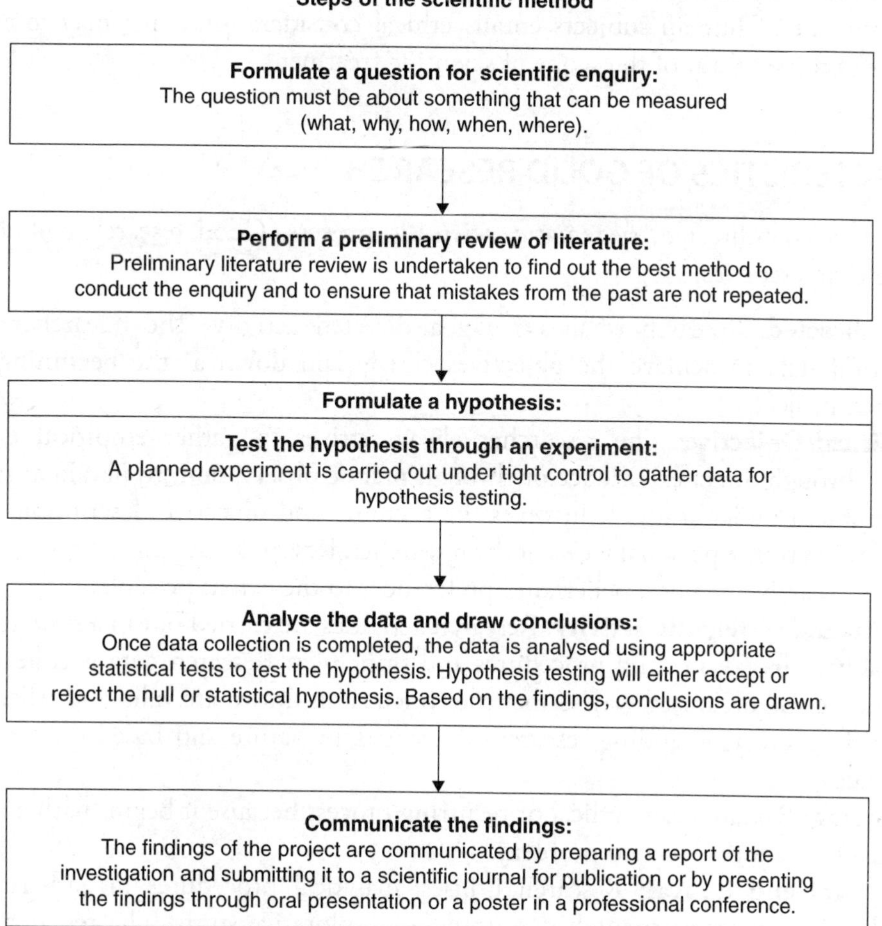

Figure 1.2 Steps of the scientific method

Advantages

1. This method is rooted in empirical and objective data.
2. The knowledge generated is unbiased and unprejudiced. Therefore, if anyone questions the information generated, they can replicate the process and determine whether the results are true or false.
3. If, on replication, different findings emerge, then the scientific method provides an opportunity to explore and exhaustively study such discrepancies.

Limitations

1. The experimenter has to work under controlled conditions; therefore, this method produces artificial knowledge that may not be applicable in real situations.
2. Some nursing phenomena cannot be subjected to scientific treatment and hence cannot be studied using this method.
3. Involvement of human subjects entails ethical considerations; this may move some nursing problems out of the scope of scientific treatment.

CHARACTERISTICS OF GOOD RESEARCH

Research is a goal-directed, systematic, scientific process. Good research embodies the following characteristics:

- **Goal-directed**: Research is always a goal-directed activity. The researcher collects empirical data to achieve the objectives clearly laid down at the beginning of the research project.
- **Empirical/Objective**: The researcher always strives to gather empirical evidence, either through direct experience or through precise observation, to obtain answers for the problem under study. It involves the accurate and objective description of facts, uncoloured by the personal views of the researcher. Research data should not be affected by the researcher's values, beliefs and preferences to the extent possible.
- **Logical and systematic activity**: Research activities are carried out in a systematic and logical way, based on valid procedures and principles. Research data is collected in a systematic and organised way so that the conclusions drawn are valid and reliable. Any scientific enquiry, including research, is realistic in nature and based on a reason or rationale.
- **Recurring**: Research is a cyclical or recurring process because it begins with a problem and leads to another related problem.
- **Analytical and critical**: Research utilises analytical procedures in gathering data, whether it is an experimental, descriptive or explorative study. The researcher must dig deep into an idea and analyse the problem critically so that relevant data can be gathered in order to arrive at the ultimate truth.
- **Control:** This is an essential feature of any experimental study. Extraneous factors that are not under direct study can influence the relationship between the variables (dependent and independent) in which the researcher is interested. These factors must be controlled to nullify their effect on the variable of interest (dependent variable). Control is a unique feature of experimental research.
- **Replicability**: Research design and procedures are replicated to enable the researcher to arrive at valid and conclusive results.
- **Patient and unhurried activity**: Research is a slow and unhurried activity. It should not be conducted in a haphazard manner.

- **Reproducibility**: Flawlessly designed and conducted research produces results that can be reproduced if someone wants to test them.
- **Accuracy**: There is no place for inaccuracy in research. Carefully planned research based on strong methodology yields accurate information.
- **Originality**: Good research is original, in the sense that it tackles something new or something old from an interesting or different angle not thought of before.
- **Training investigators**: The necessary knowledge and skills must be imparted to data collectors to avoid inaccurate data collection.

EVOLUTION OF NURSING RESEARCH IN THE WEST—IMPORTANT DATES

- 1853–56: Florence Nightingale collected data about morbidity and mortality among the soldiers of the Crimean War. She then used statistics to analyse the data. She also used graphs to depict the findings of her research. 'The Lady with the Lamp' strove to base nursing practice on research findings.
- 1859: Nightingale published *Notes on Nursing: What it is and what it is not.*
- 1900: *American Journal of Nursing* was first published.
- 1922: Sigma Theta Tau International Honor Society of Nursing founded.
- 1924: First doctoral programme in nursing started.
- 1936: Sigma Theta Tau International formed.
- 1947: Nuremberg code came into existence.
- 1950: American Nurses Association (ANA) adopted a code of ethics.
- 1952: *Nursing Research* published; ANA-sponsored research conferences conducted; ANA Commission on Nursing Research formed.
- 1960s: Shift of focus to practice-oriented research; first nursing research journals published; Declaration of Helsinki adopted by World Medical Association in 1964.
- 1970s: Standards for clinical practice developed.
- 1973: First Nursing Diagnosis Conference conducted; several other research journals started.
- 1978: Initial focus on qualitative research.
- 1982–83: Communication and Utilization of Nursing Research (CURN) project initiated.
- 1983: ANA Center for Research for Nursing established.
- 1986: National Institutes for Health (NIH) National Center for Nursing Research (NCNR) started; awards/grants given to support nursing research and training.
- 1989: Agency for Health Care Policy and Research (AHCPR) established.
- 1993: National Institute for Nursing Research (NINR) established.
- 1994: *Qualitative Health Research* began publication.
- 1997: Canadian Health Services Research Foundation established with federal funding.
- 2000: NINR issued funding priorities for 2000–04; annual funding exceeded $100 million; The Canadian Institute of Health Research launched; *Biological Research for Nursing* began publication.

- 2000: Indian Council of Medical Research (ICMR) released *Ethical guidelines for biomedical research in human subjects.*
- 2001: Nurse anesthetists gained independent prescriptive authority.

EVOLUTION OF NURSING RESEARCH IN INDIA—IMPORTANT DATES

- 1910: Trained Nurses Association of India (TNAI) began publishing *Nursing Journal of India.*
- 1955: A paper titled *Need for nursing research in India* presented by Ms Margaretta Craig at the International Council of Nurses (ICN) meet in France.
- 1960: MSc Nursing programme started by RAK College of Nursing, New Delhi; included independent thesis work by MN students with Research as a separate subject.
- 1966: Research section established by TNAI.
- 1966: TNAI conducted Nurses Time Utilisation Study.
- 1971: TNAI conducted a research study on the socioeconomic status of nurses in India.
- 1981: *Health research: A community-based approach* by Dr Farrell and Dr Bhaduri published by the WHO.
- 1982: College of Nursing, Bangalore organised a national conference on *Nursing Research in India: Prospect and Retrospect*—the first conference of its kind; stimulated the rapid pace of research in nursing sciences.
- 1984: A major breakthrough took place when University Grants Commission sponsored a workshop on *Teaching nursing research to nursing college teachers* at Bangalore; conference accessible to all faculty of nursing in India.
- 1984: WHO sponsored a workshop on 'Nursing process' at Leelabai Thackersey College of Nursing, SNDT, Mumbai.
- 1986: MPhil programme in Nursing started at RAK College of Nursing, Delhi; Research introduced in graduate nursing programmes by Indian Nursing Council.
- 1994: Indian Society of Psychiatric Nurses (ISPN) founded under the guidance of Dr K Reddemma, to provide a platform for discussion and deliberation on evidence-based practice, to create awareness and to translate research findings in MH nursing practice.
- 1996: MPhil and PhD Nursing programmes started at MAHE, Manipal.
- 2000: Society of Midwives–India established, with a mission to strengthen midwifery and achieve safe motherhood through promotion of research in midwifery.
- 2000: *Indian Journal of Continuing Nursing Education* published, with Ms Punitha Ezhilarasu from CMC College of Nursing Vellore as editor.
- 2002: Revised syllabus of General Nursing and Midwifery (2002) and Post Basic BSc Nursing (2005) incorporated Research as a separate subject.
- 2002: First national conference organised by ISPN at NIMHANS Bangalore on the theme *Child Psychiatric Nursing.*
- 2004: Publication of *Nightingale Nursing Times*, a journal featuring nursing research articles, started under the editorial guidance of Mr Prabhu Deva.

- 2005: National Consortium for PhD in Nursing established under the leadership of the Indian Nursing Council, seven leading nursing institutions of India, WHO and the Rajiv Gandhi University of Health Sciences, Bangalore. Mr T Dilip Kumar, President of Indian Nursing Council; Dr Asha Sharma, Vice President, Indian Nursing Council; Dr Manju Vasta, Principal, AIIMS College of Nursing, New Delhi; Dr K Reddemma, HOD and Professor in Nursing, NIMHANS; and Dr Sandhya Gupta, Secretary, Indian Nursing Council played a pivotal role in the development of doctoral research in India.
- 2009: Central Institute of Nursing and Research established by TNAI.
- 2009: ISPN published its first issue of *Indian Journal of Psychiatric Nursing* in March, with Dr Sandhya Gupta as editor.
- 2010: Baba Farid University of Health Sciences, Faridkot started a PhD programme under the faculty of Nursing Sciences.

Nursing Research during Nightingale's Era (1859)

Research in nursing began with Florence Nightingale. Her *Notes on Nursing* highlighted her early interest in the environmental factors responsible for promoting physical and emotional wellbeing. Her most widely known research contribution was the analysis of factors affecting soldier mortality and morbidity during the Crimean War. Based on her meticulous analyses and presentations, she was successful in effecting some changes in nursing care and, more generally, in public health. She was also a good statistician, which helped her in data analysis.

Nursing Research in the Twentieth Century

In the 1900s, most studies focused on nursing education—educational preparation and clinical experience of nursing students. Limited platforms were available to publish these studies, though *American Journal of Nursing* began publishing in 1900. At this time, there was lack of research in nursing practice. Advances in nursing research took place in the 1960s, with the publishing of *International Journal of Nursing* and *Canadian Journal of Nursing* in 1963.

By the 1970s, a number of research studies were conducted by nurses in areas such as teaching, curriculum and nursing practice. This was when nursing research also expanded internationally. *Journal of Advanced Nursing*, the premier international journal of nursing research, began publication in the United Kingdom in 1976.

The first volume of *Annual Review of Nursing Research* was published in 1983. These annual reviews include summaries of current research evidence in selected areas of research practice and encourage utilisation of research findings. In 1986, the National Center for Nursing Research (NCNR) at the National Institutes of Health (NIH) came into existence in the USA. The purpose of NCNR was to promote and financially support research projects and training related to patient care.

In 1993, the National Institute of Nursing Research (NINR) was started in the USA. In 1986, the NCNR had a budget of $16 million, whereas in the year 1999, the budget for NINR had grown to about $70 million. Journals were established during the 1990s in response to the growth in clinically oriented research and interest in EBP among nurses, including clinical nursing research, clinical effectiveness and outcome management for nursing practice.

Nursing Research in the Twenty-first Century

The commencement of the twenty-first century witnessed a spurt in nursing research globally. Numerous scientific platforms came into existence where nurses could communicate their research findings. Online journals, open-access journals and the peer review system improved the quality of nursing research. National and international conferences also boosted nursing research by providing a platform where nurses could share their research papers.

India too witnessed accelerating growth in nursing research in the last few decades. In the year 1959, the Master of Nursing programme was started in RAK College of Nursing. Dr Mary Ferguson, with other pioneers, conducted studies on the nursing and non-nursing functions of nursing personnel. In 1976, Dr Marie Farrell and Dr Aparna of RAK College of Nursing conducted seminars on nursing research to strengthen nursing research in India. In 1988, RAK College of Nursing was designated a world health collaboration centre for nursing development. The PhD in Nursing programme was started at RAK CON in 1992. Nursing education has flourished in an unprecedented manner throughout India.

CONCEPT OF EVIDENCE-BASED NURSING PRACTICE

Evidence-based practice (EBP) has emerged with the development and advancement of research activities in the nursing sciences. It refers to a practice of nursing based on evidence and not on traditions, beliefs and subjective perceptions. Evidence from research, clinical expertise and patient preferences are incorporated while making decisions about the nursing care of individual patients. Most nursing professionals seek to ensure that their care is effective, compassionate and meets the needs of patients. Therefore sound research evidence that presents feasible practices is always preferable. EBP aims to provide high-quality patient care based on research and knowledge rather than because 'this is the way we have always done it', or based on traditions, beliefs, myths, intuition or outdated textbooks.

Sackett et al. (2000) defined evidence-based practice as the process of clinical decision-making by integrating the best research evidence with clinical expertise and the patient's values. In other words, the process of EBP influences clinical decision-making in light of the best available research evidence, clinical expertise and patient preferences, in the context of the available resources.

Haynes et al. (2002) maintain that EBP is a framework for 'answering clinical questions' by evaluating and incorporating the best clinical knowledge relating to the patient's state, clinical setting and clinical circumstances.

With the emergence of new and relevant evidence, EBP is continually evolving and having an effect on clinical practice decisions to promote optimal patient care. Under the influence of EBP, nurses have an obligation to access the latest evidence, apply this in practice, and lead others to use it appropriately. Moreover, EBP has occupied a distinct place among the five core competencies that all health professionals should possess to meet the needs of the twenty-first century healthcare system.

Importance of EBP in Nursing Practice

Nursing care directly influences the patient outcome. Therefore, EBP is the need of the hour due to the obligation of quality care to society. The importance of EBP in nursing practice can be briefly summarised as follows:

- It leads to high-quality patient care and better patient outcome.
- It lifts the status of the profession as a scientific discipline.
- It keeps practice current and relevant.
- It increases the confidence of the nurses in decision-making.

Steps Involved in the Practice of EBP

1. Identify the problem situation that requires clinical decision-making.
2. Search for the available evidence.
3. Critique the evidence for validity, impact and applicability.
4. Integrate the knowledge gained into practice.
5. Develop clinical guidelines/protocols.
6. Evaluate the effectiveness of change.

Barriers to Implement EBP

The barriers to EBP have been explored by numerous research studies, some of which are as follows:

- Lack of knowledge about how to critique scientific articles
- Lack of education about the research process—as most nurses in India study Auxiliary Nursing and Midwifery (ANM)/General Nursing and Midwifery (GNM)
- Lack of awareness about research or EBP
- No support from administrators
- Lack of time to critique research literature
- Non-availability or difficulty in accessing research articles and journals
- Complexity of research reports that is not easily understood by the nurses due to lack of knowledge regarding research and statistics
- Feelings of being overwhelmed by the complexity of the EBP process

- Lack of time to search and read research articles
- Difficulty in changing current practices
- Lack of competent mentors

ETHICS IN NURSING RESEARCH

Ethics is the branch of philosophy that provides arguments about what is wrong and right in a given situation. In other words, ethics refers to moral principles that should be considered while making decisions. Nursing is a profession whose activities revolve around human beings; therefore, most research in nursing employs human beings as study participants who have values, beliefs and rights. Nurses are professionally obliged to protect these values, beliefs and rights while conducting research. Secondly, in most nursing research, the participants are usually vulnerable in some way—only people with actual or potential health problems would fall within the scope of nursing.

Consideration of ethical principles in research involving human participants came into existence after some cases of violation of these principles were reported during Nazi rule in Germany and thereafter in some studies conducted in the USA. Recently, in India, a major violation of ethics in research came to light when a drug trial was conducted on human subjects in Delhi; similarly, in Madhya Pradesh, a breach of ICMR ethical guidelines was reported from a drug trial. Therefore, it was felt that there should be some guidelines which could be used to protect human rights and safeguard people from the harmful effects of clinical trials on human beings.

The Nuremberg Code came into existence in 1947 after the exposure of Nazi atrocities during the Second World War and was amended in 1989. Several other international codes of ethics were developed—the most notable being the Declaration of Helsinki, adopted by the World Medical Association in 1964. The Council for International Organizations of Medical Sciences (CIOMS) and the WHO also proposed guidelines in 1983 and adopted them in 1993. Progress was made in nursing when the American Nurses Association (ANA) developed ethical guidelines of conduct in 1995 which were revised in 1997. India too did not remain unaffected—the Indian Council of Medical Research (ICMR) developed a 'Policy statement on ethical consideration involved in research on human subjects'; thereafter, a 'consultative document on ethical guidelines on biomedical research involving human subjects' came into existence in 1997. The ICMR released the *Ethical guidelines for biomedical research in human subjects* in 2000.

The Belmont Report endorsed by the National Commission for the Protection of Human Subjects of Biomedical and Behavioural Research (USA) has served as an archetype for many ethical guidelines adopted by several disciplines such as sociology, psychology and nursing. The broad ethical principles outlined by this report are as follows:

- Principle of beneficence
- Principle of respect for human dignity
- Principle of justice

Principle of beneficence: This is the first ethical principle that should be considered before embarking on a research project. The underlying maxim of beneficence is *Above all, do no harm*. This means that society must be benefitted by the research or, at the very least, the researcher must not harm the subjects. Any research that can cause physical, social or psychological harm to the human participants and have no potential benefit to society must not be undertaken. The principle of beneficence has many dimensions:

- Freedom from harm
- Freedom from exploitation
- Benefit from research
- Risk–benefit ratio

Any research project that might harm human subjects in any way, whether physical, psychological, social or economic, must be carefully analysed. The researcher should channelise her efforts to minimise harm and establish a risk–benefit ratio. If the harm to study participants is expected to be of a serious nature, it is strongly recommended that the project be discarded. Freedom from harm also entails that research be conducted only by qualified researchers and that dangerous equipment is not utilised during the research process.

Information provided by the human subjects is private and confidential. Therefore, it is unethical to exploit the subjects on the basis of the information they provided during the study. For example, during a project, if a researcher comes to know that a particular subject is a cocaine abuser, then the subject should not be made liable to criminal proceedings on the basis of this information. Similarly, the participants should not be subject to sexual or any other form of violation by the researcher during and after their participation in a research project. Consideration of this ethical principle is especially important for qualitative research because the psychological distance between the researcher and participant diminishes, making the participant more vulnerable to the researcher.

The nurse researcher should ascertain the risk–benefit ratio for the proposed research project on the basis of background information and methodology of the research problem under study. It is always desirable that there should be more benefit (in terms of knowledge gain and improved intervention) and less harm to the individual, as well as to society, by conducting any clinical trial. While determining the risk–benefit ratio, the researcher should ask herself, 'Would I continue with this project if one or all my family members or relatives were a part of the study?'. The researcher should take every step to minimise risk and maximise benefit from the research. When the risk is minimal, the researcher can proceed with the project, taking every possible effort to further minimise the risk at every step.

It is not possible for a qualitative researcher to analyse the risk–benefit ratio at the outset because of lack of information about the area of study. Therefore, they need to be more aware of this ethical issue.

Principle of respect for human dignity: Respect for human dignity is the second ethical principle as per the Belmont Report; it has also been given due consideration in the ANA ethical guidelines. The dimensions of this principle are as under:

- Right to self determination
- Right to full disclosure

The dignity of the prospective study participants can be protected by the right of self determination. The researcher is required to pay due respect to the dignity of the human beings as well as to their capability to make decisions in their own interest. They should be allowed to decide freely whether to participate in the study as well as to ask questions and clarify information as and when required without the threat of any penalty or prejudicial treatment. They should be allowed to quit the study at any point of time without any threat. The right to self disclosure also entails that prospective study participants not be subject to coercion, either positive (reward) or negative (penalty), to take part in the research study.

The right of full disclosure entails that the prospective study participants be provided with the fullest information required to help them decide whether to take part in the study or not. Information related to the nature of the study, its objectives, risks arising due to participation, benefits of the study, process of data collection, and so on should be fully disclosed to them.

These two dimensions are the main constituents on which informed consent is based.

Principle of justice: This is the third ethical principle and encompasses the right to fair treatment and the right to privacy of the research participants.

The researcher must respect and protect the right to fair treatment of the study participants by selecting them without any discrimination so that the risk and the benefit of the study are shared equally. Cultural and other forms of diversity need to be respected by the researcher. Study participants should not be subjected to prejudicial treatment on the grounds that they have declined to participate in the study or withdrawn from the study after initially agreeing to participate. Nursing care of the patient/participant must not be compromised by the nurse researcher who plays the dual role of nurse and researcher. Further, participants should have access to the researchers whenever they want to clarify any information. All the contracts/agreements signed by the researcher and the participants should be respected and, above all, the participants should be treated graciously and with consideration at all the times.

The prospective participants have the right to expect confidentiality of the information provided by them to the researcher. As far as possible, the researcher should strive to achieve anonymity of data. Anonymity occurs when even the researcher is not able to relate the data to specific participants. However, if anonymity is not possible, efforts should be made to keep the data under strict confidence. Identification information of the participant should be collected only when essential; otherwise, the researcher should assign a code number to each participant.

Informed consent: Informed consent, preferably a written one from the prospective participants, has become an essential requirement in nursing research. It implies that the study participants have been provided with all the necessary information related to the study, enabling them to consent to participate voluntarily or decline such participation.

However, obtaining informed consent before the commencement of the study may pose an ethical dilemma for the researcher in some situations because the participants may become conscious of the study goals and objectives during the process of informed consent and change their behaviour accordingly. Sometimes, a research project may involve children, mentally challenged patients, unconscious patients or any other person who cannot legally make decisions; in such situations, informed consent should be sought from the legal guardian of the concerned participant. **Assent** is the term used instead of consent when the underage child or adolescent freely chooses to participate in a study.

The material provided to participants should be in their preferred language and at their reading level. The information contained in the informed consent form is outlined as follows:

- Study objectives
- Actual and potential risks involved in the study
- Benefits of the study that are anticipated for the participants directly, and for the public more generally through increased knowledge
- Nature of participation—when the researcher fails to adequately inform potential research participants about the full nature of the research, thereby preventing them from making an informed decision about their participation, it is called deception
- Data collection procedure
- Number of data collection points
- Withdrawing participation any time and withholding information
- Compensation
- Contact information of the researcher
- Time duration of data collection
- Confidentiality pledge—no information/data will be divulged to others
- Anonymity—noone, including the researcher, can link the subjects with the data they provided
- Ongoing opportunities for further discussions or clarifications of any aspect of the study
- Sample size and sampling technique

Format of Informed Consent

Title of the study:
Include the study title.

Researchers:
Include the names of all researchers (student(s) and faculty) including their contact details (email address and/or office phone number).

Purpose of the research:
Include a statement about the purpose of the research. Also indicate how the research will be conducted, presented and reported.

What you will be asked to do in the research:
Include a statement regarding the role and/or responsibilities of the research participants. Include a statement regarding the estimated time commitment for participation. If incentive will be offered, indicate it here.

Risks and discomfort:
Include a statement regarding any real or perceived risks or potential discomfort that may result from participation in the research. If there is a possibility of harm or discomfort, it must be described and alleviation methods must be indicated.

Benefits of the research and benefits to you:
Include a statement regarding any benefits of the research as well as the benefits to the research participants.

Voluntary participation:
Include the following text: "Your participation in the research is completely voluntary and you may choose to stop participating at any time. A participant's decision not to continue participating will not influence their relationship or the nature of their relationship with researchers or with staff either now or in the future".

Withdrawal from the study:
Include a statement: "You may stop participating in the study at any time, for any reason, if you so decide. Your decision to stop participating, or to refuse to answer particular questions, will not affect your relationship with the researchers, or any other group associated with this project. In the event that you withdraw from the study, all associated data collected will be immediately destroyed wherever possible".

Confidentiality:
Indicate whether or not the interview documentation/recording of the participant will be associated with identifying information. Indicate how the data will be collected (e.g., handwritten notes, video/audio tapes, digital device). Indicate how the data will be stored, who will have access to it, and how it will be stored securely. Indicate how long the data will be stored and whether or not it will be destroyed after the study, and how it will be destroyed. If the data will not be destroyed, indicate where and how it will be archived.

Include the following required text: "Confidentiality will be provided to the fullest extent possible".

Questions about the research:
Indicate that if a research participant has questions about the research in general or their role in the study, that they should contact the researcher or their supervisor. Provide the supervisor's name and telephone number and/or email address. Include the following required text: "This research has been reviewed and approved by the Institutional Review Board and conforms to the standards of the Indian Council of Medical Research ethics guidelines".

Legal Rights and Signatures:

Include the following required text:

I ______________________ consent to participate in ___________ (*study title*) ______________ conducted by _______(*investigator's name*)__________.

I have understood the nature of this project and wish to participate. I am not waiving any of my legal rights by signing this form. My signature below indicates my consent.

Signature

Date

Participant name ______________________________

Signature

Date

Principal Investigator name _________________________

Signature

Date

Witness name ______________________________

Optional: Additional consent

If you require additional consent (e.g., for video/audio recording, to waive anonymity, to authorise the use photographs, to use associated data) include checkboxes or request additional signatures.

In a qualitative study, however, the researcher is usually uncertain about the risks and benefits involved in the study, the duration of data collection, and the sample size at the outset. Therefore, this information cannot be communicated clearly by the researcher to the participants. The qualitative researcher must continuously negotiate with the participants for consent as the study unfolds in the field—this type of informed consent is known as **process consent** and is taken as and when required.

RESEARCH PROCESS: QUANTITATIVE RESEARCH

Scientific research is a systematic process that focuses on being objective and gathering a multitude of information for analysis so that the researcher can come to a meaningful conclusion. While conducting research, the researcher must follow certain steps in a logical manner so that the objectives of the research study can be achieved with fewer hurdles and minimum utilisation of resources. The quantitative research process can be broadly categorised into the following phases:

- Conceptual phase
- Design and planning phase
- Empirical phase
- Analytic phase
- Disseminating phase

Conceptual Phase

This is the phase in which the researcher conceives a problem/topic/question that needs some clarification or answer. It is the initial phase of a research project and includes the following steps/activities by the researcher.

1. **Formulating the research problem**: Formulating a good researchable problem is itself a research for the beginner researcher, especially for undergraduate and postgraduate students. A good research problem should lead to improvement in patient care, provide a basis for theory development or generate knowledge required for the continuous growth of the profession. But how does one obtain a good research problem? A number of gateways, discussed later in this book, can be used to formulate a research problem. After conceptualising the problem, it should be refined and delimited with the help of review of literature so that the researcher can focus on the area that needs clarification.
2. **Review of literature**: This is important during conceptualisation of the research problem as it will provide more insight to the researcher about the problem under investigation. The researcher will come to understand what is known and what requires further investigation. It will provide an orientation to the methodology to be used for investigation. It will also help the researcher refine the problem and result in a good problem statement.
3. **Undertaking fieldwork**: Clinical fieldwork provides the real-life experience of the problem. It also provides an opportunity to the researcher to discuss the conceptualised problem with clinical and research experts who may provide new perspectives of the clinical trends. The researcher can also better understand the study population and the setting in which the research will be conducted. Sometimes, clinical fieldwork may be the starting point for a research project.
4. **Defining the terms**: The different terms used should be clearly defined by the researcher so that any ambiguity in meaning can be eliminated.

Designing and Planning the Methodology

In this phase, the researcher determines the methods and procedures to be used to address the research questions under study. The tasks that have to be carried out during this phase are as follows.

1. **Selecting the research design**: Research design is the blueprint or overall plan or architectural backbone of a study for obtaining answers to the research question. Selection of appropriate design is crucial for obtaining an objective answer to the research question under study. The nature of the research question provides a broad lead for the selection of the design. The researcher should strive for control of extraneous variables that may contaminate the study results by providing alternative explanations for the result of the study.

> For example, a researcher wants to know the prevalence of anemia among antenatal mothers attending the antenatal clinic of a selected hospital in Jalandhar, Punjab.
>
> In this case, the research question itself provides the lead that it should be a non-experimental study. Further, as the researcher is only interested in stating the rate of prevalence of anemia, it will be a descriptive study.

2. **Specifying the protocols for the intervention**: Intervention/Experimentation is an essential part of any experimental study. If the researcher undertakes a study that involves experimentation then she should specify the intervention in detail. The researcher should give due consideration to these questions while describing the intervention:
   - What exactly will you do? If it is a nursing procedure, outline the steps of the procedure.
   - Who will administer the intervention? You or someone else?
   - Specify the time duration of the intervention.
   - Specify the frequency of the intervention.
   - If the intervention has to be provided more than once, specify the interval at which it will be provided.
   - Where will the intervention be provided?
   - What equipment/instruments will be needed for the intervention?
   - Specify the points of data collection.

   Answers to these questions will result in a detailed protocol for intervention which is essential for maintaining uniformity of the intervention for all subjects. This step is not required for non-experimental studies.
3. **Specifying the population**: In this step, the researcher must specify the population in which she is interested. Population in research refers to the aggregate of the elements, objects and subjects that fulfil specified criteria and in which the researcher is interested. The researcher should outline the attributes of interest.

> For example, a researcher may specify 'myocardial infarction' and 'resident of Punjab' as attributes of interest. In this case, all patients of Punjab state with myocardial infarction will become the study population.

4. **Determining the sampling plan**: As it is almost impossible or rarely possible to study the entire population with limited resources, the researcher should select a subset of the population—termed the sample. While selecting a sample for the study, the key is that it should be representative of the entire population. If the sample is not representative of the entire population, the results of the study will not be generalisable to all the population; rather, it will be useful only for the selected sample. Unfortunately, there is no known method of sampling that guarantees the representativeness of the sample. However, probability sampling methods are considered to be good as they provide an equal chance to all members of the population to be selected for the study sample. In this step, the researcher should answer the following questions:
   - *Size of the study sample*: Novice researchers may consult a statistician for estimation of sample size for their study. For this, they will require findings from previous similar studies and the objectives of the current study. The size of the study sample will depend on certain factors, discussed later in the book; however, the general rule is to keep the sample size as large as possible to ensure representativeness of the sample.
   - *Method of sampling*: The researcher must decide on the method of sampling, whether to adopt probability sampling or opt for non-probability sampling.
   - *Procedure to recruit study subjects*: The steps used to recruit a subject for the study must be outlined.
5. **Identifying, developing and selecting tools for data collection**: Research tools are required to gather the necessary data or information to answer the research question. Data collection tools may be structured, semi-structured or unstructured, depending on the research paradigm in which the researcher is interested. In quantitative studies, tools are structured or semi-structured, whereas in qualitative studies, they are unstructured. The researcher should search for standardised tools for a particular variable of interest and, if available, she should use them after obtaining prior permission from the owner. Sometimes, the researcher may have to construct her own tools for data collection, depending on the data needs of the study. The following types of data collection measures can be used by the researcher while selecting appropriate tools for the study:
   - Bio-physiological measures—useful in most clinical studies
   - Self reported—questionnaires
   - Observation
   - Interview
6. **Developing a data collection plan**: Research should outline the activities in a logical way necessary for data collection. These steps should be followed consistently with every research participant. For example, if a researcher is conducting a study on the 'prevalence of obstructed sleep apnea and associated quality of life among stable congestive heart failure patients attending the OPD of HDHI Ludhiana'. In this quantitative, non-experimental study, the researcher decides to use the following tools for data collection:

- Structured socio-demographic sheet—to collect the socio-demographic data of the study subject
- Structured clinical profile sheet—to collect the clinical data of the subjects
- Modified Berlin Questionnaire—to assess the presence of obstructed sleep apnea in the study subject (a standardised tool)
- Kansas City Cardiomyopathy Questionnaire—to assess disease-related quality of life of the study subject (a standardised tool)

The researcher develops a detailed data collection plan (Fig. 1.3).

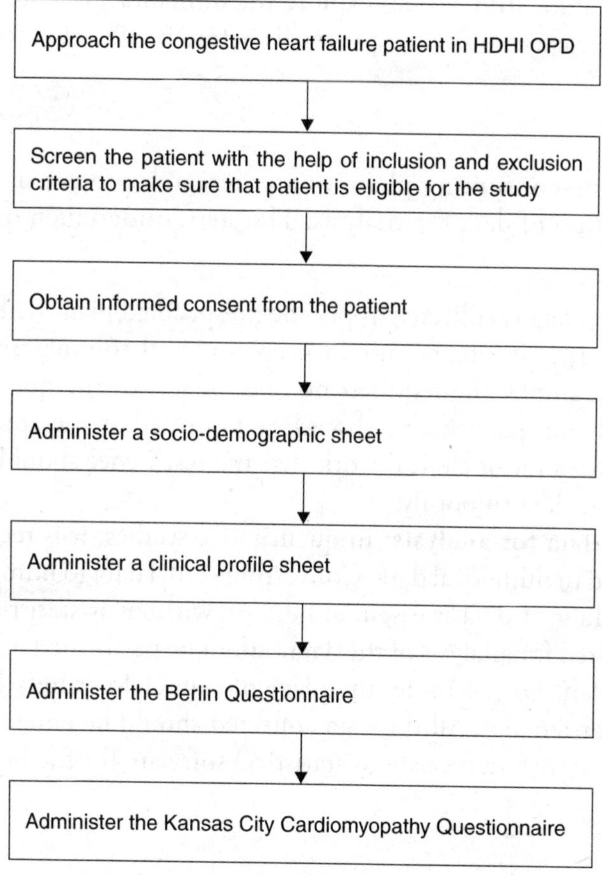

Figure 1.3 Data collection plan

7. **Ethical considerations**: After finalising the study protocols and before starting actual data collection or pilot study, the researcher should carefully and systematically consider the ethical aspects of the study. The researcher should determine the risk–benefit ratio and judge various aspects against the ethical principles outlined earlier in this chapter. The researcher should obtain ethical permission from the institutional

Ethics Committee; if the concerned institution does not have such a committee, the researcher can submit a synopsis to an independent Ethics Committee.

8. **Pretesting/Pilot study**: If the researcher plans to use a questionnaire for data collection, pretesting of the tool before actual data collection is advisable, even if it is a standardised tool. Pretesting will enable the researcher to determine whether respondents understand questions clearly or whether there is any item objectionable to the participants. The researcher should modify the tool accordingly. After finalising the tool, the researcher should check its reliability. If she has some concerns about the overall study plans, she can undertake a pilot study, which is a small-scale version of the actual study. Pilot studies help explore the difficulties in conducting the study so that the researcher can modify her protocols before final data collection.

Empirical Phase

This is the most time-consuming phase of any research project. It involves collection of data and preparation of data for analysis. The steps undertaken during this phase are as follows.

1. **Collecting data**: Data is collected as per the prespecified plan, with the help of reliable and valid tools. The researcher should keep ready all the material required for data collection. For example, the required number of sets of the questionnaire should be prepared beforehand; participants should be informed at the appropriate time. Data collection requires a lot of clerical work that the researcher should prepare for, so that she can gather the data smoothly.
2. **Preparation of data for analysis**: In quantitative studies, it is required that all verbal data be translated to numerical data. Converting verbal data to numerical form is known as 'coding'. Coding of data is essential because without it statistical or mathematical operations required for analysis of the data cannot be performed. Coding should follow a prespecified plan. For example, the place of stay (1 for rural; 2 for urban); gender (1 for male; 2 for female). All the data collected should be entered into a spreadsheet so that it can be transferred easily to statistical software for further analysis.

Analytic Phase

In this step of the research process, the researcher analyses the data to obtain answers for the questions under study. Analysis of data is necessary because the raw data alone cannot provide the answers. Analysis tools can range from simple mathematics to sophisticated statistical procedures/tests.

Interpreting the findings: This involves drawing conclusions from the analysed data and determining their implications. The researcher should attempt to explain the findings in the context of previous literature or prespecified conceptual framework. In experimental studies, if the hypothesis is supported, the researcher can easily explain the result because the findings are consistent with the preconceived idea. However, if the hypothesis is rejected, the researcher must make a strong case against inconsistencies in findings in previous literature.

Dissemination Phase

Though the researcher obtains answers to the research questions after the data is analysed and the findings are interpreted, the task is not complete until she communicates the findings of the study to the nursing community. This phase includes steps of communicating the research findings and utilising the findings in nursing practice.

1. **Communicating the findings**: Research is useless if the findings are not disseminated among the professional community. Therefore, the task is not complete until the reseacher communicates the results to the nurse practitioners. A number of platforms provide opportunities to the researcher to communicate the findings of the research. Research journals are considered a better avenue to publish original research articles as they have a wider reach in the professional community. Given below is a list of communicative channels to disseminate the results of research:
   - Write a thesis, term paper
   - Publish the research article in a professional journal
   - Present the findings orally at local, national or international conferences
   - Perform poster presentation at a conference
   - Publish on the internet
   - Write an article in a newspaper or magazine
2. **Utilising the findings in nursing practice**: The researcher should explore ways of using the research findings in nursing practice. A framework should be provided, explaining how the findings can be integrated into practice to improve existing clinical care.

RESEARCH PROCESS: QUALITATIVE RESEARCH

Quantitative research proceeds in a linear fashion, in which the researcher follows predefined steps. However, qualitative research typically unfolds in the field and the researcher must make numerous decisions and revisit the research process in a circular fashion. The unique features of qualitative research are simultaneous data collection and analysis. Based on the findings of data analysis, the researcher must make decisions about various aspects of the study. The researcher herself may not know in advance how the study will proceed in the field. Therefore, the qualitative research process cannot be described in a linear fashion. However, the main activities undertaken by the qualitative researcher are as follows.

Conceptual Phase

This involves the following activities:

1. **Selecting a research problem**: As with quantitative studies, in this research paradigm, the researcher selects a broad topic/area for the study. Qualitative studies are usually conducted to explore a phenomenon about which little is known. Unlike in quantitative studies, research questions in qualitative studies are kept broad-based which can be refined to some extent in the field.
2. **Review of literature**: There are two schools of thoughts about the review of literature in qualitative studies. One school suggests that review of literature not be undertaken at the outset of the study because it may result in biased interpretation of the phenomenon by the researcher. They suggest that the researcher undertake a full-fledged review of literature after data collection, to understand the phenomenon more realistically. The other school of thought suggests that the qualitative researcher undertake a review of literature at the outset of the study. Further, they claim that the initial review is helpful to develop insights into the problem; the researcher would also become familiar with what is already known about the phenomenon.
3. **Selecting and entering the research setting**: The next step is to explore the availability and accessibility of the prospective study participants. Based on the study requirements, the researcher must select the appropriate setting where study participants are available. Sometimes, it may be difficult to obtain access to prospective study participants; to overcome this, the researcher must use interpersonal skills to influence the gatekeepers of the particular community. Most of the planning related to research projects is undertaken in the study setting itself.

Research Design

The quantitative researcher has a predetermined research design, whereas in qualitative study, the design emerges when the researcher collects and analyses data from the field. Sometimes, a researcher may plan this in advance, when she is working with some specific qualitative research traditions, which are as follows:

- Phenomenology
- Ethnography
- Grounded theory
- Hermeneutics
- Historical research

1. **Ethical considerations**: Here, the researcher interacts and observes the study participants very closely. This means that more effort should be taken to protect the rights of the participants so that they cannot be harmed in any way by the researcher. Informed consent in qualitative studies is usually ongoing and the researcher must negotiate with the participant as and when consent is required as per the data needs of the study.
2. **Sample**: Sample size determination is usually undertaken in the field as data collection progresses. Sample size decisions are governed by the data needs of the study. Typically, a qualitative researcher collects data up to the point of data saturation (no new

information can be obtained by recruiting more subjects). Usually, the sample size is small as the researcher is not concerned with the generalisability of the result but tries to explore the phenomenon to the fullest extent. Therefore, participants are recruited for the study up to the point of data saturation.

3. **Data collection tools**: The quantitative researcher usually collects data using structured tools that provide limited information. However, qualitative researchers strive to collect more detailed information. Therefore, they require unstructured or semi-structured tools that enable participants to express their views or experience to the fullest extent. Field notes, diary, log book, unstructured interview and unstructured observation are all used for data collection in qualitative studies.

Analytic Phase

Data is analysed when it is collected in the field. Socio-demographic information may be analysed in the same way as in quantitative studies. However, detailed information must be processed in a way unique to qualitative research. The researcher should identify the themes and categories that emerge from the data and present it along with appropriate verbatim accounts. Data analysis is a time-consuming job because the researcher has to read and re-read the information; and listen to the tape-recorded interview again and again to find the themes and categories. Nowadays, statistical software has been developed to analyse qualitative data; however, their use is limited due to high cost.

Dissemination Phase

Findings can be communicated in the same way as in quantitative research.

CHAPTER SUMMARY

- Research in nursing evolved predominantly when nursing education became a part of higher education and sought its own body of knowledge, different from that of medicine.
- Without the enormous store of scientific evidence generated through systematic enquiry (research), no profession can be considered as a science.
- The ultimate purpose of nursing is to provide high-quality patient care. Clinical practice without research is practice based on tradition, without any scientific basis.
- Nursing education can use innovative teaching and learning strategies and evaluation tools developed and tested by research.
- The word *research* is made up *re* and *search*, which means searching again and again to obtain information or facts to solve a problem.
- Scientific research can be defined as a systematic and objective attempt to provide answers to certain questions.

- Problem-solving is a method of knowledge generation for systematically solving a problem of interest. This method is a logical process that follows certain steps to produce answers or solutions to the problem of interest:
  - *Step 1: Identify the problem*
  - *Step 2: Analyse the problem*
  - *Step 3: Develop the solutions*
  - *Step 4: Implement the solution*
  - *Step 5: Evaluate the results*
  - *Step 6: Standardise the solution*
- The scientific method is the most respected method of knowledge generation as it yields objective data which is widely accepted by the professional community.
- Characteristics of the scientific method:
  - *Order and control*
  - *Empirical*
  - *Generalisation*
  - *Theory development*
- Steps of the scientific method:
  - *Formulate a question for scientific enquiry*
  - *Do a preliminary review of literature*
  - *Formulate a hypothesis*
  - *Test the hypothesis through an experiment*
  - *Analyse the data and draw conclusions*
  - *Communicate the findings*
- The limitations of the scientific method are that some nursing phenomena cannot be subjected to scientific treatment and hence cannot be studied using this method.
- Characteristics of good research:
  - *Goal-directed activity*
  - *Empirical*
  - *Logical and systematic activity*
  - *Recurring*
  - *Analytical and critical*
  - *Control*
  - *Replicability*
  - *Patient and unhurried activity*
  - *Reproducibility*
  - *Accuracy*
  - *Originality*
- The commencement of the twenty-first century witnessed an expansion in nursing research globally. Numerous scientific platforms have come into existence where nurses can communicate their research findings.
- Evidence-based nursing practice refers to the practice of nursing that is based on evidence and not on traditions, beliefs and subjective perceptions.

- Lack of knowledge about how to critique scientific articles, lack of education about the research process, lack of awareness about research or evidence-based practice, no support from administrators and lack of time to critique research literature are some important barriers to evidence-based practice.
- The broad ethical principles outlined by the Belmont Report are as follows:
  - *Principle of beneficence*
  - *Principle of respect for human dignity*
  - *Principle of justice*
- The quantitative research process can be broadly categorised into the following phases:
  - *Conceptual phase*
  - *Design and planning phase*
  - *Empirical phase*
  - *Analytic phase*
  - *Disseminating phase*
- Quantitative research proceeds in a linear fashion in which the researcher follows predefined steps. However, qualitative research typically unfolds in the field and the researcher must make numerous decisions and revisit the research process in a circular fashion.

EVALUATE YOURSELF

Long Answer Questions

Q1: Define nursing research. Explain the quantitative research process in detail.

Q2: What are the methods of knowledge generation? Explain the steps of the scientific method of knowledge acquisition.

Q3: What are the characteristics of good research? Explain the need for research in nursing.

Q4: What are the ethical principles used in nursing research? Explain in detail.

Q5: Write a short note on informed consent.

Short Answer Questions

Write short notes on:

1. Research process
2. Problem-solving process
3. Need for research in nursing
4. Ethics in nursing research
5. Evidence-based practice

Multiple Choice Questions

Q1: A limitation of the problem-solving method is that:
(a) Results are inaccurate (b) Results have limited generalisability
(c) Results are less reliable (d) None of the above

Q2: Control is an essential feature of:
(a) Experimental study (b) Descriptive study
(c) Qualitative study (d) Historical study

Q3: *Nursing Journal of India* was started in the year:
(a) 1905 (b) 1910
(c) 1915 (d) 1920

Q4: Evidence-based nursing practice refers to the practice of nursing that is based on:
(a) Evidence and not traditions, beliefs and subjective perceptions
(b) Traditional knowledge and skills acquired from senior colleagues
(c) Evidence generated through non-scientific methods
(d) Both A and B

Q5: Which of the following is/are the barrier/s to evidence-based practice in nursing?
(a) Availability of competent mentors
(b) Availability of time to critique research literature
(c) Lack of time to search and read research articles
(d) All of the above

Q6: Principle of beneficence includes:
(a) Freedom from harm (b) Right to self determination
(c) Right to full disclosure (d) Right to fair treatment

Q7: Principle of respect for human dignity includes:
(a) Right to self determination (b) Right to full disclosure
(c) Right to fair treatment (d) Freedom from harm

Q8: Principle of justice includes:
(a) Right to fair treatment (b) Right to privacy
(c) Both A and B (d) Right to fair treatment

Q9: Formulating research problems is a step of which phase of the quantitative research process?
(a) Conceptual phase (b) Design and planning phase
(c) Empirical phase (d) Analytic phase

Q10: The qualitative research process proceeds in a:
(a) Linear fashion (b) Circular fashion
(c) Zigzag fashion (d) None of the above

Answers

1. b	**2.** a	**3.** b	**4.** a	**5.** c
6. a	**7.** a	**8.** c	**9.** a	**10.** a

FURTHER READING

Barrow J. 1991. *Theories of Everything*, Oxford University Press.

Burns N, Grove S. 2001. *The Practice of Nursing Research: Conduct, Critique, and Utilization, 4th ed.* WB Saunders Company: Philadelphia.

Fink R, Thompson CJ, Bonnes D. 2005. Overcoming barriers and promoting the use of research in practice. *Journal of Nursing Administration* 35 (3):121–129.

Funk SG, Champagne MT, Wiese RA, Tornquist EM. 1991. Barriers to using research findings in practice: The clinician's perspective. *Applied Nursing Research* 4 (2): 90–95.

Haynes RB, Devereaux PJ, Guyatt GH. 2002. Clinical expertise in the era of evidence-based medicine and patient choice. *Evidence-Based Medicine* 7: 36–38.

ICMR (Indian Council of Medical Research). 1997. *Consultative Document on Ethical Guidelines on Biomedical Research Involving Human Subjects* (draft). ICMR: New Delhi.

Kuhn T. 1962. *The Structure of Scientific Revolutions,* University of Chicago Press.

Newhouse R, Dearholt S, Poe S, Pugh LC, White KM. 2005. Evidence-based practice: A practical approach to implementation. *Journal of Nursing Administration* 35 (1): 35–40.

Polit DF, Beck CT. 2003. *Nursing Research: Principles and Methods, 7th ed.* Lippincott Williams & Wilkins: Philadelphia.

Pravikoff DS, Tanner AB, Pierce ST. 2005. Readiness of US nurses for evidence-based practice. *American Journal of Nursing* 105 (9): 40–51.

Sackett DL, Haynes RB. 1995. On the need for evidence-based medicine. *Evidence-Based Medicine* 1: 5–6.

Sackett DL, Rosenberg WMC, Gray MJA, Hayes RB, Richardson WS. 1996. Evidence-based medicine: What it is and what it isn't. *British Medical Journal* 312: 71–72.

Sackett DL, Straus SE, Richardson WS, Rosenberg W, Haynes RB. 2000. *Evidence-based medicine: How to practice and teach EBM,* Churchill Livingstone: London.

Unattributed. *Research in 'Dictionary' tab.* Merriam Webster (m-w.com).

Wilson EB. 1952. *An Introduction to Scientific Research.* McGraw-Hill.

Research Problem/Question

Chapter overview

- Definition of terms
- Introduction to research problems
- Identification of the research problem
- Sources of research problems
- Characteristics of a good problem statement
- Evaluation of the research problem
- Research questions, objectives and variables
- Assumptions, limitations and delimitations
- Hypothesis—definition, characteristics, types, testing and errors in testing

"Far better an approximate answer to the right question, which is often vague, than an exact answer to the wrong question, which can always be made precise".

—JW Tukey (1962)

DEFINITION OF TERMS

Research problem A perplexing situation that needs to be resolved to improve nursing practice, or a state of difficulty that needs to be resolved. According to Robert Gerber, "A research problem is the situation that causes the researcher to feel apprehensive, confused and ill at ease". It is something that perturbs the researcher and which needs to be resolved by scientific enquiry.

Research objectives Specific statements intended to be achieved in a research project. They should be specific, measurable, feasible and tangible.

Research question An interrogative statement that subsequently leads to the development of the problem statement. Empirical data is used to derive the answer for the research question. For example, in 'a study to evaluate the effectiveness of the training programme on the knowledge, attitudes and practice of Basic Life Support techniques among students of Class 9 from selected schools in Punjab', the researcher may have asked the following questions before arriving at the problem statement:

- Can students of Class 9 learn and retain BLS knowledge and practice the techniques?
- What is the attitude of Class 9 students towards BLS after exposure to the training programme?
- Has the training programme improved the BLS performance of Class 9 students?

Hypothesis A statement of the predicted relationship between two or more variables. It is the scientific estimate based on the available literature which explains how two or more variables are related to each other.

For the example given earlier, the researcher can formulate the following hypotheses:

- H_1: There will be a significant difference in the knowledge, attitudes and practice of Class 9 students who receive BLS training and those who do not, as measured by the structured knowledge questionnaire, attitude scale and observation checklist at 0.05 level of significance.
- H_2: There will be a significant relationship between the knowledge, attitudes and practice of Class 9 students who receive BLS training and those who do not, as shown by the structured knowledge questionnaire, attitude scale and observation checklist at 0.05 level of significance.

Assumptions Statements that are taken for granted. They are believed to be true without any valid proof; however, unlike a hypothesis, they are not subjected to testing based on the data collected in a study.

For example, any descriptive study that involves a paper and pencil tool for data collection assumes that 'the information provided by the study participants is true'. However, there is no evidence or proof that the information provided by the study participants is indeed true; nor can it be tested by the data.

Delimitations The boundaries predefined by the researcher at the beginning of a research project. These are choices made by the researcher that list the things that will not be done during the course of the study—the population that will not be studied, the methodological procedure that will not be used, the literature that will not be reviewed. The researcher is required to provide reasons for these delimitations.

Limitations Shortcomings or weaknesses of the study that are beyond the control of the researcher. These are conditions/influences that place restrictions on the methodology, result and conclusions of a study. As the researcher cannot control these conditions, it is necessary that she explore and acknowledge the same in the research report so that the reader is aware of the same. While exploring the limitations, a researcher needs to focus on these areas:

- Analysis
- Tools and techniques of data collection
- Sample
- Time constraints

Operational definition Variables that are defined operationally to explain how they will be measured in a study. The operational definition of variables differs from the standard/theoretical definition. It incorporates the operation/action/procedure/manoeuvre required to measure them in a study. For example, consider the variable 'obstructed sleep apnea'. The standard definition is that it is apnea that occurs during sleep due to obstruction of the airways. However, in a research study, it can be defined operationally as 'apnea that occurs during sleep due to obstruction of the airways as evaluated by the Berlin Questionnaire'. Similarly, in another study, it may be defined as 'apnea that occurs during sleep due to obstruction of the airways as evaluated by overnight polysomnography'. The operational definition of a variable may vary from study to study.

Population The aggregate of subjects/objects in which the researcher is interested. It can be of two types:

- *Target population*: The aggregation of subjects/objects for which the researcher intends to generalise the findings of the study.
- *Accessible population:* A portion of the target population that is accessible to the researcher as a pool of subjects from which the sample is selected.

Sample A subset of the population that represents the entire population.

INTRODUCTION TO RESEARCH PROBLEMS

Identifying and formulating the research problem statement is the first step of the research process. Stating the research problem clearly is a challenging task, especially for the novice researcher. It entails more than just choosing a topic for the research project—it involves delving into an idea of interest so that the researcher can arrive at a statement for which data collection and analysis is feasible.

It may begin at the broader level, but through successive steps, is pared down to reveal a narrower focus and a more workable idea. The process can be likened to a Russian matryoshka doll, where the largest doll can be opened to reveal a smaller doll, which contains another smaller doll, and so on till we reach the smallest doll nestled in the centre of the whole object. Similarly, a researcher needs to peel away a general idea to reach a more specific and workable research problem.

IDENTIFICATION OF THE RESEARCH PROBLEM

Identification of a good researchable problem is essentially a research itself. Novice researchers face a lot of difficulty in searching for a good research problem. However, by using a systematic approach, anyone can discover a research problem that is not only researchable but which can also satisfy the scientific temperament of the profession. The novice researcher should initially focus on a broad area of interest, but it should not be too broad. The broader the problem, the more difficult it is to narrow down. The researcher must narrow her focus as she moves from the more general to the more specific. When this happens, several possible problems may emerge.

Madsen's criteria can also be used to kick-start this journey. It involves the following:

- **Sustain interest and stimulate the imagination**: The researcher must be imaginative and interested in a phenomenon. She should ask a lot of 'Why', 'How' and 'What' questions relating to the phenomenon. She should also reconsider a question for which there exists no answer in the literature or which has caused conflict among previous researchers.
- **Within the competency range**: After the researcher obtains an idea of the type of question to be used for the study, she should consider whether her expertise as a nurse qualifies her to undertake this question for scientific enquiry.
- **Having the potential to make a contribution to the body of knowledge**: She should then consider whether the selected query/problem/question will make a significant contribution to the body of knowledge of the nursing profession.
- **Based on an obtainable data**: The researcher should check if data collection is feasible for the selected scientific enquiry (Fig. 2.1).

At the end of this, she should script a single sentence that summarises her ideas; for example: *My study is about the effect of ginger juice on the reduction of morning sickness among primigravidae.*

The example about congestive heart failure and sleep apnea can be broken down thus: The researcher identified 'congestive heart failure' as her broad area of interest. Then, during the review of literature, she discovered that congestive heart failure patients frequently experienced sleep-related problems. She then further narrowed down the problem and chose the aspect 'sleep quality of congestive heart failure patients' as her specific area of interest. It is interesting that the researcher could identify a descriptive, experimental or explorative study from this research idea, as described below.

- *Scenario 1: Exploratory survey method:* The researcher is concerned about the sleep quality of patients with congestive heart failure and is interested in exploring the factors responsible for the same. The researcher can plan an explorative survey to find out the factors influencing sleep quality among congestive heart failure patients.
- *Scenario 2: Experimental method:* The researcher is concerned about the sleep quality of patients with congestive heart failure and she plans to conduct an experiment to test whether the sleep quality of such patients can be enhanced.

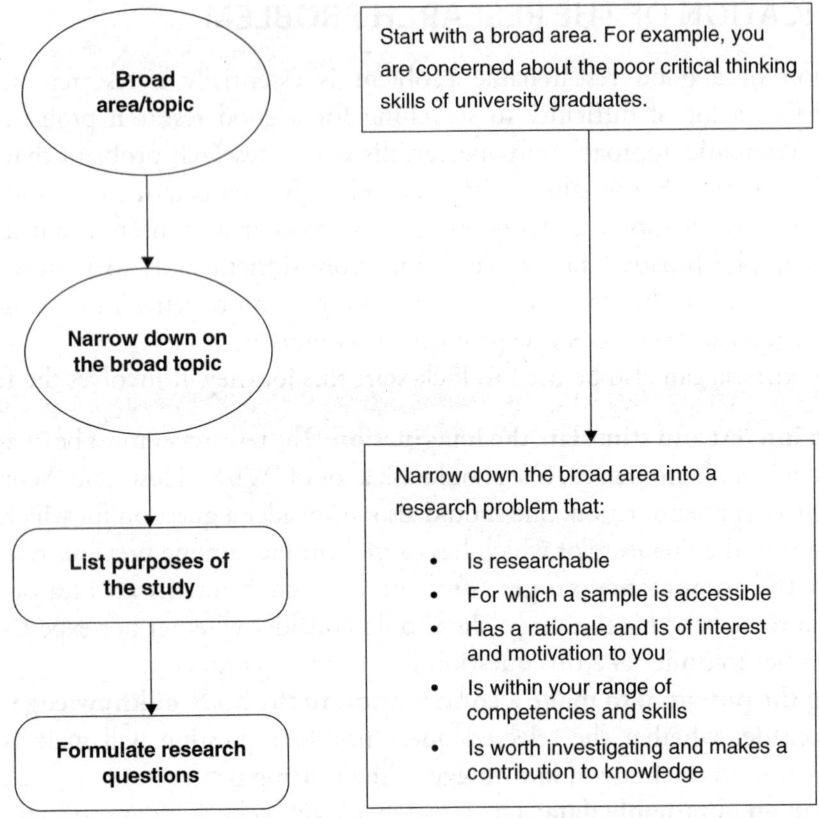

Figure 2.1 Steps in identification of the research problem

- *Scenario 3: Descriptive survey method:* The researcher may simply want to describe various aspects of the sleep quality of patients with congestive heart failure. She may administer the Kansas City Cardiomyopathy Questionnaire to a sample of congestive heart failure patients and describe various aspects of sleep quality in these patients.

SOURCES OF RESEARCH PROBLEMS

Good researchable problems in nursing can be generated from many sources. Novice researchers can explore these sources on their journey to identify a research problem.

- **Professional experience**: Nurse Practitioners may have encountered some practice-related problems that may be researched to generate evidence for nursing practice. Traditionally, nursing care protocols are transferred from an experienced nurse to a novice nurse, and there is scope for each of these protocols or procedures to be evaluated for their scientific merit. Therefore, professional experience is an important source of problems that can be researched to generate scientific evidence for nursing practice.

The researcher must ask herself 'Why am I performing this procedure in this particular way? Is there any scientific evidence for this? Can I change some steps to make it more scientific?'. These questions may help the researcher arrive at a research problem.

- **Journal articles**: Original research, review articles and case reports published in professional journals highlight areas for future research. Sometimes, individual research articles recommend a topic for future research or the novice researcher could replicate a study published in a journal in her local setting.

  Tip: Postgraduate nursing students are advised to go through the latest issues of journals of their speciality as this will familiarise them with the latest trends and areas of research in that speciality.

- **Magazines and periodicals**: Some nurse researchers feel that publications other than professional journals contain only diluted articles written for the general public. This is true to some extent, but these articles tend to eliminate technical jargon and are often good sources of research problems and hypotheses. These articles often provide interesting perspectives on complex problems and may raise questions that nurse researchers can pursue.
- **Supervisor/Guide**: Another source of research problems is the academic advisor, supervisor or guide. They are better aware of the questions and problems in an area of speciality and can provide a better research problem.
- **Funding agencies**: Funding agencies are another good source of research topics. Government and non-government organisations frequently send out announcements of funding for research topics. National consortium for PhD in Nursing, Trained Nurses Association of India, Sigma Theta Tau International Honour Society of Nursing, American Nurses Association and Indian Council of Medical Research are pioneer organisations that throw light on future areas of research in nursing and medicine. They also provide funds for the research planned within their area of interest. Professional research organisations also publish summaries that offer a close look at the main areas of research in various fields. These summaries are often useful for obtaining information about research topics, as they survey a wide variety of studies.
- **Interest and motivation**: The researcher should pick a topic that is of interest to her, because projects require a lot of effort and if the topic is not interesting, sustaining motivation will become difficult and the project may be derailed.
- **Data archives**: Data archives, such as the Royal College of Nursing archives, National Database of Nursing quality indicator, ANA database and Nurses Archives are valuable sources of ideas for researchers.
- **Social problems**: Social problems that affect the health of people can also be considered for research by nurse scholars. For example, the emerging trend of teenage sex, use of tobacco, female feticide, child marriage, delivery at home in rural India and obesity are some social problems linked to the health status of people. These topics can be explored by nurse researchers.

- **Gaps in literature**: The nurse researcher should look for gaps in the nursing literature and fill the same by undertaking research. She should become a good reader and explore in depth a particular topic of interest, till she finds her research problem.
- **Theories**: Nursing theories arise from research and also act as a source of problems for research. Hypotheses can be generated from nursing theories which can then be tested by research. Deductions are made based on the theory. Hypotheses are developed and tested empirically.

CHARACTERISTICS OF A GOOD PROBLEM STATEMENT

A good problem statement should:

- Identify the key variables under study
- Define operationally the key terms and variables of the study
- Define a concept in terms of the operations or processes used to measure or manipulate the concept (operational definition)
- Describe the nature of the population of interest
- Guide the reader and the researcher through the study
- Clarify exactly what the researcher wants to establish or solve (objectives)
- Be limited to a specific question or set of subquestions (research questions)
- Not be very long or very short (ideally the title should be 12–15 words long)

For example: *A randomised control trial on the efficacy of transparent film dressing versus pressure dressing for the prevention of bleeding and discomfort among patients who underwent coronary angiography at selected hospitals in Nagpur.*

Format of the Research Problem Title

The research problem title should include the following elements:

- Type/Design of the study
- Main purpose of the study
- Population under study
- Setting of the study

Consider the following example: *An experimental study* (design of the study) *to assess the comparative efficacy of heparin saline and normal saline flush for maintaining patency of intravenous lines* (primary purpose of the study). *among patients admitted to DMCH, Ludhiana* (population and setting of the study).

EVALUATION OF THE RESEARCH PROBLEM

Once the research problem is finalised, it is subjected to a critical evaluation by the research committee of the college to determine its merit. To evaluate a research problem, it is compared to the criteria given in the box below.

R—Researchability
R—Relevance
F—Feasibility (Resources + Time + Expertise + Ethical Considerations + Subjects)
N—Novelty
S—Significance

The 'RRFNS' approach to evaluate a research problem is examined in detail.

Researchability An important criterion for the evaluation of a research problem, researchability is the extent to which a research problem is researchable and can be resolved through analysis and interpretation of data derived from a research study. If the selected research problem is not researchable, there is no scope to proceed with that project. A topic might prove unsuitable for investigation simply because the question being asked has no answer, or at least cannot be answered with the available facilities and information. A topic may not lend itself to productive research if it requires collecting data that cannot be measured reliably and in a valid manner. In addition, the researcher should determine whether variables can be defined and measured.

Relevance The research problem should have professional relevance and improve the practice of clinical nursing, nursing education, administration or research (methodological study). A research problem lacking professional relevance cannot be considered appropriate as it does not increase the body of professional knowledge. For example, a nurse researcher is interested in exploring the variety of costumes used by Indians—this cannot be considered a good research problem in nursing science as it lack professional relevance.

Significance The significance of a research problem is determined by its merit, that is, whether the results will have practical or theoretical value. The researcher should ask herself 'Will the results add to the information already available in the field?', 'Is the problem important to patients, nurses or society?', 'Who will benefit from the knowledge generated'. If a study does not provide a positive answer to these questions, it has little value beyond the experience the researcher acquires from conducting it. This does not mean that all research has to be ground-breaking. Many investigators, however, waste a lot of valuable time trying to develop grand projects when in fact the smaller problems are of more concern to the consumers.

Feasibility The feasibility of a research problem should be analysed in terms of the cost, time, expertise, ethical principles and availability of subjects.

- In many cases, the cost of a research study is the sole determinant of its feasibility. A researcher may have an excellent research problem, but if the costs are exorbitant, the project must be abandoned. Therefore, the researcher needs to create an itemised list of all the materials, equipment and other facilities (computer, laboratory time, technical equipment, photocopier and transportation) required before beginning the project. If the costs are higher than what the researcher can afford, she should try to acquire financial aid from funding agencies, local governments and other groups that subsidise research projects.

- Research studies must be designed in such a way that they can be completed in the time available.
- The researcher must carefully analyse whether the project may cause any physical or psychological harm to the subjects under evaluation. Will they be required to answer embarrassing questions that may create adverse reactions? Is there any possibility that exposure to research conditions will have lasting effects?
- Researcher expertise in the problem area as well as in the statistical methods that will be used to analyse research data is also an important determinant of the feasibility of the project.
- Availability of the research subject within the given time frame is another important criterion. The researcher should also decide whether administrative permission can be obtained so as to not hinder access to the records required to collect data for the study.

The researcher can use the following checklist to assess the overall feasibility of her research project.

Feasibility criteria	Yes	No
Do you have enough funds/financial assistance to meet the monetary requirements of the project?		
Is there any violation of ethical principles in the project?		
Will you be able to collect the required data in the given time frame?		
Are the desired number of subjects available within the given time frame for the study?		
Do you have the required expertise in the given problem area as well as in the required statistical operations?		

RESEARCH QUESTION

The research question is the starting point of the study. It is a question that can be answered directly through data analysis. The researcher must critically analyse the research problem, data collection tools and research design to generate questions that can be answered by the research study. However, sometimes research questions are formulated first and the data collection tools and research design are finalised later.

Characteristics of a Good Research Question

A well-articulated research question has the following qualities:

- It is clear, uncomplicated and can be easily understood by others.
- It should state the relationship between two or more variables.
- It should mention variables that are measurable.
- It can be answered in the available time frame and with the available resources.

The research questions determine the population to be studied, the setting for the study, the data to be collected and the time period for the study. A clear and concisely stated research question is the most important requirement for a successful research project. Hulley and colleagues have suggested the 'FINER' criteria for the development of a good research question.

- **F**easible: A good research question should be feasible in terms of time, money, researcher expertise and availability of subjects.
- **I**nteresting: It should be of interest to the researcher.
- **N**ovel: It should be intended to explore a new concept or idea for the profession.
- **E**thical: It should comply with ethical principles of nursing research.
- **R**elevant: It should be of relevance to scientific knowledge/theory as well as to organisational, health or social management and policy.

Another useful format for the development of a specific research question is the PICOT format:

P	Population (patients)	■ What are the specifics of the patient population that you want to study?
I	Intervention (for intervention studies only)	■ What is the intervention that you intend to study?
C	Comparison group	■ What is the main alternative to compare with the intervention (placebo or no intervention)?
O	Outcome of interest	■ What do you intend to accomplish, measure, improve or affect?
T	Time	■ What is the time interval for follow-up to assess the outcome?

Knowing the specific population of interest, intervention (and comparator) and outcome of interest may also help the researcher identify an appropriate tool for data collection. The PICOT approach helps generate a question that aids in protocol development, suggesting inclusion and exclusion criteria and identifying the groups of patients to be included.

Types of Research Questions

A research project can consider three basic types of questions.

Descriptive research questions These are appropriate when the researcher wants to describe the phenomenon of interest. For example, the researcher may want to find out the proportion of teachers who support the teaching of Basic Life Support in secondary school. In this situation, she is only interested in describing how many teachers are in support of teaching BLS in secondary school.

Statistical tests used to answer descriptive questions:

- Mean, median and mode
- Frequency tables
- Histograms, line graphs

Relational research questions When the researcher wants to know the relationship between two or more variables, relational research questions are appropriate. For example, the researcher wants to find out the proportion of male and female teachers who support the teaching of Basic Life Support in secondary school. In other words, she is interested in studying the relationship between gender and the preference for teaching BLS in secondary school.

Statistical tests used to answer relational questions:

- Simple correlation
- T-test
- ANOVA

Causal research questions Causal research questions are appropriate for experimental research study. Here, the researcher wants to know whether one or more variables (independent variables) cause or affect one or more outcome variables (dependent variables). For example, the researcher conducts a workshop for a group of teachers to determine whether their opinion about teaching Basic Life Support to secondary school students has changed.

RESEARCH OBJECTIVES

After deciding on the problem title and research questions, the researcher needs to determine the research objectives—an important element of the problem statement. Research objectives define the specific aims of the study and are clearly stated in the introduction of the research protocol. They are important because they guide the development of the study protocol, design of the study and play a role in sample size calculation and determining the usefulness of the study. Study objectives should be focused on outcomes that are important to patients and be clinically relevant.

Characteristics of Good Research Objectives

Research objectives should be 'SMART'—they should be specific, measurable, attainable, realistic and time-bound:

- **Specific**: The research objectives should be specific, clarifying the what, when and how of the research problem.
- **Measurable**: They should be measurable—the researcher must be able to decide/quantify to what extent the objectives have been achieved.
- **Attainable**: The researcher must be able to attain the specified objective. Objectives that are not attainable, in terms of resources and the expertise of the researcher, cannot be considered as good objectives.
- **Realistic**: The researcher should be able to obtain the level of change reflected in the objectives.
- **Time-bound**: The objectives should be accomplished in the specified time frame.

The researcher must ensure that each specific objective begins with the word 'to'.

Consider the following example: *An experimental study to evaluate the effectiveness of the training programme on the knowledge, attitudes and practice of Basic Life Support techniques among Class 9 students in selected schools of Punjab.*

Here, the objectives of the study are:

- **To** develop and implement the BLS training programme for students of Class 9
- **To** assess and evaluate the knowledge, attitudes and practice of students of Class 9 regarding BLS before and after implementation of the training programme
- **To** find the relationship between the knowledge, attitudes and practice of BLS among students of Class 9 before and after implementation of the training programme
- **To** determine the association between the knowledge, attitudes and practice of Class 9 students regarding BLS for selected demographic variables before and after the administration of the training programme
- **To** find the association between the knowledge, attitudes and practice of Class 9 students regarding BLS for selected anthropometric variables before and after the administration of the training programme

These objectives are specific, measurable, attainable, realistic and time-bound and hence can be considered as appropriate objectives for the given research problem.

RESEARCH VARIABLES

A variable is a construct that is deliberately and consciously invented or adopted for a scientific purpose. For example, 'assertiveness' is a construct based on observations of presumably assertive and less assertive behaviour or having a value of less or more. It is so defined and specified that it can be observed and measured, for example, by administering an assertiveness test. Constructs are used in theoretical schemes and are related to other constructs.

A variable is a characteristic/property that varies from one subject/object to another. It is a symbol to which numerals of values are assigned. For example, the symbol 'height' is assigned a set of numerical values which may range from 50 to 200 cm. In the case of the variable 'literacy', there are only two possible values, i.e., literate (1) and illiterate (2); such variables are called **dichotomous variables**. Other examples of two-value variables are citizen–noncitizen, rural–urban and so on. Besides dichotomous variables, some variables are polytomies, for example, religion—Hinduism, Islam, Christianity, Buddhism, Jainism, etc.

Variable can be classified in many ways, but the two most common methods are as follows:

Independent and dependent variables

An independent variable (IV) is the presumed cause of a change in the dependent variable (DV). The independent variable is also known as the 'intervention', 'experiment', 'cause' or 'predictor', while the dependent variable is also known as the 'effect', 'outcome' or 'criterion' variable. The independent variable is the antecedent while the dependent variable is the consequent.

Consider the following example: *A randomised control trial to assess the efficacy of pomegranate juice in reducing blood pressure among hypertensive patients in a selected community of Bhopal, MP.*

In this study, the intervention/experiment/independent/cause variable is 'pomegranate juice', while the dependent/outcome/effect/consequent variable is 'blood pressure'.

Tip: The classification of variables as independent or dependent is used in all experimental and case control studies. The novice researcher should not use this classification in descriptive and exploratory studies as variables will not be manipulated in these studies.

Continuous and categorical variables

Continuous variable (also called ordinal variable) is used extensively in nursing research. It is measured on an ordered set of values within a certain range. For example, an attitude scale towards Basic Life Support may have values ranging from 16 to 80.

A categorical variable (also called nominal variable) involves two or more subsets or categories. Each categorical variable is further divided into subsets according to the characteristics that the variable is supposed to measure. For example, the variable socio-economic class (SES) may consist of three categories such as high SES, middle SES and low SES.

Other types of variables

- **Research variables**: In a descriptive/explorative study, all the variables of interest are known as research variables.
- **Demographic variables**: These are related to and describe the demographic profile of the study sample. For example, age, socio-economic status, religion, occupation, gender, professional experience and professional qualifications.
- **Extraneous variables**: These denote the extraneous situations or conditions that compete with the independent variable to have an effect on the dependent variable. Extraneous variables should be carefully identified and controlled by the researcher so that possible alternative explanations for the change in the dependent variable can be eliminated. There are several mechanisms of control of extraneous variables, such as matching and control group.

For example: *A randomised control trial to assess the efficacy of pomegranate juice in reducing blood pressure among hypertensive patients in a selected community of Bhopal, MP.* In this study, which variables can be identified as extraneous variables? Which variables also have an impact on blood pressure? After critically analysing the situation and performing an in-depth literature review, the researcher can specify that the following are extraneous variables:

- Current use of antihypertensive drugs
- Any other method of treatment adopted by the study participant (Ayurveda, Homeopathy, etc)
- Recent change in lifestyle during the study period
- Recent change in dietary habits during the study period

As mentioned earlier, these extraneous variables need to be controlled so that the researcher can clearly establish the relationship of pomegranate juice and blood pressure without any other possible alternative explanations.

Operational Definition of Variables

According to Bridgman (1927), "Operational definition means that variables used in the study must be defined as they are used in the context of the study and be publicly observable. This is done to facilitate measurement and to eliminate confusion". For example, if the researcher states that she will be studying self-esteem among patients who had undergone radical mastectomy, she should be able to explain what 'self-esteem' means in the study.

However, it should be borne in mind that not all variables are directly observable. For example, learning, memory, reasoning, and so forth cannot be observed directly. Therefore, they have to be measured in such a way that the researcher can make a convincing case for the existence of these invisible variables (Mitchell and Jolley 1988). For example, though learning cannot be seen directly, its effect on the knowledge score can be observed, i.e., learning can be operationally defined as an increase in the knowledge score. Thus, if it is observed that students improve their knowledge score after educational intervention, it can be concluded that learning has occurred. Similarly, operational definitions can be provided for such intangible variables such as attitudes, assertiveness, anxiety, and so forth.

Tips for developing research questions, hypotheses and objectives for research studies

- Inculcate the habit of asking questions as a scholar.
- Cultivate a habit of in-depth reading about a topic. Undertake a detailed literature review to enhance knowledge base and fluency with the topic.
- Keep track of recent technological advances and current trends in the area of interest.
- Consult with experts, mentors and colleagues to obtain valuable inputs that will be helpful in identifying and refining the research questions.
- Use FINER criteria to develop the relevant research questions.
- Ensure that necessary inputs are present in the research questions as per the PICOT format.
- Formulate a research hypothesis from the research question.
- Formulate clear and well-defined specific research (if needed) objectives.
- Ensure that the research question and objectives are answerable, feasible and clinically relevant.

ASSUMPTIONS

Most descriptive and exploratory studies require a statement of the underlying assumptions of the study. An assumption is a statement that is accepted as true or certain without any valid proof; in other words, these are taken for granted in a study. Assumption is synonymous with supposition or presupposition, belief, expectation, conjecture or speculation. These assumptions should be explicitly stated in the first chapter of the thesis/dissertation. Assumptions are usually made about the following:

- **Assumption about instruments**: The researcher assumes that the instrument/tool being used is a valid and reliable instrument to measure the variables under investigation.
- **Assumption about the methodology**: The researcher assumes that the methodology adopted for the study is appropriate to the problem being addressed and the purpose of the study.
- **Assumption about the participants**: The researcher assumes that participants are representative of the population and respond to questions honestly or participate without biasing the study results.

- **Assumption about the analysis**: Every statistical test has certain requirements. For example, parametric statistical tests (such as Pearson correlations, ANOVA) require normally distributed data. Therefore, the researcher is required to assume that the data will be normally distributed. If the data is not normally distributed, non-parametric procedures such as Spearman Rho should be used instead of the Pearson correlation coefficient.
- **Assumption about the power to detect**: Before conducting the analysis, the researcher assumes that the statistical tests selected and the size of the sample are sufficient to detect significant relationships if they actually exist in the population.
- **Assumption about the result**: The researcher assumes that the results are generalisable beyond the sample to the target population. Finally, it is assumed that the results of the study will be relevant to the professionals.

LIMITATIONS AND DELIMITATIONS

Limitations are the weaknesses/shortcomings of a study over which the researcher has no control, whereas delimitations are those elements of the study over which the researcher can exercise control and about which specific decisions can be taken.

The delimitations of a study are the boundaries that are predefined by the researcher in the beginning phase of a research project so that the goals do not become impossibly large. These are the choices made by the researcher that explain what will not be done—the population that will not be studied, the methodological procedure that will not be used, the literature that will not be reviewed, and so on. The researcher is required to mention the reasons for not carrying out these items and also clearly list the other options available and the reasons why these options were not selected (for example, practicality, interest or relativity).

The limitations of a dissertation are the potential weaknesses in a study that are beyond of the control of the researcher. As the researcher cannot control these conditions, it becomes necessary for her to explore and acknowledge the same in the research report so that the reader is made aware of these shortcomings before utilising the research findings. Limitations of a dissertation are typically reported in the discussion section of the thesis. Every research study has certain limitations that arise because of sample size, data collection tools, statistical tests and so on.

- **Limitations related to the instrument:** Research instruments are limited by their reliability and validity.
- **Limitations related to the methodology:** The results of a study are limited by how well the adopted research methodology has addressed the problem and purpose. The methodology adopted may increase or decrease the chances of finding an answer to the question under study.
- **Limitations related to analysis:** The results of the study are limited by the power of the statistical test to find statistical significance. The chosen statistical test must have

sufficient power to detect significant difference if they exist in the population. *G Power* is a free software program designed to determine the power of statistical tests.

- **Limitations related to the participants:** The study is limited by how well the study sample represents the entire population. In addition to this, the study results are limited by the honesty of the study subjects and their non-biased involvement (i.e., not changing their response/behaviour because they are aware that they are participating in a study).
- **Limitations related to the result:** The generalisability is limited by how well the sample represents the population. The study is also limited by the usefulness of the results to the professionals.

Consider the example: *Prevalence of obstructive sleep apnea–associated risk factors, and the quality of life among patients with congestive heart failure in India—a cross-sectional survey.*

The author delimited this study to:

1. Congestive heart failure patients seeking treatment in the OPD of a specific hospital because it was not feasible for her to collect data from other hospitals.
2. The use of the modified Berlin Questionnaire to detect OSA.

The limitations of the study were highlighted in the discussion section of the research article as follows:

The present study is limited in several ways. First, the cross-sectional data cannot actually demonstrate causal connection between variables; rather, they show statistical associations that may be consistent with several causal formulations. Second, we used the convenience sampling method, which reduces the generalisability of results. Third, we did not use polysomnography, which is a criterion standard to detect OSA. As a result, findings regarding OSA were solely dependent on self-report than the estimate of OSA. Finally, participants in the present study may not be representative of all people with CHF; in particular, those who were not coming for regular follow-up were at highest risk of OSA.

HYPOTHESIS

A hypothesis is a tentative prediction or explanation of the relationship between two or more variables. The relationship between the independent and the dependent variable is described using a connective phrase such as 'more than', 'greater than' or 'less than' or 'no different from' or 'the same as'.

Hypothesis statements are not wild guesses on the part of the researcher; rather they are educated predictions based on rationale and existing research findings. Hypotheses are generated from nursing theories. They are developed in the beginning phase of the project because their purpose is to guide the study. A hypothesis may lead the researcher to the research design, tools, data collection and analysis. Research questions are often attempts to refute/validate theories through the testing of hypotheses.

Characteristics of a Good Hypothesis

A good hypothesis must be based on a good research question. It should be simple, specific and stated in advance (Hulley et al. 2001). Following are the characteristics of a good research hypothesis:

Hypothesis should be simple: A simple hypothesis contains one independent and one dependent variable; for example, positive family history of hypertension increases the risk of developing the condition in first-degree relatives. Here, the single independent variable is positive family history of hypertension and the outcome variable is hypertension. A complex hypothesis contains more than one predictor variable or more than one outcome variable; for example, positive family history and stressful life events are associated with an increased incidence of hypertension. Here, there are two predictor variables, i.e., positive family history and stressful life events, and one outcome variable, i.e., hypertension.

Hypothesis should be specific: There should be no ambiguity about the subjects and variables, or about how the test of statistical significance will be applied in a specific hypothesis. The hypothesis must use concise operational definitions that summarise the approach to measuring variables. Often, these details may be included in the study proposal and may not be stated in the research hypothesis.

Hypothesis should be stated in advance: The hypothesis must be stated in writing during the proposal stage. This will help keep the research effort focused on the primary objective and create a stronger basis for interpreting the study's results, as compared to a hypothesis that emerges as a result of inspecting the data. The habit of post-hoc hypothesis testing (common among researchers) comprises using third-degree methods on the data (data dredging) to yield something significant. This leads to overrating of the occasional chance associations among variables in the study.

Types of Hypotheses

Null/Statistical hypothesis The word null means nothing or zero. A null hypothesis states that there is **no relationship** between two or more variables. The null hypothesis is the formal basis for testing statistical significance. By starting with the proposition that there is no association, statistical tests can estimate the probability that an observed association could be due to chance. For example, there is no difference in critical thinking skills between men and women or there is no relationship between socio-economic status and academic performance. Such a hypothesis is denoted by the symbol H_0, which means:

- The researcher does not expect the groups to be different
- The researcher does not expect the variables to be related

Null/Statistical hypothesis

$H_0: \mu_1 = \mu_2$ OR $H_0: \mu_1 - \mu_2 = 0$

In other words:

- The mean for the control group (μ_1) is equal to the mean for the experimental group (μ_2).
- The mean for the control group (μ_1) minus the mean for the experimental group (μ_2) is equal to zero.

The null hypothesis is often the reverse of what the researcher actually believes in and it is put forward to allow the data to contradict it.

Alternative/Research hypothesis The alternative hypothesis (H_1) is the opposite of the null hypothesis. It depicts the relationship between variables as believed in/expected by the researcher. It states that there is a relation/association between two or more variables. For example:

- H_1: There will be a significant difference between the knowledge, attitudes and practice of Class 9 students who receive BLS training and those who do not receive this training as measured by a structured knowledge questionnaire, attitude scale and observation checklist at 0.05 level of significance.
- H_2: There will be a significant relationship between the knowledge, attitudes and practice of Class 9 students who receive BLS training and those who do not receive this training as measured by a structured knowledge questionnaire, attitude scale and observation checklist at 0.05 level of significance.

The alternative hypothesis cannot be tested directly; it is accepted by exclusion if the test of statistical significance rejects the null hypothesis. For example, the alternative hypothesis for the study discussed earlier is that there are differences in the CPR knowledge mean scores between the control group and the experimental group, represented by the following notation:

$$H_a: \mu_1 \neq \mu_2$$

H_a: The alternative hypothesis may be that the mean scores between the experimental and control groups are not the same.

$$H_a: \mu_1 > \mu_2$$

H_a: The alternative hypothesis may be that the mean scores of the experimental group are higher than the mean scores of the control group.

H_a: $\mu_1 < \mu_2$

H_a: The alternative hypothesis may be that the mean scores of the experimental group are lower than the mean scores of the control group.

The research hypothesis is developed from the research question and then the main elements of the study—sampling, intervention, comparison and outcome variables—are summarised in a form that establishes the basis for testing and statistical significance. For example, a research study comparing lecture cum discussion with LCD versus lecture cum discussion without LCD on learning the human circulatory system among BSc Nursing first year students. The experimental group would be lecture cum discussion with LCD and the control group would be lecture cum discussion without LCD. The investigative team would first state a research hypothesis. This could be expressed as a single outcome (for example, lecture cum discussion with LCD leads to better learning of the human circulatory system) or potentially as a complex/composite outcome; that is, more than one outcome (for example, lecture cum discussion with LCD leads to both improved immediate learning and improved learning retention).

One- and two-tailed alternative hypotheses A one-tailed (or one-sided) hypothesis specifies the direction of the association between the predictor (independent) and outcome variables (dependent). The prediction that students with previous exposure to the CPR course will have a higher pretest mean CPR knowledge score than students with no exposure to the CPR course is a one-tailed hypothesis. A two-tailed hypothesis states only that an association exists; it does not specify the direction. The prediction that students with previous exposure to the CPR course will have a different knowledge score, either higher or lower, than those with no exposure to the CPR course is a two-tailed hypothesis. (The word 'tail' refers to the tail ends of the statistical distribution, such as the familiar bell-shaped normal curve that is used to test a hypothesis).

A one-tailed hypothesis has the statistical advantage of permitting a smaller sample size as compared to that allowed in a two-tailed hypothesis. It is noteworthy that one-tailed hypotheses are not always appropriate; some researchers believe that they should never be used. However, they are appropriate when only one direction for the association is important or meaningful. An example is the one-sided hypothesis that a drug has a greater frequency of side effects than a placebo; the possibility that the drug has fewer side effects than the placebo is not worth testing. A two-tailed hypothesis should be used unless there is strong justification for using a one-tailed hypothesis. As Bland and Altman stated, "One-sided hypothesis testing should never be used as a device to make a conventionally non-significant difference significant". Whatever strategy is used, it should be stated in advance; otherwise, it would lack statistical rigor.

Simple versus complex hypothesis A simple hypothesis contains one independent variable and one dependent variable. For example, the post-test knowledge score of the experimental group will be higher than the control group at 0.05 level of significance.

A complex (multivariate) hypothesis predicts the relationship between three or more variables.

For example: *There will be a significant association between the knowledge, attitudes and practice and the selected demographic variables of Class 9 students who receive the BLS training programme and those who do not receive the training, as measured by a structured knowledge questionnaire, attitude scale and observation checklist at 0.05 level of significance.*

Directional versus non-directional hypothesis A directional hypothesis predicts the direction and nature of the relationship between the two variables. For example, green grass juice will reduce the cholesterol levels of the subjects in an experimental group as compared to those in a control group. A non-directional hypothesis does not specify the nature of the relationship between the variables. For example, there is a relationship between the use of green grass juice and the cholesterol levels of obese patients.

Hypothesis Testing

The purpose of hypothesis testing is to confirm or refute the statement that the observed findings did not occur by chance alone but rather, they occurred because there was a true difference in the outcomes because of the intervention under study. A hypothesis (for example, digoxin is associated with an increased incidence of bradycardia among patients with congestive heart failure) is either true or false in the real world. Because the investigator cannot study all of the population, she must test the hypothesis in a sample of the target population. No matter how much data a researcher collects, she can never absolutely prove or disprove the hypothesis (Hulley et al. 2001).

For hypothesis testing, the researcher begins by presuming the null hypothesis—that there is no association between the independent and outcome variables in the population. Based on the data collected in the study sample, the investigator uses statistical tests to determine whether there is sufficient evidence to reject the null hypothesis in favour of the alternative hypothesis (that there is an association in the population). The standard for these tests is shown as the level of statistical significance (also known as alpha).

The null hypothesis for the preceding research hypothesis would then be that there is no association between digoxin and bradycardia among congestive heart failure patients at a 0.05 level of significance. At the end of the study, the null hypothesis is tested statistically. If the findings of the study are not statistically significant, the researcher cannot reject the null hypothesis. If the findings are significant, then she can reject the null hypothesis and accept the alternate hypothesis (i.e., there is a difference in bradycardia prevalence between those CHF patients who take digoxin and those who do not).

Steps in hypothesis testing

1. State the null hypothesis clearly with the level of significance.

2. Determine the statistical test (parametric versus non-parametric) as per the level of measurement (ratio, ordinal, nominal, continuous) of the variables of interest as stated in the null hypothesis.
3. Calculate the test value.
4. Check the test value with the test table and identify whether the *p* value is above or below the pre-decided level of significance.
5. If the *p* value for the test is below the level of significance, the results are statistically significant or otherwise.
6. If the results are significant, the researcher can reject the null hypothesis and accept the research hypothesis.

Errors in hypotheses testing

Type I and type II errors Sometimes, purely by chance, a sample may not be representative of the population. Thus, the results in the study sample will not reflect veracity in the population, and the random error will lead to an erroneous inference. A type I error (false-positive) occurs if an investigator rejects a null hypothesis that is actually true in the population; a type II error (false-negative) occurs if the investigator fails to reject a null hypothesis that is actually false in the population. Though type I and type II errors can never entirely be avoided, the investigator can reduce the likelihood of their occurrence by increasing the sample size (the larger the sample, the lower the likelihood that it will differ substantially from the population). False-positive and false-negative results can also occur because of bias (observer bias, instrument bias, recall bias) in the study.

Alpha beta and power After data collection is completed, the investigator uses statistical tests to determine whether or not to reject the null hypothesis in favour of its alternative. However, there is a chance of type I and II errors in hypothesis testing. The investigator can establish the maximum chance of making type I and type II errors in advance. The probability of committing a type I error (rejecting the null hypothesis when it is actually true) is called **α (alpha)**, also known as the level of statistical significance.

If the study of digoxin and bradycardia is designed with $\alpha = 0.05$, for example, then the investigator has set 5% as the maximum chance of incorrectly rejecting the null hypothesis (and erroneously inferring that the use of digoxin and the incidence of bradycardia are associated with patients with congestive heart failure). This is the level of reasonable doubt that the investigator is willing to accept when she uses statistical tests to analyse the data after the study is completed.

The probability of making a type II error (failing to reject the null hypothesis when it is actually false) is called **β (beta)**. The complement of beta ($1 - \beta$) is called the power of the study. It specifies the probability of observing an effect in the sample (if one of a specified effect size or greater exists in the population).

If β is set at 0.10, then the investigator has decided that she is willing to accept a 10% chance of missing an association of a given effect size between digoxin and bradycardia.

This represents a power of 0.90, i.e., a 90% chance of finding an association of that size. For example, suppose that there really would be a 30% increase in the incidence of bradycardia if the entire population took digoxin. Then, 90 times out of 100, the investigator would observe an effect of that size or larger in her study. This does not mean, however, that the investigator will be absolutely unable to detect a smaller effect; just that she will have a likelihood of less than 90% of doing so.

Ideally, alpha and beta would be set to zero in a study. This would eliminate the possibility of false-positive and false-negative results. However, in practice, they are made as small as possible. Sample size determination aims to choose an adequate number of subjects to maintain alpha and beta at acceptably low levels, without making the study expensive or difficult. However, reducing alpha and beta usually requires increasing the sample size.

Many studies set alpha at 0.05 and beta at 0.20 (a power of 0.80). The conventional range for alpha is between 0.01 and 0.10; and for beta, between 0.05 and 0.20. In general, the investigator should choose a low value for alpha when the research question is of a type that makes it particularly important that a type I (false-positive) error be avoided, and she should choose a low value of beta when it is especially important to avoid a type II error.

***P* value** When the data is analysed using parametric and non-parametric tests, such tests determine the *P* value. It is the probability of obtaining the study results by chance if the null hypothesis is true. The null hypothesis is rejected in favour of the alternative hypothesis if the *P* value is less than alpha, the predetermined level of statistical significance (Daniel 2000). 'Non-significant' results are those with *P* value greater than alpha. However, it does not imply that there is no association in the population; rather, it only means that the association observed in the sample is small compared with what could have occurred by chance alone. For example, an investigator might find that men with a family history of hypertension are twice as likely to develop stroke as those with no family history, but with a *P* value of 0.09. This means that even if family history and stroke were not associated in the population, there is a 9% chance of finding such an association due to random error in the sample. If the investigator had set the significance level at 0.05, she would have to conclude that the association in the sample was 'not statistically significant'. It might be tempting for the investigator to change her mind about the level of statistical significance ex post facto and report that the results 'showed statistical significance at $P < 0.10$'. A better choice would be to report that the 'results, although suggestive of an association, did not achieve statistical significance ($P = .09$)'. This solution acknowledges that statistical significance is not an 'all or none' situation.

Effect size The chance that a study will be able to detect an association between an independent variable and a dependent variable depends on the actual magnitude of that association in the population. Effect size refers to the magnitude of the effect of the independent variable on the dependent variables. If it is large (such as a 90% increase in the incidence of bradycardia in people who are on digoxin), it will be easy to detect it in the sample. Conversely, if the size of the association is small (such as a 2% increase in bradycardia), it will be difficult to detect in the sample. Unfortunately, the actual magnitude of the association may not be known by the researcher. Therefore, she must choose the size of the association that she would like to be able to detect in the sample. This quantity is known as the effect size.

Selection of an appropriate effect size is the most difficult aspect of sample size planning. Sometimes, the investigator can use data from other studies or pilot tests to make an intelligent guess about a reasonable effect size. When there is no data that can be used to estimate it, she can choose the smallest effect size that would be practically/clinically meaningful; for example, a 10% increase in the incidence of bradycardia. However, sometimes even a 1% increase in incidence would be highly important. Thus, the choice of effect size is always somewhat arbitrary, and considerations of feasibility are often overriding.

CHAPTER SUMMARY

- In simple terms, a research problem is a question that needs to be answered to improve the nursing practice, or it is a state of difficulty that needs to be resolved.
- Research objectives are the specific statements intended to be achieved in a research project. They should be specific, measurable, feasible and tangible.
- A research question is an interrogative statement derived from the problem statement.
- Hypothesis is the statement of the predicted relationship between two or more variables. It is a scientific guess based on the available literature that explains how two or more variables are related with each other.
- Assumptions are statements that are taken for granted. They are believed to be true without any valid proof.
- The delimitations of a study are the boundaries that are predefined by the researcher in the beginning phase of a research project. These are the choices made by the researcher which explain what will not be done during the course of the study.
- Limitations are shortcomings or weaknesses of the study which are beyond the control of the researcher. These are the conditions/influences that place restrictions on the methodology, result and conclusions of a study.
- The operational definition of variables differs from the standard/theoretical definition. It incorporates the operation/action/procedure/manoeuvre required to measure them in a study.
- Population is the aggregate of subjects/objects in which the researcher is interested. It is of two types:
  - *Target population is the aggregation of the subject/objects to which the researcher is intended to generalise the findings of the study.*
  - *Accessible population is the portion of the target population that is accessible to the researcher as a pool of subjects from which the sample is recruited.*
- The sample is the subset of the population that represents the entire population.

- The problem statement should include the following elements: type of the study/ design of the study; main purpose of the study; population under study; setting of the study.
- Many sources can generate good researchable problems in nursing: professional experience, journal articles, magazines and periodicals, funding agencies, data archives, social problems, gap in literature and nursing theories.
- Researchability, relevance, feasibility (resources + time + expertise + ethical considerations + subjects), novelty and significance are the criteria used to evaluate a research problem.
- A good research question should be feasible, interesting, novel, ethical and relevant.
- Research questions can be of different types: descriptive, relational and causal.
- Research objectives define the specific aims of the study and are clearly stated in the introduction of the research protocol.
- Research objectives should be 'SMART'—specific, measurable, attainable, realistic and time-bound.
- A hypothesis should be simple, specific and stated in advance at the outset of the study.
- A null hypothesis states that there is no relationship between two or more variables. It is the formal basis for testing statistical significance.
- A directional hypothesis predicts the direction and nature of the relationship between the two variables.
- A non-directional hypothesis does not specify the nature of the relationship between the variables.
- A type I error (false-positive) in hypothesis testing occurs if an investigator rejects a null hypothesis that is actually true in the population; a type II error (false-negative) occurs if the investigator fails to reject a null hypothesis that is actually false in the population.
- The probability of committing a type I error is called α (alpha) which is also known as is the level of statistical significance.
- The probability of making a type II error is called β (beta). The complement (1 – β) is called the power of the study.
- A variable is a characteristic/property that varies from one subject/object to another.
- An independent variable (IV) is the presumed cause of a change in the dependent variable (DV). An IV is also known as the intervention, experiment, cause and predictor. The DV is also known as the effect, outcome or criterion variable.
- A continuous variable (also called ordinal variable) is capable of taking on an ordered set of values within a certain range.
- A categorical variable (also called nominal variable) may be made up of two or more subsets or categories.
- Extraneous variables are the extraneous situations or conditions that compete with the independent variable to have an effect on the dependent variable.

EVALUATE YOURSELF

Long Answer Questions

Q1: What are the sources of research problems in nursing? Explain the criteria for a good research problem.

Q2: Formulate study objectives for the following study title: "A descriptive study to assess the quality of nursing care in selected hospitals of Ahmadabad, Gujarat".

Q3: What do you mean by hypothesis testing? Explain the process of hypothesis testing with an example.

Q4: What is the power and effect size of a study? Explain with examples.

Q5: Explain the target and accessible populations in a research study with examples.

Q6: Explain the types of variables with examples.

Short Answer Questions

Write short notes on:

1. Hypothesis
2. Sample
3. Population
4. Limitations
5. Delimitations
6. Target population
7. Accessible population
8. Variables
9. Assumptions

Multiple Choice Questions

Q1: Dichotomous variable is:

(a) Literacy
(b) Educational status
(c) Occupation
(d) All of the above

Q2: The effect size is

(a) Magnitude of effect of independent variable on dependent variable
(b) Magnitude of effect of dependent variable on independent variable
(c) Magnitude of effect of extraneous variable on dependent variable
(d) a and c

Q3: Hypothesis is:
(a) Predicted relationship between two or more variables
(b) Established relationship between two variables
(c) Power of the study
(d) Effect size of the study

Q4: Null hypothesis is also known as:
(a) Statistical hypothesis
(b) Simple hypothesis
(c) Complex hypothesis
(d) Directional hypothesis

Q5: The alpha of a study is set to 0.05. This means:
(a) There is a 5% chance of committing a type I error
(b) There is a 95% chance of committing a type I error
(c) There is a 5% chance of committing a type II error
(d) There is a 95% chance of committing a type II error

Q6: One-tailed hypothesis is also known as:
(a) Non-directional hypothesis
(b) Directional hypothesis
(c) Complex hypothesis
(d) Both a and b

Answers

1. a **2.** a **3.** a **4.** a **5.** a **6.** b

FURTHER READING

Bland JM, Altman DG. 1994. One- and two-sided tests of significance. *BMJ* 309:248.

Brian Haynes R. 2006. Forming research questions. *J Clin Epidemiol* 59: 881–86.

Daniel WW. 2002. Hypothesis testing. In: *Biostatistics, 7th ed.* John Wiley and Sons, Inc., New York, pp. 204–294.

Freedman B. 1987. Equipoise and the ethics of clinical research. *N. Engl. J. Med.* 317: 141–145.

Guyatt G, Rennie D. 2002. *User's guide to medical research: A manual for evidence-based clinical practice, 3rd ed.* AMA Press Printing, Chicago.

Hanson BP. 2006. Designing, conducting and reporting clinical research. A step by step approach. *Injury* 37: 583–594.

Hulley S, Cummings S, Browner W, *et al.* 2007. *Designing clinical research, 3rd ed.* Lippincott Williams and Wilkins, Philadelphia.

Hulley SB, Cummings SR, Browner WS, Grady D, Hearst N, Newman TB. 2001. Getting ready to estimate sample size: Hypothesis and underlying principles. In: *Designing clinical research – An epidemiologic approach, 2nd ed.* Lippincott Williams and Wilkins, Philadelphia. pp. 51–63.

Medawar PB.1969. *Induction and intuition in scientific thought.* American Philosophical Society, Philadelphia.

Popper K. 1976. *Unended Quest.* An Intellectual Autobiography. Fontana Collins, pp. 42.

Sackett D, Strauss S, Richardson W, *et al.* 2000. *Evidence-based medicine: How to practice and teach evidence-based medicine, 2nd ed.* Churchill Livingstone, Edinburgh.

Wulff HR, Pedersen SA, Rosenberg R. 1986. Empirism and Realism: A philosophical problem. In: *Philosophy of Medicine.* Blackwell Scientific Publications, Oxford.

3 Review of Literature

Chapter overview

- Introduction to review of literature
- Definition of literature review
- Purpose of literature review
- Sources of literature review—primary and secondary; electronic and printed
- Process of review of literature
- Writing a review of literature
- Review format

INTRODUCTION TO REVIEW OF LITERATURE

Review of literature is an important step carried out by scholars to explore the relevant data/facts in a particular area of interest. By conducting a comprehensive review of literature, the researcher becomes familiar with the existing body of knowledge on that subject and can identify gaps and plan research studies to fill the same. Most textbooks on nursing research identify review of literature as the second step in the quantitative research process; however, it is equally true that it can serve as the starting point for a research project. It deals with the analysis of a body of literature in order to classify it according to themes or categories. A literature review often forms part of a larger research project, such as within a thesis (or major research paper), or it may be an independent written work, such as a synthesis or systematic review paper.

DEFINITION OF LITERATURE REVIEW

According to Fink, review of literature is, "The process of reading, analysing, evaluating and summarising scholarly material about a specific topic. The results of this may be compiled in a report or may serve as part of a research article, thesis or grant proposal".

According to Beanland et al., "It should be a broad, comprehensive, in-depth, systematic and critical review of scholarly publications, unpublished scholarly print material, audiovisual material and personal communications".

The material to be reviewed typically includes scholarly journals and books, authoritative databases and primary sources. Sometimes, it includes newspapers, magazines, other books, films, and audio and video tapes, and other secondary sources.

Literature review should provide an overview of what has been researched, who the key experts/authors are, what questions have been explored, what tools/instruments have been used, and what methods and methodologies are appropriate and useful for the particular research project. According to Queensland University, "A literature review is an evaluative report of information found in the literature related to the selected area of study. The review describes, summarizes, evaluates and clarifies this literature. It gives a theoretical base for the research and helps to determine the nature of research".

The University of Toronto states that, "A literature review is an account of what has been already established or published on a particular research topic by accredited scholars and researchers".

PURPOSE OF LITERATURE REVIEW

During a research project, the researcher needs to make many decisions relating to various aspects of the project. Review of literature helps the researcher make an informed decision by providing relevant information to the researcher. Some of the important purposes served by literature review are discussed here.

- **Generating an idea for research**: An in-depth literature review helps the researcher identify the gaps in the literature, inconsistency in the results of studies, conflicting findings and unexplored areas; this can lead to the development of research problems. The recommendation section of a journal article throws light on areas of future research. It also provides information about areas of prior scholarship so that duplication of effort can be avoided.
- **Refining the research questions**: While performing a literature review, the researcher may come across unanswered questions related to an area of enquiry. The research questions can be further processed by incorporating valuable inputs from previous studies.
- Review of literature provides **insight into what is already known** and what needs to be explored in an area of interest.
- The researcher can determine **whether a study should be replicated** in her institutional settings with a different group of subjects.
- **Conceptual framework** is an important aspect of all nursing research studies. Literature review supplies the researcher with information about which theory or conceptual model is best applicable for a selected research problem. The researcher can find out which conceptual framework had been used by previous studies in similar areas.

- In-depth literature review helps a researcher **develop interventional protocols** for an experimental study.
- With the help of literature review, the researcher can **define the key variables** of her study.
- Review of literature can make the researcher **aware of the extraneous variables** which need to be controlled.
- It helps the researcher **decide on the best research approach** and design for her study. The researcher may come across various designs used in previous studies and can judge which design has the potential to best answer the research question.
- **Data collection tools and techniques** can be explored through systematic literature review. The researcher can identify which are the reliable and valid standardised tools to measure the variable of interest, which tool can be used unchanged or whether the tool needs to be modified for her study group and setting.
- It helps the researcher **formulate a hypothesis** for the newly developed research problem.
- It assists the researcher in **developing a new data collection tool** to measure a concept when a valid and reliable tool is not available.
- It provides **background data** which is used to discuss the findings of the study and helps in discovering implications and recommendations.

SOURCES OF LITERATURE REVIEW

Literature can be obtained from two main sources, classified as primary and secondary.

Primary sources are the primary accounts provided by witnesses of an event. It is considered a fundamental document relating to a particular subject. It is written by the person who conducted the research study or discovered a fact. All original research articles published in journals or electronic databases may be considered as primary sources.

Secondary sources are descriptions prepared by someone other than the original researcher. It includes documents or any other publications which discuss information originally presented elsewhere. Secondary sources are accessible as physical objects or electronically in databases on the internet.

Primary and secondary sources can be further classified as electronic and print sources.

Electronic Sources

Computer-assisted literature search has revolutionised the review of literature. General literature search can be achieved using a number of search engines:

WebCrawler	Info.com	ChaCha
Lycos	Yahoo! Search	Blackle.com
Yandex	Ask.com	DuckDuckGo
Google	Live Search	Bing

These search engines can provide useful general information, but for nurse scholars, the most relevant literature will be found in nursing databases. Some important nursing databases are listed here.

CINAHL plus with full text It is a leading database used by most nurse researchers. It includes scholarly journal articles about nursing and allied health sciences. It indexes more than 950 journals and publications of American Nurses Association and National League for Nursing. It contains material such as books, pamphlets, dissertations, conference proceedings, professional practice standards, nurse practice acts, critical paths, and research instruments from 1982 to the present. This database includes 420,000 records from biomedicine, management, behavioural sciences, health sciences, education and consumer health literature. It is accessible at http://www.cinahl.com.

MEDLINE® database Medical Literature Analysis and Retrieval System Online is another electronic source of literature review commonly used by nurses and other healthcare professionals. It is accessible through PubMed online. It is widely recognised as the premier database for bibliographic coverage of biomedical research. It covers more than 11 million records and more than 4300 journals.

PubMed This is the National Library of Medicine's (NLM) premier database of scholarly citations covering nearly 4500 journals published in the US and more than 70 other countries. The PubMed database includes scholarly journal articles about health and medicine, nursing, audiology and biology and many other areas. Every week, new citations are updated in the database. It is available at http://www.pubmed.com.

MedlinePlus It is the NLM's website for consumer health information. It is available at http://www.medlineplus.gov.

Registry of nursing research Sigma Theta Tau International Honor Society of Nursing provides access to this database through its Virginia Henderson International Nursing Library. Access has been designed so as to make it easier for users to explore evidence and scientific findings from more than 2200 research article abstracts and conference abstracts. Free access to this database is available at http://www.nursinglibrary.org.

Cochrane database of systematic reviews Cochrane database is a leading source of systematic reviews of primary research in human healthcare and policy. It includes systematic reviews of experimental studies and provides information about various interventions relating to prevention, treatment and rehabilitation of a specific disease and other problems in health sciences. A reader can judge whether an intervention is feasible or not for a specific problem. It is a unique collection of known evidence in a particular area of interest. Each systematic review, as compared to other forms of literature reviews, are more in-depth and comprehensive and address a specific question which reduces the chances of bias and subjectivity and increases the reliability of the review. It also incorporates references of all the trials related to an intervention. Intervention, methodology, diagnostic test accuracy and overviews of reviews are the four types of review published in this database. The impact factor of this database was 5.939 in the year 2013, which is very high. It can be accessed at http://www.cochranelibrary.com/.

HaPI Health and Psychosocial Instruments is a leading source of a variety of different types of data collection instruments (i.e., questionnaires, checklists, index measures, coding schemes/manuals, rating scales, projective techniques, vignettes/scenarios, tests) in the fields of health, psychosocial sciences, nursing, sociology, organisational behaviour, communication and public health. It can be accessed at http://bmdshapi.com/.

Health reference centre academic This database provides over 160 full-text journals in medicine, nursing, alternative medicine and consumer health. It also includes overviews of clinical topics, and abstracts for more than 1500 additional titles on patient and consumer health information.

R2 digital library This is a web-based database from Rittenhouse Book Distributors. This platform provides access to many medical, nursing and allied health books content from key publishers in the field. It offers the best selection of up to date, health sciences–focused, cross-referenced content. The R2 Digital Library offers exclusive access to health science ebooks and pass-through access to PubMed, MeSH, CINAHL and Precision Search from Doody Enterprises. It can be accessed at www.r2library.com.

Scopus It is a unique abstract and citation database of scientific journals, books and conference proceedings. It delivers a comprehensive overview of research output in the fields of science, technology, medicine, social sciences, and arts and humanities. There are 55 million records, 21,915 titles and 5000 publishers in this database. It provides smart tools to track and analyse research articles. Citation overview/tracker facilitates tracking of citations over time for a set of authors or documents. Analyze results helps assess trends in search results. It also helps to explore how many citations an article or author has received. It can be accessed at www.scopus.com.

EBSCOhost online research databases This is the leading database of scholarly research articles and an ebook provider in the field of health sciences. It has more than 375 full-text and secondary research databases and more than 300,000 ebooks. EBSCO provides access to world-class content in all subject areas including magazine and journal articles. It serves thousands of libraries and other institutions with premium content in every subject area. It can be accessed at www.ebscohost.com.

AgeLine This is a database of literature exclusively related to the segment of population aged 50 and above. The various types of literature available in this database include social gerontology, ageing-related content from the health sciences, psychology, sociology, social work, economics and public policy. It indexes over 600 journals, books, book chapters, reports, dissertations and consumer guides. This database addresses ageing issues from the individual, national and global perspectives. It was previously freely available through the American Association of Retired Persons; at present, it is available on subscription through EBSCOhost. It can be accessed at http://www.ebscohost.com/ACADEMIC/ageline.

Alt health watch This database offers full-text articles from more than 190 international, and often peer-reviewed, journals. Periodicals, peer-reviewed journals, academic and professional publications, magazines, research reports and association newsletters focused on complementary, alternative and integrated approaches to healthcare are available. It can be accessed at http://www.ebscohost.com/academic/alt-healthwatch.

ERIC A free literature search may be carried out at http://www.eric.ed.gov.

Psyc INFO It includes scholarly articles on psychology, medicine, psychiatry, education, social science, business and organisational behaviour. It covers academic paper, research, journal articles, dissertations, books and technical reports from over 45 countries and in more than 30 languages. It may be accessed at http://www.psychinfo.com.

Dissertation abstracts online Abstracts of Master's and doctoral theses are available in this electronic database.

Sociological abstracts This includes scholarly journal articles from sociology and other social and behavioural sciences.

Health STAR **(Health services technology administration and research)**

Radix **(Nursing and managed care database)**

ETOH **(Alcohol and Alcohol Problems Science Database)**

Rndex **(Nursing and managed care database)**

AIDSLINE **(AIDS Information On-Line)**

CancerLit **(Cancer Literature)**

EMBASE **(the Excerpta Medica database)**

Online journals

- Journal of Clinical Nursing (http://onlinelibrary.wiley.com/journal/10.1111/%28ISSN%291365-2702)
- Japan Journal of Nursing Sciences (http://onlinelibrary.wiley.com/journal/10.1111/(ISSN)1742-7924)
- Journal of Symptoms and Signs (http://www.intermedcentral.hk/index.php?journal=jss)

- Journal for Specialists in Pediatric Nursing (http://onlinelibrary.wiley.com/journal/10.1111/(ISSN)1744-6155)
- Journal of Advanced Nursing (http://onlinelibrary.wiley.com/journal/10.1111/(ISSN)1365-2648)
- Journal of Cardiovascular Nursing (http://journals.lww.com/jcnjournal/pages/default.aspx)
- AACN Advanced Critical Care (http://journals.lww.com/aacnadvancedcriticalcare/pages/default.aspx)
- International Journal of Nursing Studies (http://www.journals.elsevier.com/international-journal-of-nursing-studies)
- International Nursing Review (http://onlinelibrary.wiley.com/journal/10.1111/(ISSN)1466-7657)

Printed Sources

Printed research summaries may be located from published abstracts such as Nursing Research Abstract, Psychological Abstracts, Dissertation Abstract International and Masters Abstract International. Several national and international journals can be used to review research-related literature. Following are the main national and international journals:

- The Nursing Journal of India
- International Journal of Nursing Care
- International Journal of Nursing Education
- Journal of Cardiovascular Nursing
- Journal of Advanced Nursing
- Journal of Symptoms and Signs
- Nursing Research
- Nursing Sciences Quarterly
- Applied Nursing Research
- Advances in Nursing Sciences
- Clinical Nursing Research
- American Journal of Nursing
- International Journal of Nursing Studies
- Journal of Nursing Administration

REVIEWING LITERATURE

The process of reviewing includes:

- Searching for literature
- Sorting and prioritising the retrieved literature
- Analytical reading of papers
- Evaluative reading of papers

- Comparison across studies
- Organising the content
- Writing the review

Searching for literature Before starting the literature review, the researcher should be clear about the keywords that will be most helpful in retrieving the relevant literature from a known source. Most research abstracts mention keywords at the end. These can be used by the researcher while performing an online literature search. On entering the keywords in the search box, links to the relevant existing literature are displayed. Novice researchers are advised not to use the words 'of', 'and', 'both' and any other connecting phrase as keywords as these may render the literature search less effective.

The literature search can be performed for hard copies from a research library; the researcher must refer to the library indexing system or catalogue to retrieve the literature of interest.

Sorting and prioritising the retrieved literature Once the researcher has gained access to online sources of literature, she will find many research articles, most of which may not be of use. She needs to go through the abstracts (appear at the beginning) of the article to determine their usability for the study. Articles are sorted and arranged in the order of priority for full reading and review.

Analytical reading of the papers This step includes an analytical, in-depth reading of all the relevant articles as per the set priority. The researcher should immerse herself in the related literature and obtain insights about the research problem.

Evaluative reading of the papers Evaluative reading of the papers is undertaken to judge the strength and limitations of the relevant literature.

Comparison across the studies Research studies are compared to identify the variations and different strategies used by researchers. The researcher must compare the studies on the basis of research methodology adopted, research designs, sample size, population, inclusion criteria, exclusion criteria, variables, tools and techniques of data collection, results, statistical tests used and so forth.

For example, Table 3.1 compares the prevalence of obstructed sleep apnea (OSA) in patients with congestive heart failure (CHF) across various studies.

Organising the content Relevant research papers should be organised in a predefined order. The contents of the papers should be extracted in the researcher's own words and should be shown in chronological order or by relevance in the thesis.

Writing a review of the literature Before writing a review of the literature, the researcher should undertake certain steps:

1. *Clarify important questions*: The novice researcher should clarify the following from the supervisor:

Table 3.1 Global prevalence of OSA in CHF patients

S. No.	Authors	Country	Prevalence (%)	Sample	Technique*
1.	Ferric et al.	New Zealand	53	CHF out-patients	PSG**
2.	Jawahri	USA	12	Male patients with systolic HF	PSG
3.	Tremela et al.	France	25	LVF, NYHA II, III	PSG
4.	Roebuck et al.	Australia	28	Patients with severe CHF	PSG
5.	Oldenburg et al.	Germany	36	Stable CHF patients	Polygraphy
6.	The present study	India	18	Stable CHF patients	Questionnaire
			8	Healthy controls	
7.	Sharma et al.	India	13.7	General population	Questionnaire and PSG
8.	Udwadia et al.	India	7.5	General population	Questionnaire

**Technique used for the diagnosis of OSA*
*** Polysomnography*

- How many sources should she include?
- What types of sources (books, journal articles, websites) should she use?
- Must she summarise, synthesise or critique sources by discussing a common theme or issue?
- Should she evaluate the sources?
- Should she provide subheadings and other background information, such as definitions and/or a history?

2. *Find models*: The researcher should look for other literature reviews in the area of interest or in the discipline, and read them to get a sense of the type of themes she might want to check for in her own research or ways to organise the final review.
3. *Narrow down the topic*: There are hundreds or even thousands of articles and books on most areas of study. The narrower the topic, the easier it will be to limit the number of sources the researcher needs to read in order to obtain a good survey of the material.
4. *Find a focus*: A literature review, like a term paper, is usually organised around ideas, not the sources themselves, as an annotated bibliography would be organised. This means that the researcher will not just list the sources but elaborate on each in detail, one at a time.
5. *Consider organisation:* Having now obtained a focus and having narrowed it down to a thesis statement, the researcher should consider the most effective way of presenting

the information. She should specify the most important topics and subtopics that the review needs to include and also the order in which they should be presented. In short, she should develop an organisation for the review, both at a global and at a local level.

REVIEW FORMAT

There is no any standardised format for review of literature and it may vary from one discipline to another. Whatever the format for review literature, it should provide a rationale for engaging in primary research; it should also be self-contained. An original research article published in a journal usually does not have a separate section for literature review; therefore, the author of the article presents it in the background and introduction section of the article. However, the review of literature is a separate chapter in BSc Nursing and MSc Nursing which is arranged as an introduction, middle (body) and conclusion. The review of literature should critically analyse the published literature through comparison and classification. Here, the format of review literature used in postgraduate nursing thesis is discussed.

Introduction Here, the researcher should define or identify the general topic or area of concern. This would provide a context for reviewing the literature. The introduction should specify the reasons for reviewing the literature and explain the organisation of the review (sequence). The researcher should state what literature is and is not included (the scope of review).

Body The body is the main section in which research papers or other types of literature (reviews, theoretical articles, case studies) are arranged in groups according to common themes such as qualitative versus quantitative studies, specific purpose or objective, chronology, etc. The individual research studies should be summarised with as much or as little detail as each merits, according to its comparative significance in the literature. Strong 'umbrella' sentences should be used at the beginning of paragraphs, and brief 'so what' summary sentences at intermediate points in the review will assist readers in understanding comparisons and analyses. The researcher should proceed from the general view of the research to the specific problem of interest.

Chronological approach: This means studies that have been published most recently will be presented first, followed by other studies in chronological order. For instance, the studies published in 2013 will be presented first, followed by those published in 2012 and so on. The disadvantage of this system is that there is relatively no continuity among subjects.
Thematic approach: Such reviews are organised around a topic or issue, rather than the progression of time. However, chronology may still be an important factor in a thematic review while more authentic thematic reviews tend to move away from chronological order.
Methodological approach: This approach differs from the other two in that the content of the material is not the focusing factor. Instead, the focus is on the methods of the researcher.

Conclusion The conclusion of a review of literature should summarise the main contributions and evaluate the current 'state of the art' literature reviewed. Major flaws or gaps in research, inconsistencies in theory and findings, and areas or issues pertinent to future study should be highlighted. Some insight must be provided into the relationship between the central topic of the review and the larger scope of study, such as a discipline or a profession.

Novice researchers must understand the importance of writing a good review of literature. Table 3.2 depicts the differences between what constitutes a good review and a bad review of literature.

Table 3.2 Differences between good and bad review of literature

Good review of literature	Bad review of literature
■ Has appropriate breadth and depth	■ Is constructed in an arbitrary way
■ Is a synthesis of available research	■ Is confined to description
■ Is a critical evaluation	■ Is an annotated bibliography
■ Uses rigorous and consistent methods	■ Is narrow and shallow
■ Has clarity and conciseness	■ Is confusing and longwinded

Example of a bad review Obstructed sleep apnea has many consequences. Patidar, Sukh and Choudhary (2009) found that it is a problem of obese people that can lead to hypertension, stroke, diabetes, excessive daytime sleeping (leading to automobile crash), myocardial infarction and even death. They also found that the prevalence of OSA is similar in men and women. Their research was a survey of 100 men and women residents of a selected community in New Delhi. Sharma's study on OSA lists many problems caused by OSA. In his excellent book, Varma (2005) gives a long list of consequences that OSA victims have suffered.

Example of a better review OSA patients suffer a range of health consequences, from excessive daytime sleepiness and road traffic accidents to stroke, hypertension and diabetes (Patidar, Kaur and Saini 2014, Ahir 2001, Kaur and Patidar 1999). For example, Patidar, Kaur and Saini (2014) noted that 60% of OSA patients were suffering from hypertension and diabetes.

CHAPTER SUMMARY

- Review of literature refers to the process of reading, analysing, evaluating and summarising scholarly material about a specific topic. The results may be compiled in a report or may serve as part of a research article, thesis or grant proposal.

- It should be a broad, comprehensive, in-depth, systematic and critical review of scholarly publications, unpublished scholarly print material, audiovisual material and personal communications.
- Identification of a research problem, development or refinement of research questions, finding out gaps or inconsistencies in the body of knowledge, identification or development of clinical interventions to test through empirical research, identification of suitable design and data collection methods for a research study, and provision of insight about how others have defined and measured key variables are some important purposes of review of literature.
- Literature can be reviewed from two main sources: primary and secondary.
- Primary sources are the fundamental documents relating to a particular subject or idea. Often, they are first-hand accounts written by a witness or researcher at the time of an event or discovery.
- Secondary sources are documents or recordings that relate to or discuss information originally presented elsewhere.
- CINAHL Plus with full text is a database that deals exclusively with nursing and includes scholarly journal articles about nursing and allied health sciences.
- PubMed is the National Library of Medicine's (NLM) premier database of scholarly citations covering nearly 4500 journals published in the US and more than 70 other countries.
- Sigma Theta Tau International Honor Society of Nursing provides access to Registry of Nursing Research, a database, through its Virginia Henderson International Nursing Library.
- Writing a review of literature starts with clarification of important questions and proceeds through model finding, narrowing the topic, finding a focus and considering the organisation (introduction, body and conclusion).

EVALUATE YOURSELF

Long Answer Questions

Q1: Define review of literature. List the purposes of the literature review.

Q2: Explain the process of review of literature step by step. How will you organise the review of literature in your thesis? Explain with an example.

Q3: What are the sources of literature review? Explain with examples.

Q4: List the important electronic and print databases used by nurse researchers for review of literature.

Q5: What important questions will you ask while evaluating the review of literature?

Short Answer Questions

Write short notes on:

1. Primary and secondary sources of review literature
2. Electronic search for review
3. Steps of literature review
4. Online journals in nursing
5. Need for review of literature

Multiple Choice Questions

Q1: Which of the following is a nursing and allied health sciences database?

(a) CINAHL Plus (b) Pub Med
(c) Medline Plus (d) All of the above

Q2: HaPI stands for

(a) Health and Psychosocial Instruments
(b) Hazardous Psychological Illness
(c) Harmful Psychological Instruments
(d) Health and Psychiatric Illness

Q3: Which of the following is exclusively related to a population of 50 years and above?

(a) Elderly line (b) AgeLine
(c) Old age line (d) Helpline

Q4: Psyc INFO includes scholarly articles related to

(a) Psychology (b) Medicine
(c) Psychiatry (d) All of the above

Q5: Health STAR stands for

(a) Health services technology administration and research
(b) Health sector technology administration and revolution
(c) Health service techniques administration and response
(d) Health service technology augmentation with research

Answers

1. a **2.** a **3.** b **4.** d **5.** b

FURTHER READING

About.com Grammar and Composition glossary (http://grammar.about.com/od/il/g/literaturereviewterm.htm retrived on 14/03/2013)

Afolabi M. 1992. The review of related literature in research. *International Journal of Information and Library Research* 4(1): 59–66.

Anson CM, Schwegler RA. 2000. *The Longman Handbook for Writers and Readers, 2nd ed,* Longman, New York.

Bourner T. 1996. The research process: Four steps to success. In: *Research methods: Guidance for postgraduates,* Greenfield, T (ed), Arnold, London.

Bruce CS. 1994. Research student's early experiences of the dissertation literature review. *Studies in Higher Education* 19(2): 217–229.

Caspers JS. 1998. Hands-on instruction across the miles: Using a web tutorial to teach the literature review research process. *Research Strategies* 16(3): 187–197.

Cooper HM. 1989. Integrating research: *A guide for literature reviews, 2nd ed,* Sage Publications, Newbury Park, California.

CQ University Library. *Literature Review Tutorial.* (http://libguides.library.cqu.edu.au/litreview)

Jones R, Bizzaro P, Selfe C. 1997. *The Harcourt Brace Guide to Writing in the Disciplines,* Harcourt Brace, New York.

Lamb SE. 1998. *How to Write It: A Complete Guide to Everything You'll Ever Write,* Ten Speed Press, Berkeley, California.

Leedy PD. 1997. *Practical research: Planning and design, 6th ed,* Merrill, Upper Saddle River, NJ.

Libutti P, Kopala M. 1995. The doctoral student, the dissertation, and the library: A review of the literature. *Reference Librarian* 48(5): 5–25.

Mauch JE, Birch JW. 2003. *Guide to the successful thesis and dissertation: A handbook for students and faculty, 5th ed,* Marcel Dekker, New York.

Rosen LJ, Behrens L. 2000. *The Allyn and Bacon Handbook, 4th ed,* Allyn and Bacon, Boston.

Taylor D. University of Toronto. *The Literature Review: A Few Tips on Conducting It.* (http://www.writing.utoronto.ca/advice/specific-types-of-writing/literature-review)

Troyka, LQ. 2002. *Simon and Schuster Handbook for Writers,* Prentice Hall, Upper Saddle River, NJ.

Research Approaches and Designs

Chapter overview

- Introduction to research approach/design
- Definitions of research design
- Factors influencing selection of design
- Types of research approaches—quantitative, qualitative, pragmatic and action
- Quantative research design—experimental: true experiments, quasi-experiments, pre-experiments; non-experimental: descriptive and exploratory, comparative study, case control study, prospective and retrospective
- Validity of research design
- Qualitative research design—historical research, grounded theory, ethnography, phenomenology
- Other research designs—case study, secondary data analysis, meta-analysis, evaluation research, focus group interviews

INTRODUCTION TO RESEARCH APPROACH/DESIGN

When the research questions have been finalised by the researcher, she should select the research approach/design that will be most suitable for answering the questions. Research design is the overall blueprint of a research study specified by the researcher to undertake a study of interest. Classification of research designs is based on the type of approach used by the researcher.

Definition of Research Design

Research design is referred to as a master plan that specifies the procedure for data collection and analysis, selection of participants and how and when treatment conditions will be implemented in a research study. The term research design is used interchangeably with research methodology.

Research design is defined as a blueprint of study that specifies various procedures such as research approach, sampling method, process of randomisation, setting of the study, treatment condition, tools and techniques for data collection and analysis use to obtain answers to the research questions and for testing hypotheses. Fig. 4.1 highlights the components of a research design.

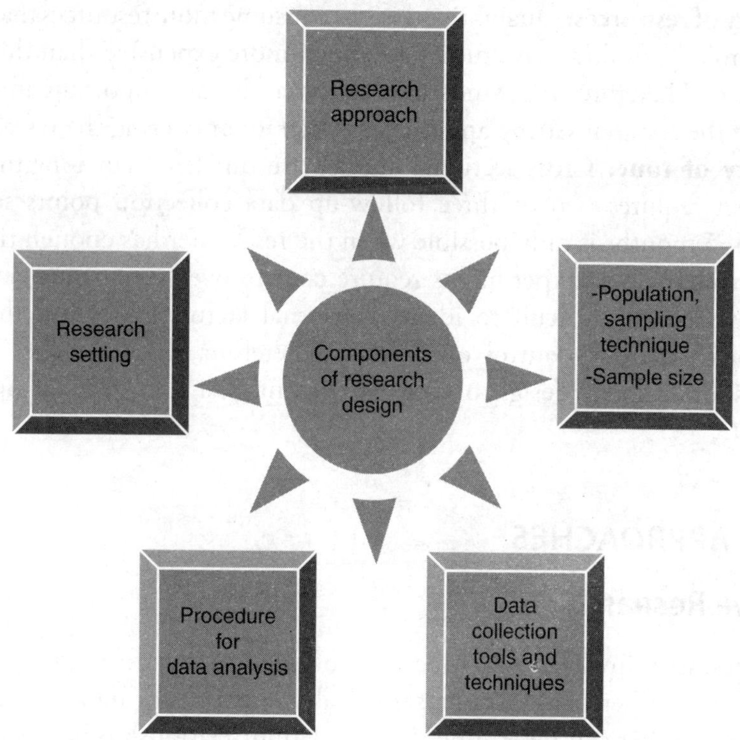

Figure 4.1 Components of research design

The researcher makes decisions about these components of research design after carefully analysing the pros and cons of every selection so that answers to the research questions can be obtained objectively and accurately. Various factors are considered during this decision-making process.

Factors influencing selection of design

- **Purpose of the study:** This may focus on description, exploration and/or prediction of phenomena and experimentation to establish causal relationship between independent and dependent variables. Accordingly, the researcher must select a descriptive, explorative or experimental design for the study.
- **Nature of the problem under investigation:** Whether the problem requires experimentation or if a simple observation will be sufficient. Accordingly, the researcher will select either experimental design or observational study.

- **Availability of subjects:** Whether the targeted subjects/patients are easily accessible and available in sufficient number. How much time it will take to recruit the required number of participants. Answers to these questions will assist the researcher in selecting the appropriate sampling strategy and sample size. For example, if a patient suffering from a rare disease is the study participant, the researcher should choose the snowball sampling technique or a small sample size for the study.
- **Availability of resources:** Qualitative designs consume more resources than quantitative studies. Similarly, multicentre studies are much more expensive than those conducted in one place. Therefore, the funds available may be an important influence in the selection of the research setting and the approach for answering the research questions.
- **Availability of time:** Cross-sectional studies are quicker than longitudinal studies. Studied that requires two or three follow-up data collection points separated by a period of 4–5 months is only possible when the researcher has enough time to invest.
- **Control mechanisms:** Experiments require control over extraneous factors. In some situations, it is very difficult to identify external factors and select the appropriate mechanism to exercise control over them. Therefore, the researcher should either select quasi-experiment design or pre-experiment design instead of opting for true experiment.

RESEARCH APPROACHES

Quantitative Research

Quantitative research involves the collection of data in the form of quanta/numbers that enable the researcher to undertake statistical operations for data analysis. Using this approach, the researcher can determine the association/relationship between two or more variables. For example, people with congestive heart failure may have increased prevalence of obstructed sleep apnea, as compared to their healthy counterparts. Quantitative researchers need to take care to avoid bias, opinions and attitudes which may affect the study results.

The quantitative researcher operates in a predetermined manner and sequence. Sample size, sampling technique, population, independent variable, dependent variables, extraneous variables, control, research variables, statistical tests, data collection tools and techniques are considered, prepared and controlled in advance.

Qualitative Research

Unlike in quantitative research, qualitative research is focused on gaining a rich and complex understanding of people's lived experience, culture and human behaviour. Qualitative research is less concerned with the generalisation of findings to the larger population. Neither the sample size nor the other features mentioned in quantitative research are predetermined; rather, these decisions are made in the field as the study unfolds.

Data collection and analysis takes place simultaneously in the research field itself. Data is collected in the form of verbatim accounts on the basis of observation and interaction with the participants. Data is not converted to numerical form and is therefore not amenable to statistical operations.

Interviews with participants are open-ended, giving them the opportunity to liberally explore their point of view towards a phenomenon. This may mean adopting a less formal and more open-ended approach, which is less narrow and more exploratory than that used in quantitative research. The researcher is free to go beyond the initial response that the participant gives and to ask why, how, in what way, etc. In this way, subsequent questions can be tailored to the response already given. Data is collected to the level of saturation (no new information can be obtained by recruiting more study participants), which in turn determines the sample size.

Sample size is usually small in qualitative research because the methods used in data collection are time- and labour-intensive. Also, a large number of people are not required for the purposes of statistical analysis or to make generalisations from the results.

Table 4.1 Differences between qualitative and quantitative research

Qualitative research	Quantitative research
Quality research assumes that there is no single reality; it varies by person and time. Truth is complex and dynamic, leading to many realities.	Quantitative research believes that there is only one reality. Truth is absolute; multiple truths are not possible.
It is considered a soft science.	It is considered a hard science.
It is subjective, inductive, dialectic and holistic in nature.	It is objective and reductionist in nature.
Emphasis is on understanding the meaning of phenomena.	Emphasis is on quantising phenomena.
Unstructured data collection tools are used.	Structured data collection tools are used.
It is concerned with uniqueness of data.	It is concerned with generalisation of data.
Goal is to generate theory.	Goal is testing of theory.
Research questions are broad.	Research questions are narrow and specific.
It uses process consent (ongoing, dynamic).	It uses informed consent.
Theoretical sampling is used.	Probability or non-probability sampling is used.

Mixed Methods Approach/Pragmatic Approach

The pragmatic approach is a blend of the quantitative and qualitative approaches. Pragmatic researchers use any of the methods, techniques and procedures typically associated with quantitative or qualitative research. Data analysis depends on the nature of the variable to be analysed. However, it is sometimes possible to convert qualitative data into quantitative data and vice versa, though transforming quantitative data into qualitative data is not very common. Triangulation is a common feature of mixed method studies; this refers to the use of a variety of data sources (data triangulation), of several different researchers (investigator triangulation) and of multiple methods to study a research problem (methodological triangulation).

Participatory Approach/Action Research

Sometimes, researchers aim to bring about positive changes in the lives of the research subjects belonging to marginalised or vulnerable groups, or try to give these groups a voice. Participatory research aims for some kind of reform; therefore, it is important that they involve the study group in the research at all stages of the research process. The researchers are required to interact informally with the study group or even live amongst them. Research participants are termed co-researchers in recognition that the study is not simply about them but also by them.

The researcher is required to adopt a less neutral position than that which is usually required in scientific research. This is why this type of research has been criticised for not being objective. However, it is noteworthy that for some groups of people, this approach is necessary as otherwise the thoughts, feelings or behaviour of the group members could not be fully understood.

RESEARCH DESIGNS

Quantitative Research Designs

Quantitative research designs are summarised in Fig. 4.2.

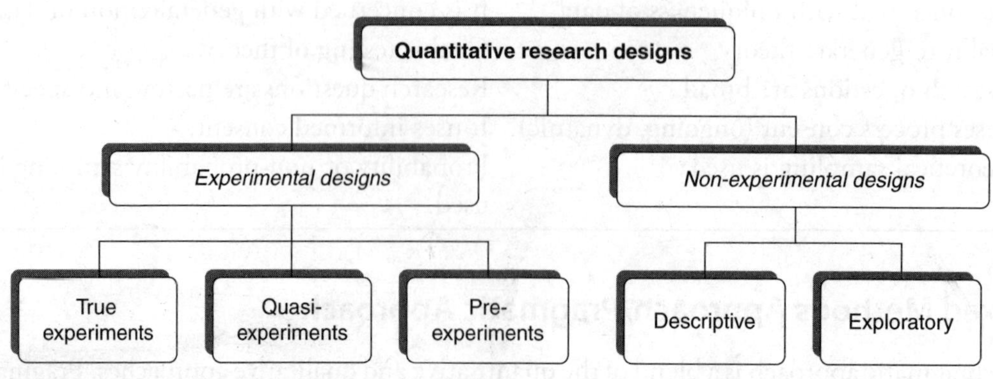

Figure 4.2 Quantitative research designs

Experimental research

Experimental research aims to test the effectiveness of an intervention in which control is practiced over all the factors that can affect the result of an intervention. In this kind of research, the researchers are active agents who manipulate the independent variable so as to affect the dependent variable, and subsequently determine its effect.

Experimental research is further classified into three categories: true experiment, quasi-experiment and pre-experiment.

True experiment This has three essential characteristics, depicted in Fig. 4.3.

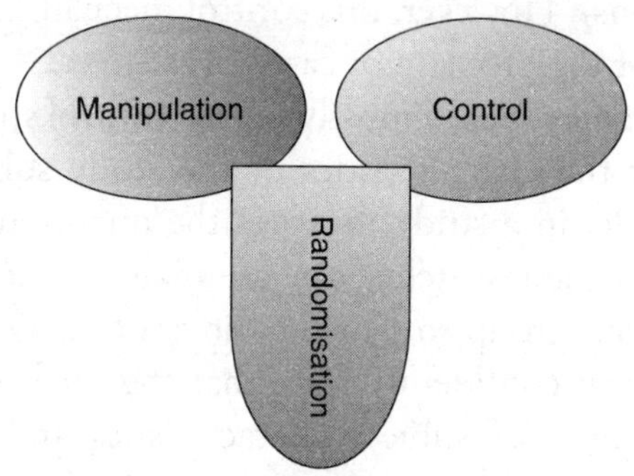

Figure 4.3 Essential characteristics of true experiment

- **Manipulation** refers to the experiment, independent variable (IV) or intervention. The researcher is interested in observing the effect of IV on the dependent variable (DV). All experimental research studies essentially have this feature.
- **Control** is the second essential criteria for true experiments. Here, researchers are interested in observing the cause and effect relationship between the independent and dependent variables. However, many external factors can compete with the IV to affect the DV. Therefore, it is necessary for the researcher to control these extraneous factors/conditions/variables to nullify their effect on the DV. Several mechanisms can be used to achieve control over the extraneous variables.
  - **Control group:** A control group is the product of the process of randomisation and is the most frequently used technique of control in experimental groups. The presence of a comparable control group in the experimental study ensures that, at the outset of the study, extraneous variables are equally distributed in both groups and the only difference is of the intervention provided to the experimental group. After implementation of interventional protocols, both groups are again compared in terms of outcome of interest (dependent variable) and any difference between the groups can be confidently attributed to the intervention.
  - **Cross-over design:** This is the most powerful study design in which the same patient is randomly assigned to a different ordering of treatments. As the same subject is used as the control counterpart, it eliminates all possible extraneous

situations and the best possible control is ensured. For example, Mr. S is first assigned to treatment condition A and the outcome of interest is measured. After washout period, he is assigned to treatment conditions B and again outcome of interest is measured. Now, the data of both the treatment conditions from the same person can be compared to find out which treatment condition is most effective. While studying the effect of two or more independent variables, this method of control can be exercised. For only two treatment conditions, half of the subjects are randomly assigned to treatment condition A and the half to treatment condition B. Counterbalancing is used for more than two treatment conditions to remove the ordering effect (see Table 4.4 for different treatment ordering for more than two treatment conditions). However, this control mechanism is not applicable in every situation because of the problem of carry-over effect.

- **Matching:** This strategy is used mostly in case control studies that require matching information about the characteristics of the study subjects to form comparison groups. For example, in a study to assess the quality of life of gas victims of the Bhopal gas tragedy, the researcher can use matching to form a gas victims group and a healthy persons group so that the difference between the two groups can be observed and she can confidently state that the quality of life of the gas victims is poor. The matching of subject characteristics and other factors believed to be extraneous results in the formation of two comparable groups. For matching, the researcher should have prior knowledge of the subject characteristics (e.g., age, gender, height, weight) which may have an extraneous effect on the study results. For example, if there is a 25-year-old male in the gas victim group, a healthy male of 25 years will be required for the control group. When the number of characteristics increases, pair-matching becomes a very difficult or sometimes impossible task.
- **Analysis of covariance:** This method of control is frequently used in non-equivalent quasi-experimental studies. In this study design, it is not possible to have a randomised control group; therefore, the researcher opts for a control group that is different from the experiment group. This pre-existing group difference can be analysed and removed by a statistical procedure known as analysis of covariance. It removes the effect of pre-existing group differences (extraneous variables) on the dependent variable, thereby isolating the group differences actually caused by the intervention. Pretest measures of the dependent variable provide a basis of control in this design, which is taken into account by ANCOVA to isolate the effect of covariance from that of the independent variable on the dependent variable.

- **Randomisation** is the process of random allocation of the study subjects to the experiment and control groups. It is often misunderstood by many nurse researchers and is equated with random sampling. Randomisation is not a sampling technique, rather it is the random assignment of the sample/study subjects either to the experiment or the control group. Randomisation takes place after the sample has been recruited (either by non-probability or probability method) for the study. It is the third essential criteria for true experiments. The purpose of randomisation is to create experimental and control

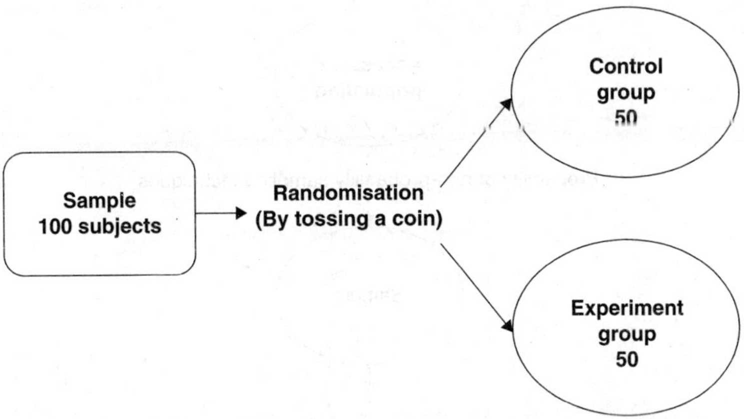

Figure 4.4 Randomisation

groups comparable in terms of extraneous variables. The process of randomisation can be undertaken by lottery method, tossing of a coin (Fig. 4.4) or over the Internet (www.randomisation.com).

True experimental designs

- **Post-test only**: In this, true experimental design data is collected only after the introduction of the intervention/independent variable to the experimental group. Data is collected on the dependent variable. No data collection is undertaken before the introduction of the experiment; therefore it is termed post-test only (Fig. 4.5).

  The post-test only design is symbolically represented as given below:

R_E: X O
R_C: ____ O
R_E: Randomly assigned Experimental group
R_C: Randomly assigned Control group
X: Intervention
O: Observation/Post-test data collection

A randomised control trial to assess the efficacy of transparent film dressing versus pressure dressing on bleeding and discomfort among patients who had undergone coronary angiography. In this post-test only study, investigators assessed bleeding and discomfort after the intervention of transparent dressing versus pressure dressing.

- **Pretest–Post-test**: This is the experimental design most widely used by researchers in nursing. It involves collection of data before and after the intervention (Fig. 4.6).

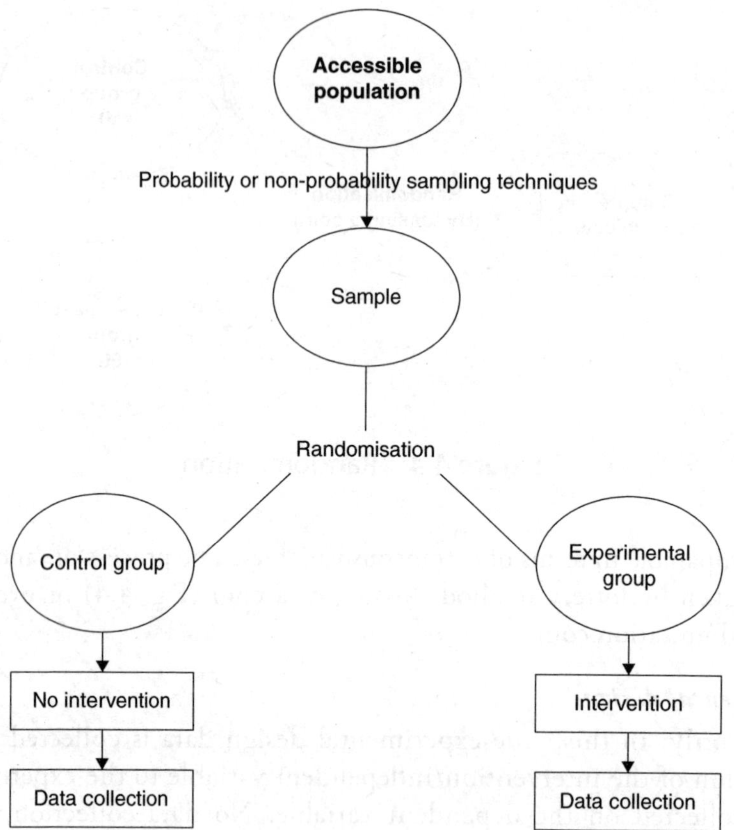

Figure 4.5 Post-test only design flowchart

The pretest–post-test design is symbolically represented as given below:

R_E: O_1 X O_2
R_C: O_3 ____ O_4
R_E: Randomly assigned Experimental group
R_C: Randomly assigned Control group
X: Intervention
O_1 and O_3: Pretest data collection from the Experimental and Control groups, respectively.
O_2 and O_4: Post-test data collection from the Experimental and Control groups, respectively.

An experimental study to evaluate the effectiveness of the training programme on the knowledge, attitudes and practice of Basic Life Support Techniques among Class 9 students in selected schools of Punjab. This study involves assessment of the knowledge, attitudes and practice of BLS among Class 9 students before and after the training.

- **Solomon four-group**: This is used to remove the effect of pretesting on the dependent variable as well, as it allows the researcher to understand the magnitude of the effect

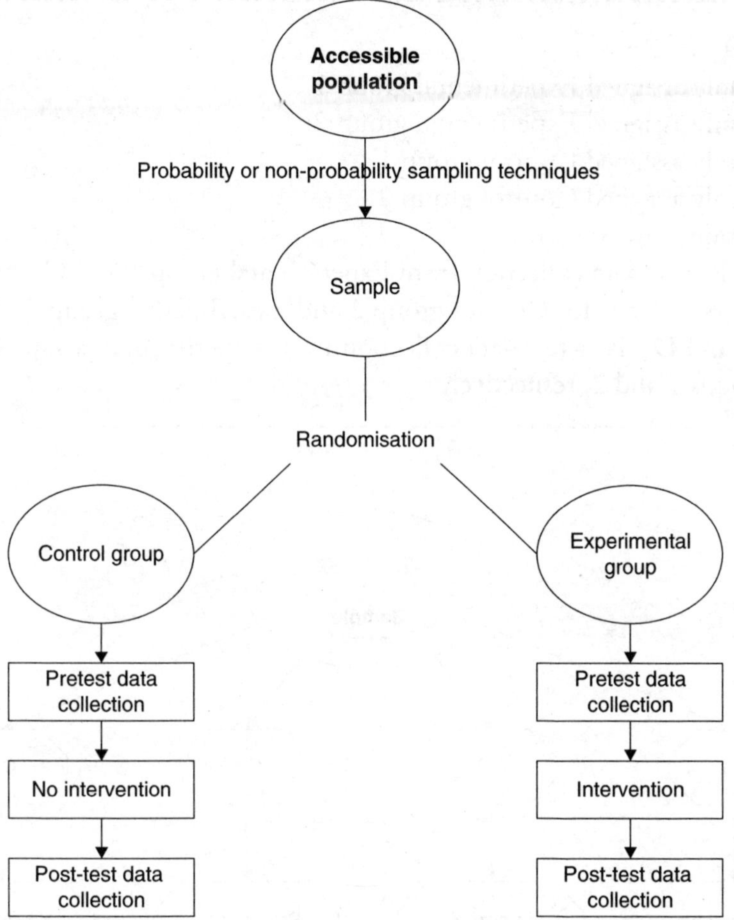

Figure 4.6 Pretest–post-test design flowchart

of pretesting on the dependent variable. For example, if respondents complete a questionnaire measuring their knowledge of BLS as a pretest, they may then subsequently decide to seek answers to a few unfamiliar questions. At the post-test, they may score better compared to how they would have scored without taking the pretest to overcome the problem of testing effect. In this design, the researcher randomly allocates the sample into four groups: two control groups and two experimental groups. Fig. 4.7 represents the Solomon four-group design.

This design is symbolically represented as under:

$\mathbf{R_{E1}: O_1 X O_2}$
$\mathbf{R_{E2}: X O_3}$
$\mathbf{R_{C1}: O_4 \_\_\_ O_5}$

R_{C2}: ____ **O_6**
R_{E1}: Randomly assigned Experimental group 1
R_{E2}: Randomly assigned Experimental group 2
R_{C1}: Randomly assigned Control group 1
R_{C2}: Randomly assigned Control group 2
X: Intervention
O_1 and O_4: Pretest data collection from Experimental group 1 and Control group 1, respectively. No pretest for Control group 2 and Experimental group 2.
O_2, O_3, O_5 and O_6: Post-test data collection from Experimental groups 1 and 2 and Control groups 1 and 2, respectively.

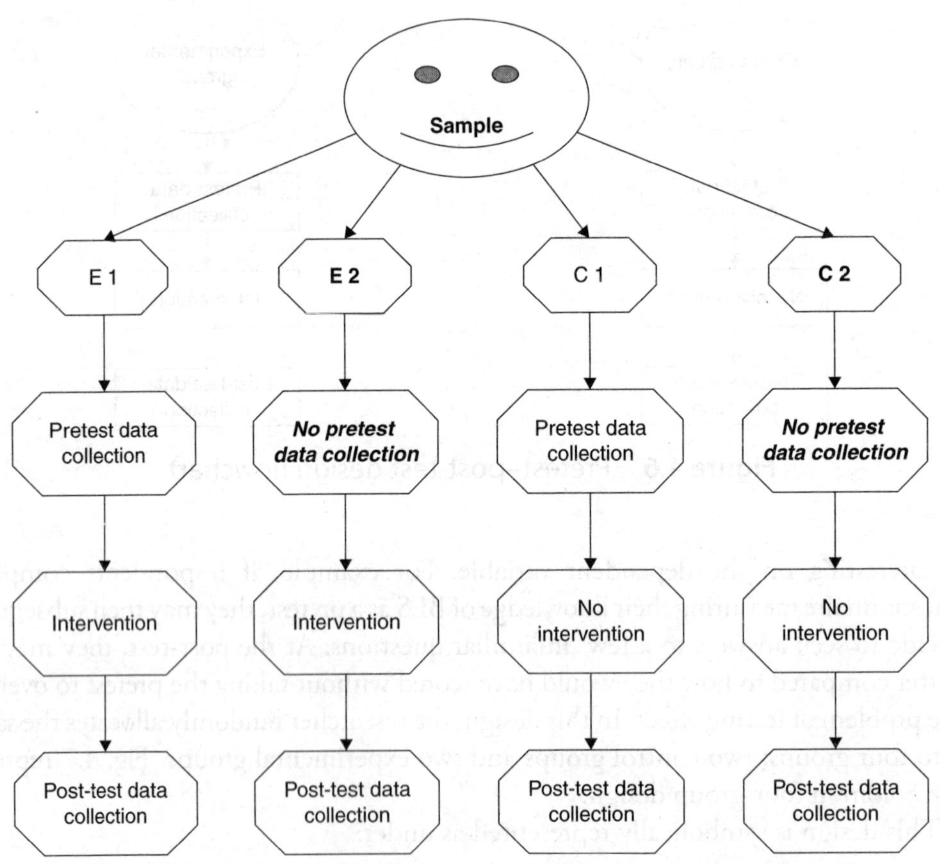

Figure 4.7 Solomon four-group design flowchart

An experimental study to assess the effect of HIV workshop on the knowledge and attitudes towards HIV among staff nurses working in a selected hospital of Mathura, UP. This study involves the risk of pretesting effect, which may contaminate the study results. Therefore, the Solomon design is required here so that the pretesting effect as well as the effect of the workshop to enhance the knowledge and attitudes of staff nurses towards HIV can be studied.

- **Factorial**: Sometimes, the researcher may want to study the effects of two or more interventions, each at at least two levels, simultaneously in a single study. In factorial design, all levels of each independent variable are combined with all levels of the other independent variables to produce all possible conditions. For example, a psychiatry nurse is interested in assessing the effectiveness of two types of psychotherapy (behavioural and cognitive) on depressive patients. At the same time, she wants to know whether long-term or short-term therapy (i.e., the levels of independent variable) is more effective. To study all this in a single study, factorial design is required. In this case, it would be called a 2 × 2 (two-by-two) factorial design because there are two independent variables, each of which has two levels. If the first independent variable had three levels, then it would be a 3 × 2 factorial design. Note that the number of distinct conditions formed by combining the levels of the independent variables is always the product of the number of levels. In a 2 × 2 design, there are four distinct conditions. In a 3 × 2 design, there are six. One way to represent a factorial design is with a design table. Table 4.2 represents a 2 × 2 factorial design in which one independent variable is the type of psychotherapy (behavioural vs. cognitive) and the other is the duration of that therapy (short vs. long) used to treat a sample of depressed people.

Table 4.2 Two-by-two factorial design

	Duration of therapy	
Type of psychotherapy	**Long**	**Short**
Behaviour	*Behaviour* therapy with *long* duration	*Behaviour* therapy with *short* duration
Cognitive	*Cognitive* therapy with *long* duration	*Cognitive* therapy with *short* duration

Factorial design provides an economic means to study two or more interventions/independent variables with two or more factors/levels in a single study. The subjects would be randomised in one of the four blocks, as highlighted in Table 4.2.

- **Cross-over**: This is used to assess the effectiveness of two or more interventions in a single study. It is the most powerful of all experimental designs as every research participant act as a control in addition to being a part of the experiment group. Each participant receives each treatment in sequence. For example, subject 1 first receives treatment A, then treatment B, then treatment C. Similarly, subject 2 might receive treatment B, then treatment A and then treatment C. On the other hand, it is important

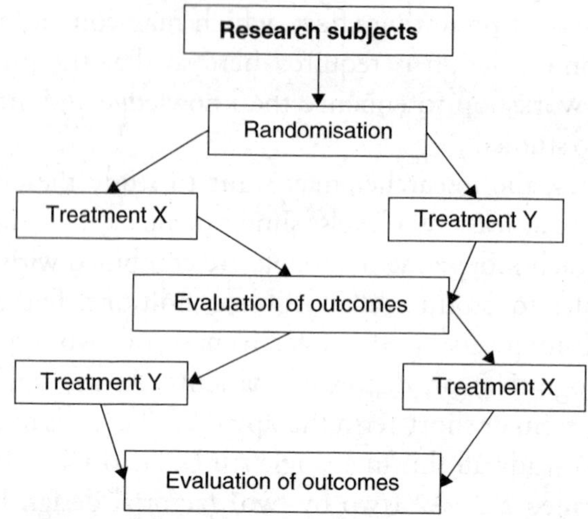

Figure 4.8 Cross-over design flowchart

in a cross-over study that the underlying condition does not change over time, and that the effects of one treatment disappear before the next is applied (Fig. 4.8).

Cross-over designs can assess 'which intervention is superior to the other', whether treatment X is better than treatment Y or vice versa. It increases the precision of estimation by removing the 'patient effect' as the same subject acts as control as well as part of the intervention group. However, cross-over design is limited in several ways. Firstly, it may be cumbersome to decide the duration of the washout period (after the subjects complete the first intervention, they must take a break, called a washout period, before they start the second treatment) so as to avoid the carry-over effect. Secondly, the assumption of no carry-over effects is difficult to test.

- **Treatment sequence**: Subjects are randomly assigned to different treatment ordering. For example, if there are two interventions A and B, then there will two different treatment orderings, as depicted in Table 4.2. Some subjects will receive treatment A first followed by treatment B. Some will receive treatment B first followed by treatment A. Further, if there are three treatments A, B and C, then there will be six possible sequences (see Table 4.3) because there are three choices available in the first period, two choices in the second, and one in the third. Similarly, if we have four treatments, there will be 24 different treatment sequences, and in case of five treatments, it will be 120.

Table 4.3 Treatment sequences with two interventions

1	2
A	B
B	A

Table 4.4 Treatment sequences with three interventions counterbalancing

1	2	3	4	5	6
A	B	C	A	B	C
B	C	A	C	A	B
C	A	B	B	C	A

- **Randomised block**: This is not only a research design but also a method of control in experimental research. Sometimes, it is difficult to control an extraneous variable while using some other common experimental designs. In randomised block design, there are two independent variables, but the second one is not subjected to manipulation (it is a naturally occurring extraneous variable that is interwoven in the design as an independent variable). For example, if gender is considered a confounding variable in an experimental study, it can be controlled by including it in the design itself, as depicted below:

Gender	**Study groups**	
	Control	**Experiment**
Male		
Female		

The above table shows a randomised block design for a nursing experiment. Subjects are assigned to blocks, based on gender. Then, within each block, subjects are randomly assigned to either control condition or treatment. For this design, 100 men get the control condition, 100 men get the intervention, 100 women get the control condition, and 100 women get the intervention.

It is known that men and women are physiologically different and react differently to intervention. This design ensures that each treatment condition (control/intervention) has an equal proportion of men and women. As a result, differences between treatment conditions cannot be attributed to gender. This randomised block design removes gender as a potential source of variability and as a potential confounding variable.

Strengths of true experimental design

- It is the most powerful method for hypothesis-testing of the relationship between an independent and a dependent variable.
- It can establish causal relationship between variables.
- It yields rich evidence for intervention effects.

Limitations of true experimental design

- They are artificial in nature (tightly controlled setting, intervention) and nothing is allowed to proceed naturally as a phenomenon.
- Control over extraneous factors is another obstacle for experimental research.
- *Hawthorne effect*: Sometimes, mere awareness among the participants that they are being studied can bring about a change in behaviour, altering the study results that do not represent the truth.

Quasi-experimental designs As mentioned in the previous section, true experiments require three essential characteristics: intervention, control and randomisation. Quasi-experimental designs lack one of these essential requirements (either control or randomisation). Therefore, it is considered slightly weaker in terms of strength of the evidence it yields as compared to true experiments. However, it provides a good platform to test an intervention in situations where control or randomisation is not possible. In the nursing sciences, most experiments are conducted using quasi-experimental designs. Quasi-experiments designs are listed as follows:

- **Non-equivalent control group design**: This design is useful when the researcher is interested in assessing the effectiveness of an intervention, but due to some reason, it is not possible to have either a control group or randomly assign the subjects to the experimental and control groups. For example, if a hospital is planning to implement a policy reform (intervention) and wants to assess its effect on job satisfaction and retention among the staff nurses. In this situation, all the staff nurses of this hospital will be part of the experimental group because they will be part of policy reform. It is not possible to divide the staff nurses into experimental and control groups because they will be affected by policy reform in that hospital. Now, how can the researcher assess its impact on job satisfaction and retention. This situation call for quasi-experimental design and the researcher can select a comparable group outside the hospital where rules and regulations are similar to some extent. The comparable group is also known as the non-equivalent control group as it is not similar to the experimental group in a number of variables of interest. However, by doing so, the researcher is unable to control all the extraneous variables affecting the dependent variables. Non-equivalent control group design can be depicted as see in Fig. 4.9.

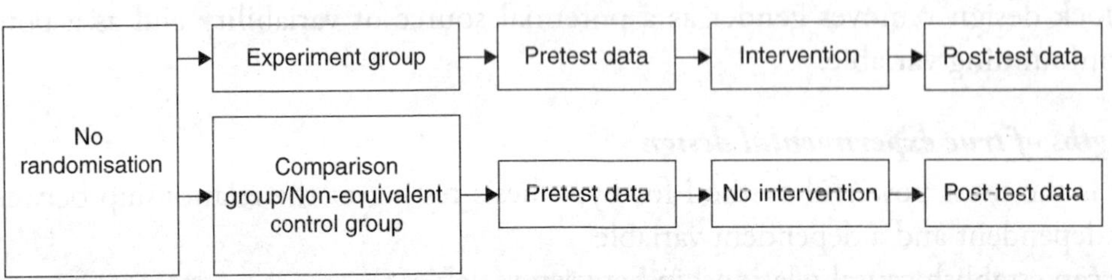

Figure 4.9 Non-equivalent control group design

For example, a quasi-experimental study to assess the effectiveness of infra-red therapy on episiotomy pain and wound healing among postnatal mothers admitted at selected hospitals of Ludhiana, Punjab.

- **Time series design**: Time series are useful to assess the long-term effects of an intervention in which at a specified interval intervention is withheld or intensified. Data is collected over the extended period of time. Usually a small group of subjects is recruited for the study which is followed to assess the effectiveness of the treatment as well as its long-term efficiency and adverse effects (Fig. 4.10).

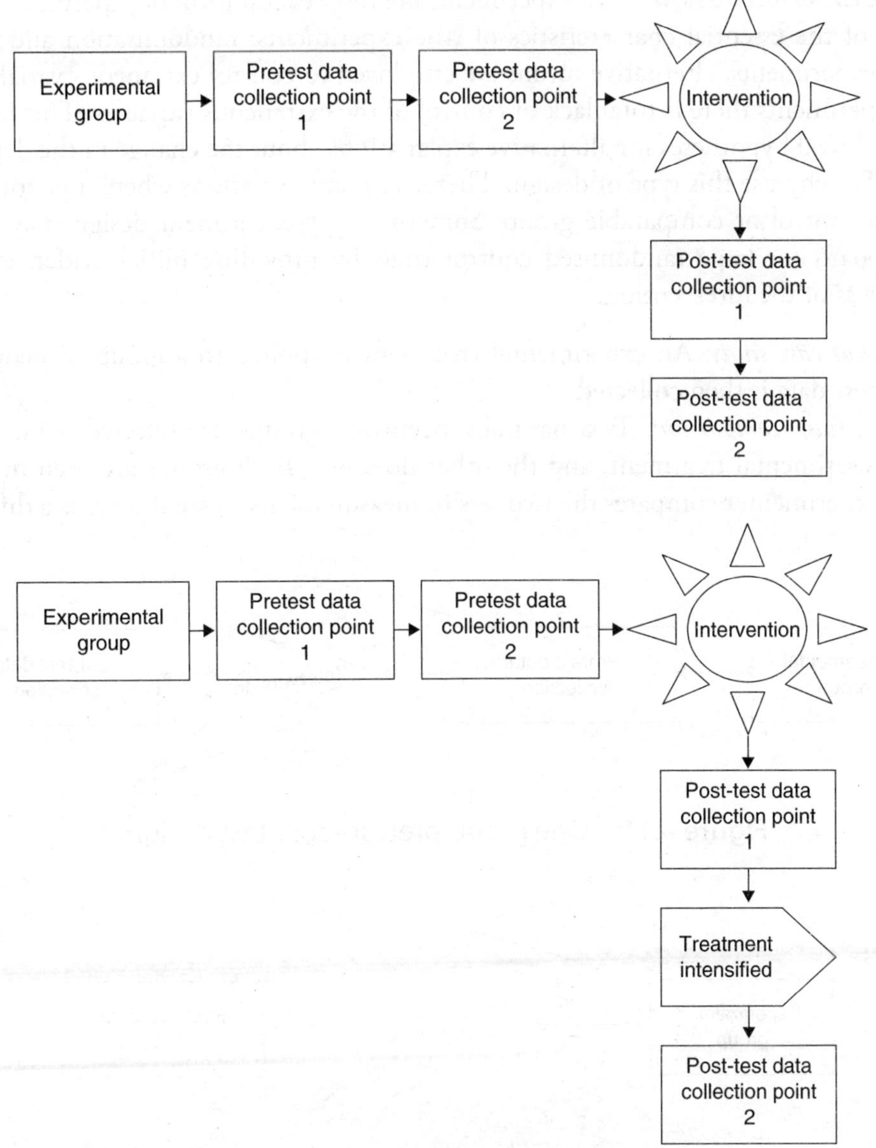

Figure 4.10 Time series design flowchart

Advantages and disadvantages of quasi-experiments Quasi-experiment designs provide feasibility to test some interventions that cannot otherwise be studied by using true experiment designs. However, because of lack of sufficient control over the extraneous variables, the evidence generated is weak as there are a number of rival hypotheses which compete with the research hypothesis (providing an alternative explanation for the change in dependent variables). However, quasi-experiments are frequently used by the nurse researcher because of their practical applicability in many situations where true experiments are not possible.

Pre-experimental design Pre-experiments are the weakest form of experiments as they lack two of the essential characteristics of true experiments: randomisation and control. In quasi-experiments, alternative means are employed to control extraneous variables, but in pre-experiments there is total lack of control of the extraneous variables. This leads to a number of rival hypotheses for alternative explanations about the change in the dependent variable. So why use this type of design? There are many situations where it is not feasible to have a control or comparable group. Sometime, pre-experiment design may serve as a springboard for large randomised control trials by providing initial evidence for the effectiveness of the intervention.

- *One-shot case study*: An experimental treatment is applied to a group of people, and post-test data is then collected.
- *Static group comparison*: Two naturally occurring groups are selected. One receives the experimental treatment, and the other does not. Both groups are then measured. The experimenter compares the two sets of measurements to see if there is a difference.

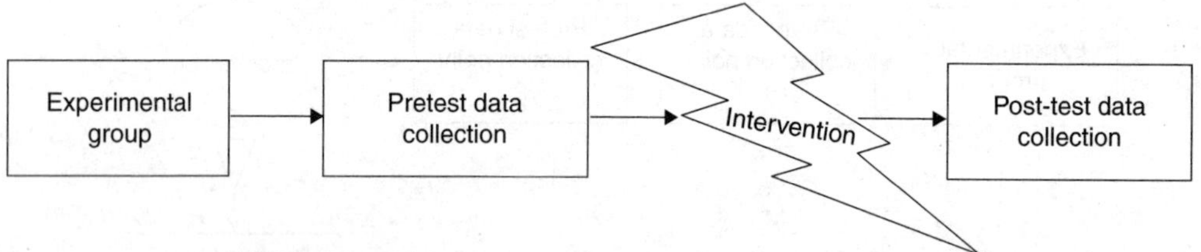

Figure 4.11 One group pretest–post-test design

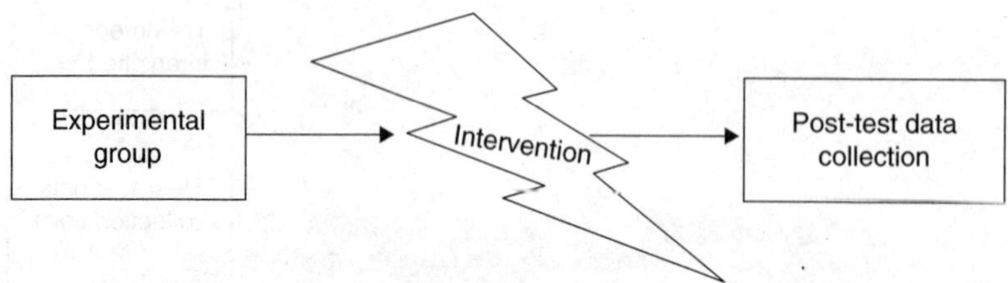

Figure 4.12 One group post-test only design

For example, the efficacy of ginger extract on the symptoms of morning sickness among antenatal mothers in Punjab, India. A pre-experimental one-group pretest–post-test design was planned for this study.

Non-experimental research

This type of design lacks all three essential characteristics of true experiments, i.e., manipulation of the independent variable, control group and randomisation. There are many situations in which it is not possible to manipulate the independent variable, either practically or because of ethical concerns. For example, if the researcher wants to study the effects of smoking among adolescents; in this case, to conduct a true experiment, the researcher will have to randomly divide the sample into the experimental group and control group. Later on, the experimental group will be asked to smoke cigarettes and the control group will not. Now, the question that needs to be addressed is whether one group can be asked to smoke cigarettes. Is it ethically acceptable? Certainly, we cannot. Then how we can study this problem? The answer gives rise to a group of designs known as non-experimental studies, in which researchers observe the variables of interest in their natural setting, as they occur or have already occurred, and try to discover the relationship among them. However, it is risky to determine causal relationship among variables in a non-experimental study.

Essential criteria for cause and effect relationship

To establish that variable A causes changes in variable B, the following conditions should be met:

- Both variable A and variable B should be related to each other.
- The researcher should be able to establish the occurrence of both variables (as variable A occurred before variable B, it caused changes in variable B).
- There should be lack of confounding variables that can suggest an alternative explanation of the relationship.

In non-experimental research designs, determination of cause–effect relationship is problematic because of lack of the third criteria. Some important non-experimental designs are as follows:

- *As per time dimension*
  - Retrospective
  - Prospective
  - Cross-sectional
  - Longitudinal
- *As per research objectives dimension*

- Descriptive
- Exploratory
- Comparative

Time

- **Retrospective design**: When the researcher identifies the *effect* first and looks back to identify the *cause*, it is termed a retrospective study. For example, the classic smoking and lung cancer study can be conducted retrospectively as well as prospectively. If the researcher chooses a retrospective design, first, she must identify patients with lung cancer as well as individuals without lung cancer to be study subjects. Thereafter, information about antecedents from both groups will be collected and compared to isolate the presumed cause for the same.
  - **Case control design**: This is a type of retrospective study in which the researcher begins with two groups of subjects, namely, case (lung cancer) and control (without cancer). Control over the extraneous variables can be exercised by using a technique known as matching. Subjects recruited in the control group are matched with cases with respect to key extraneous variables (age, gender, height and weight) so that both groups are comparable at the outset of the study.
- **Prospective design**: When the researcher identifies the cause first and looks forward to identify the effect, it is termed a prospective study. For example, the classic smoking and lung cancer study can be conducted retrospectively as well as prospectively. If the researcher chooses a prospective design, first she must identify smokers as study subjects. Thereafter, they will be followed to identify the appearance of lung cancer.

  Prospective designs are considered more powerful then retrospective designs. However, it is risky to infer causal relationship in both designs because of lack of the third criteria of a cause–effect relationship, though both designs meet the remaining two criteria.
- **Cross-sectional design**: This is a design in which there is only one point of data collection. The phenomenon of interest is captured at a given point of time. The most important advantage of cross-sectional studies is that in general they are quick and cheap. As there is no follow up, fewer resources are required to run the study.

  For example, a cross-sectional survey to assess the prevalence of anemia among adolescent girls residing in the slums of Agra, UP.
- **Longitudinal design**: This involves multiple points of data collection over an extended period of time. Participants are followed for a specified period of time in order to study the evolution of the phenomenon of interest. Attrition is one of the main concerns for the researcher while conducting a longitudinal study. They are further categorised as panel studies, trend studies and cohort studies. Panel studies involve a group of subjects believed to provide information on the phenomenon of interest. The same group of subjects is contacted several times to elicit the required information for the study. However, trend studies are aimed at studying the change in pattern in relation to a phenomenon of interest. Data gathered from a particular population is characterised

by a specific attribute, such as education level. Different subjects from the same population are recruited at different times throughout the study.

A cohort study typically involves a cohort sample, that is, a group of subjects that experiences some type of event in a selected time period, and studies them at intervals through time. For example, a group of nursing postgraduates of the same age from different nursing colleges with the same degree are studied every five years on how they have progressed. Or, a longitudinal study to assess the impact of meditation on blood sugar levels among diabetic patients.

Research objectives dimension

- **Descriptive design:** Descriptive studies involve the observation and description of the phenomenon, facts about how they are present in their natural setting. It simply describes how the variables are present and related to each other in the natural setting without manipulating anything. There are three types of descriptive studies:
  1. *Univariate*: These involve the description of a single variable of interest. The two common variants of univariate studies in the field of epidemiology are prevalence study and incidence study.

     Prevalence refers to the number of cases in the population at a given point of time. The following formula can be applied to calculate the prevalence rate of a disease.

$$\text{PR} = \frac{\text{Number of cases at a given point of time}}{\text{Number of persons at risk in the population}} \times \text{K}$$

     Here, K is a constant (the desired number using which prevalence is calculated; e.g., 100, 1000, 10,000, 100,000, etc).

     For example, a study to assess the prevalence of obstructed sleep apnea among congestive heart failure patients seeking treatment as out-patients of selected hospitals of Kochi, India.

     Incidence refers to the number of new cases within a specified time period divided by the size of the population initially at risk. For example, if a population initially contains 1000 non-diseased persons and 35 develop a condition over two years of observation, the incidence proportion is 35 cases per 1000 persons, i.e., 3.5%.

$$\text{IR} = \frac{\text{Number of new cases over the specified period of time}}{\text{Number of persons at risk in the population}} \times \text{K}$$

     Thus, incidence conveys information about the risk of contracting the disease, whereas prevalence indicates how widespread the disease is. Prevalence is the proportion of the total number of cases to the total population and is more a measure of the burden of the disease on society with no regard to time at risk or when subjects may have been exposed to a possible risk factor.

For example, a study to assess the incidence of obstructed sleep apnea among congestive heart failure patients seeking treatment at cardiac OPD from the year 2005 to 2008.

2. *Co-relational*: This is a type of non-experimental research in which two variables of interest are correlated with each other in their natural setting without manipulation of any variable. For example, the height of school children can be correlated with their dietary preferences (vegetarian, non-vegetarian). As some variables of interest cannot be manipulated because of ethical reasons, their relation with other variables must be studied in their natural setting. A co-relational study may be descriptive or explorative depending on the phenomenon under study.
3. *Comparative*: This is a type of non-experimental research in which two or more mutually exclusive groups are compared in relation to variables of interest. For example, a comparative study to assess the prevalence of attention deficit hyperactivity disorder among children of working and non-working mothers. A comparative study may be descriptive or explorative depending on the phenomenon under study.

- **Exploratory study**: Sometimes, little is known about the phenomenon of interest. In this situation, the researcher aims to explore the phenomenon, termed an exploratory study. However, to explore a phenomenon about which little is known, qualitative designs are better suited though it can also be studied quantitatively. For example, an exploratory study to assess the factors associated with domestic violence among women residing in slum areas of Bangalore, Karnataka.

Some researchers have given another classification of non-experimental designs by combining the time and research objectives dimensions, shown in Table 4.5.

Table 4.5 Combination of time and research objective dimensions

Time dimension	Research objective dimension		
	Descriptive	**Exploratory**	**Predictive**
Retrospective	RD	RE	RP
Cross-sectional	CD	CE	CP
Longitudinal	LD	LE	LP

Validity of research designs

Research designs are subject to critical analysis for strength and weakness. A powerful research design usually produces authentic results that are generalisable to the target population. However, a weaker research design is susceptible to many biases which compromise the generalisability and pose questions for the study results. The validity of a research design is discussed under two heads: internal and external.

Internal validity This is equated with the extent to which it can be inferred that the independent variable truly influenced the dependent or outcome variable. Internal validity of a study is enhanced when the researcher has placed a tight control mechanism for extraneous factors which competes with the independent variable to have an effect on the dependent variable, leading to generation of a rival hypothesis which provides the alternative explanation for change in the outcome variable. While assessing for the internal validity of a study, an evaluator must ask this question: to what extent is it possible to establish that only the independent variable caused changes in the dependent variable. If there is no other possible alternative explanation for the change in the outcome variable, the internal validity of the study is considered to be high.

Campbell and Stanley (1966) have identified six important extraneous conditions that may compromise the internal validity of a study. These extraneous conditions are also known as threats to internal validity.

- **External events:** The threat of history occurs when some external event may have caused a change in the outcome variable. The external event may have a comparable effect to the independent variable on the dependent variable. The researcher should carefully analyse the threat of history and report it in the study findings.
- **Maturation of subjects:** Maturation refers to the process occurring within subjects as a result of passage of time during the course of the study. For example, with time children mature physically and psychologically. Therefore, this threat to internal validity may surge in a study that has an extended period of data collection and the dependent variable is related with physical/psychological maturation of participants. In this situation, maturation with time other than the independent variable may be an alternative explanation for change in the dependent variable which compromises the internal validity of the study.
- **Effect of pretesting:** It is the effect of taking a pretest on the post-test score of the research participants. When an experiment is conducted to change the attitude/opinion of the participants about a sensitive issue, it is possible that the pretest may sensitise the participants to explore the issue on their own, leading to a higher score on post-test. However, the testing effect is offset in true experimental studies as both the experimental and the control group will experience the testing effect to a similar extent, making them again comparable with each other. Solomon research design may be appropriate to isolate the pretest effect from the intervention effect.
- **Instrumentation:** This threat to internal validity occurs due to change in data collection tool between two points of data collection. If we use existing tool at baseline and an updated version of the same tool at another point of data collection it will lead to effect of instrumentation.
- **Mortality:** This threat is mostly present in longitudinal studies which involve data collection over an extended period of time. If the rate of attrition is different in the groups being compared, it may lead to biased study findings as the group becomes under-representive of the subjects initially selected.

- **Selection:** This is the most prevalent threat to internal validity. When the process of randomisation is not followed to assign a subject to the experiment or control group, it will result in groups that have pre-existing differences. This pre-existing inequality can serve as a basis to provide an alternative explanation for the change in outcome variable other than the intervention. Sometimes, in experimental design, a participant may elect not to receive treatment and place themselves in the control group, leading to risk of selection bias in the study.

External validity It refers to the extent to which study findings are generalisable to the population. It is determined by the size of the sample and the sampling technique. A sufficiently large sample selected by random procedure leads to very high external validity. The results can be generalised to any population that has similar characteristics to the accessible population under study. There are many threats to external validity such as novelty effect, experimenter effect, measurement effect and expectancy effect.

- **Novelty effect:** It occurs when the researcher is testing a new intervention. The participants may become enthusiastic or unconvinced with the new treatment which affects study results. When the novelty of the treatment wears out with time, it will yield different results.
- **Experimenter effect:** The personal characteristics and behaviour of a researcher may have an effect on the behaviour and response of the study participants. The same results will not be produced with a different researcher.
- **Hawthorne effect:** Sometimes, participants change their behaviour in a particular manner because they know that they are taking part in a research project and are being observed by the researcher. It will limit the generalisability of the study findings, as in another setting the Hawthorne effect may not be present.
- **History and treatment togetherness:** When an external event takes place along with the intervention, it will influence the study results. In the absence of that event, similar results cannot be reproduced.

Qualitative Research Designs

Qualitative designs are classified as per the discipline underlying the research area of interest. Some of the important qualitative designs are discussed hereunder.

Historical research

This is the systematic study of past events to obtain an account of what happened in the past. It is not a mere accumulation of facts and dates or a description of past events. Rather, it is a dynamic account of past events which involves an interpretation of those events in an attempt to recapture the ideas that influenced them. Historical design is of particular relevance to nurses investigating the social, political, economic and historical context of decisions made that affected health or the practice of nursing at a particular period in time (Christy 1975).

Aims of historical research (based on Berg 1998)

1. To unearth the unknown, as some historical events are not recorded.
2. To answer questions about the past so as to understand the current situation.
3. To identify the relationship that the past has to the present.
4. To record and evaluate the achievements of individuals, institutions or organisations.
5. To assist in understanding the culture and social structure in which we live.

Methodology The following steps are usually undertaken to conduct historical enquiry, though there is some overlap and movement back and forth between the steps:

1. *Identification and formulation of the research problem or question:* This is the first step in any type of research, including historical research. The researcher identifies and formulates the research question. The source of historical research problems may be current issues in nursing education, the accomplishments of an individual (e.g., Florence Nightingale), an educational policy or the relationship between events.
2. *Data collection or literature review:* This step involves identifying, locating and retrieving or collecting information related to the research topic. In most historical research, the information sources are often contained in documents such as records, relics (articles of clothing, buildings, books, architectural plans, desks, or any other object that might provide useful information about the past), diaries or newspapers, photographs, and interviews with individuals who have had experience with or have knowledge of the research topic (also known as oral histories).

   These sources of information may be of two types: primary and secondary:
   a. *Primary source* is one that has direct involvement with the research question being investigated, like a diary, an original map or an interview with a person that experienced the event.
   b. A *secondary source* is one that was created from a primary source, such as books written about the event. As a rule of thumb, secondary sources are considered less useful than primary sources.
3. *Evaluation of materials*: Historical researchers are concerned with the authenticity and accuracy of the source of information because any source can be affected by a variety of factors such as prejudice, economic conditions and political climate. There are two types of evaluation criteria against which every source of information will be judged by the researcher:
   a. *External criticism*: This is the process of determining the validity, trustworthiness or authenticity of the source (to ascertain if the source is what it claims to be). The researcher seeks to establish the genuineness of a document and to address the question of whether it is authentic in what it purports to be. External criticism can be undertaken by handwriting analysis or by determining the age of the paper on which something was written.

b. *Internal criticism*: This is the process of determining the extent to which the information contained in the sources collected is reliable and authentic. This is done by positive and negative criticism (Christy 1975).
c. *Positive criticism*: This means that the researcher understands the statements and meaning conveyed in the sources in their past context, and is not altered by present-day conceptions. However, there are problems of vagueness and presentism in positive criticism. Vagueness refers to uncertainty in the meaning of the words and phrases used in the source. Presentism refers to the assumption that the present-day connotations of terms also existed in the past.
d. *Negative criticism*: This refers to establishing the reliability or authenticity and accuracy of the content of the sources used. First-hand accounts by witnesses to an event are typically assumed to be reliable and accurate. Christy (1975) notes that this involves establishing whether the author was actually present at the events (eyewitness) and whether the information can be considered true, that is, determining whether it is a primary or a secondary source.

   Historical researchers often use three techniques in handling evidence:
   - *Corroboration:* It refers to comparing documents to determine if they provide the same information. It is often used to obtain information about accuracy and authenticity.
   - *Sourcing:* It refers to identifying the author, date of creation of a document and the place it was created to establish the authenticity or accuracy of information.
   - *Contextualisation:* It refers to identifying when and where an event took place to establish authenticity and accuracy of information.

4. *Data synthesis and report preparation*: This refers to synthesising the information collected or putting the material into a narrative format of the topic selected. The process includes selecting, organising and analysing the materials collected into relevant themes to develop a contiguous and meaningful whole.

   For example, a historical study to assess the pattern of uniform change of nursing personnel in India.

Grounded theory

Grounded theory is a qualitative research tradition that emerged from the discipline of sociology. It is the most useful qualitative research design used to study social structure and social process. The term grounded means that the theory developed from the research has its roots or is grounded in the data from which it was derived.

The methodology of grounded theory was developed by American sociologists Glaser and Strauss in 1967 in the School of Nursing, University of California, San Francisco. They believed that the theory obtained by this qualitative method was truly grounded in data.

According to Glaser and Strauss (1967), "Grounded theory investigates the actualities in the real world and analyses the data with no preconceived ideas or hypothesis". It is the discovery of theory from data systematically obtained from social research.

Strauss and Corbin (1990) defined it as a qualitative research method that uses a systematic set of procedures to develop an inductively derived grounded theory about a phenomenon.

Two primary characteristics of grounded theory research design are:

- The constant comparison of data with emerging categories
- Theoretical sampling of different groups to maximise similarities and differences of information (theoretical sampling is the process of data collection whereby the analyst jointly collects, codes and analyses her data and decides what to collect next and where to find it, in order to develop the theory as it emerges (Glaser and Strauss 1967))

Types of grounded theory

- **Substantive:** It is grounded in data on a specific substantive area, such as postpartum depression, postpartum blues.
- **Formal theory:** Substantive theory, as mentioned above, serves as a springboard for developing a higher, more abstract-level formal theory from a complicated substantive grounded theory study.
- **Constructivist grounded theory:** Rooted in pragmatism and relativist epistemology, this theory assumes that neither data nor theories are discovered; rather, they are constructed by the researcher as a result of her interactions with the field and its participants. Data is co-constructed by the researcher and the participants, and coloured by the researcher's perspectives, values, positions and geographical location.

Methodological characteristics (Glaser and Strauss 1967)

- Identifying area of interest, avoiding theoretical preconceptions and using theoretical sensitivity
- Discovery of basic social processes in the data
- Simultaneous collection and analysis of data
- Creation of analytic codes and categories developed from data and not by pre-existing conceptualisations (theoretical sensitivity)
- Writing analytical memos at the stage between coding and writing
- The integration of categories into a theoretical framework
- Data collection methods—in-depth unstructured interviews and observational methods, audio/video tape recording, diaries
- The ongoing analysis informs the direction of the next interview or group of interviews and is explicitly aimed at developing theory
- Researchers will become theoretically sensitive by immersing themselves in the data and trying to understand what the participants see as being significant and important. Concurrent data collection/analysis allows the researcher to become theoretically sensitive to the data.
- Theoretical saturation of concepts is the point at which data collection and the analysis cycle can conclude. Saturation means that no additional data is found.

Analysis of data Initially, the researcher compares one interview (or other data) to another (or other comparative data). From this comparison, a theory emerges. Researchers compare the initial data to the theory, and the results are written in the margin of the notes taken as 'codes'. Codes refer to the underlying issues amongst the 'noise' in the data. During analysis of an interview, the researcher will become aware of the words and phrases that highlight an issue of importance or interest to the research; they are noted and described in a short phrase known as code (Allan 2003). Coding can be open, axial or selective.

- *Open:* It is concerned with identifying, naming, categorising and describing phenomena found in the text. Essentially, each line, sentence and paragraph is read in search of the answer to the repeated question 'what is this about and what is being referenced here?'.
- *Axial:* This involves assembling data in new ways after open coding. Axial coding is the process of relating codes to each other, via a combination of inductive and deductive thinking. To simplify this process, rather than look for any and all kinds of relations, grounded theorists emphasise causal relationships, and fit things into a basic frame of generic relationships.
- *Selective*: This involves the integration of the categories in the axial coding model. In this phase, conditional propositions (or hypotheses) are typically presented. The result is a substantive-level theory relevant to a specific problem, issue or group.

Thereafter, the researcher identifies categories from these codes. Links between categories are identified which gives rise to a core category around which the final theory develops. The core category accounts for most of the variation of data and therefore most other categories relate to it in some way.

The core category is a more highly abstracted category but must remain grounded in the data. The main categories are related to the core category and these categories show how the core category functions in the lives of participants.

Methodological Rigor in Grounded Theory

Grounded theory has its own criteria for assessing the rigour or quality of the study (Glaser 1978):

- **Fit and relevance** – to what extent do the categories relate to the data and derive from constant comparison and conceptualisation of the data
- **Workability** – the integration of the categories into the core category that emerges
- **Modifiability** – ensuring that all the concepts important to the theory are incorporated into it by the constant comparison process. A modifiable theory can be altered when new relevant data is compared to existing data.

Ethnography

Ethnography is a type of qualitative research design aimed at exploring cultural phenomena and at representing it graphically and in writing. It is a research tradition rooted in anthropology and sociology. The ethnography researcher strives to achieve rich, holistic insights into people's views and actions, as well as the nature (sights, sounds) of their habitat through detailed observations and interviews.

Ethnography is a labour-intensive task requiring the researcher to work 'in the field', in the culture under study. During the process, the researcher not only observes the culture under study but also distinguishes and understands the patterns of behaviour and function to recognise the traits that make up that culture. It is not sufficient for an ethnographer to record what she sees; rather, she must construct the research questions that would allow her to explain and interpret the culture under study.

Data collection techniques

Observation: This is one of the main research methods available to ethnographers. It is participative observation in which the researcher takes part in socio-cultural activities while observing the subjects at the same time.

Interviewing: In addition to observing a culture, ethnographers conduct interviews with members of that culture. It allows the researcher to obtain an in-depth perspective of the culture, which is not possible through observation alone.

Collecting and reading cultural artefacts: Cultural artefacts contribute to the overall understanding of the culture. The ethnographer needs to investigate the surface details of an object, research its history, or learn about people's rules and rituals for using and making the object. Researchers use the term material culture to refer to those objects, personal artefacts loaded with meaning and history, i.e., tools, musical instruments, jewellery and clothes.

Consider the following guidelines while analysing cultural artefacts:

- Begin by noticing the look, shape, size, texture and other visible qualities of the artefact.
- Explore the purpose, history and unusual features of the artefact by talking to the members of the culture.
- Notice how the members of the culture use it.
- Compare your observations of the object with descriptions and annotations from the research participants.

Finding research sites The following is an example of a list of ethnographic research sites that can be used by ethnographers:

- Temple
- Gurudwara
- Langar
- Barber shop

- A practice facility of a college football team
- Homeless shelter
- Church

Gaining access to the site This means not only being physically present at the site, but also making sure that all the people involved know that the researcher is at the site to conduct research and that they are the participants in this project. Explaining the aims and purposes of the study to everyone who is observed and interviewed will enable the researcher to have access to the members of the culture. In order to gain access to an ethnographic research site, the principles given below can be followed:

- Contact the members of the community well in advance and visit the site in person and talk to the people involved.
- If gaining access to the site depends on obtaining permission from a person who is in charge, identify and contact that person first.
- Keep a low profile as people hesitate to talk to someone who appears to be high profile. Introduce yourself to everyone involved and explain the purpose of the study and the roles of the participants as well as yours. Therefore, it is important to put the participants of the study at ease; otherwise they will not behave in a natural way.

Keeping field research notes and journals It is important that in the course of the project, the researcher makes careful notes of everything she observes (interview). Here are some of the types of information that can be recorded in the researcher's journal:

- Interview questions, answers and reflections
- Descriptions of cultural artefacts
- Research leads and ideas
- Observations and reflections on them
- Reflections on what is and is not working in the project
- Notes to self to follow up on something or to ask more questions

Several techniques can be used for taking notes in the field. As an ethnographer, the researcher can use a double-entry journal. After dividing a page of a notebook in half, in the left-hand side column, she can record her observations of a culture or its components, and in the right-hand side, record her reflections, explanation, and questions; for example, if she can write about the physical descriptions of artefacts and also reflect on their meaning for the culture under study.

Writing a research report A thick description is an ethnographic technique that allows a researcher to create an 'observation in context'. For instance, in an ethnographical study of Balinese cock-fighting, the author Clifford Geertz does not just describe what he sees before, during and after the cock fights, but also attempts to place his observations in the larger context of Balinese history, culture and social norms. Therefore, the ethnographer must include not only the observations of concrete events, people and conversations, but also mention the cultural, historical and social contexts these events are happening in.

Phenomenology

Phenomenology is the study of the nature and meaning of phenomena. The phenomenological researcher aims to provide a rich textured description of lived experience. The lived experience is a key concept and focus of investigation for phenomenology. The life-world comprises the world of objects around us as we perceive them and our experience of our self, body and relationships. It is the "locus of interaction between ourselves and our perceptual environments and the world of experienced horizons within which we meaningfully dwell together" (von Eckartsberg 1998). It can be defined as the world that is lived and experienced, a world "that appears meaningful to consciousness in its qualitative flowing given-ness, not an objective world but a humanly relational world" (Todres et al. 2006).

The phenomenologist strives to enter the consciousness of the participants towards a phenomenon. Persons who have lived through a phenomenon are interviewed by the researcher to explore all the dimensions of that experience. When people have experienced something, they tend to become conscious towards it; this is known as **intentionality**, the key area of focus in a phenomenology study. This intentionality between the person and his experience with an event or thing is explored in detail by the researcher through qualitative methods. The researcher is required to help participants express their world as directly as possible. The central question in a phenomenological enquiry is 'what is the structure and essence of the experience of this phenomenon for these people'.

For example, one significant finding in research on a woman's lived experience of having multiple sclerosis (Finlay 2003) was how she was profoundly concerned about the impact of the disease on her relationship with her children. Specifically, she was distressed by the numbness in her hands which meant that she could no longer feel the softness of her childrens' skin properly. The intentional, embodied relationship between a mother and her children was highlighted.

A phenomenologist is required to put on hold her views, opinions, assumptions or understanding of the phenomenon under study as it may distort the study findings. This is known as **bracketing**. It is required in descriptive phenomenology to ensure that the researcher is open and views the phenomenon differently as expressed by participants.

Types of phenomenology Different variants of phenomenological research have been described as per the type of phenomenon under investigation and the kind of knowledge the researcher seeks. Rather than being static, the different phenomenological approaches are dynamic and undergo constant development as the field of qualitative research as a whole evolves. There are two important schools of thought in phenomenology: descriptive and interpretive (hermeneutics).

Descriptive phenomenology is concerned with the rich description of the phenomenon of interest. It was developed by Husserl (1962). **Interpretative phenomenology** is focused on the interpretation and understanding of the phenomenon. It was developed by Heidegger (1962) who opposed the view of his professor, Husserl. The aim of heuristic enquiry is to produce a composite description and creative synthesis of the experience.

There are four aspects of lived experience in which a phenomenologist is interested:

- Lived space or spatiality
- Lived body or corporeality
- Lived time or temporality
- Lived human relation or relationality

Data collection and analysis The key quality in the data sought by phenomenologist is concreteness (Wertz 2005). Entry into a participant's world is necesary to have full access to his experiences. The researcher aims to experience the phenomenon through in-depth conversation, as it was experienced by the participant. The most common methods for data collection include in-depth conversation/interview, use of narratives in interviews, diaries, participant observation and reflective diaries. The data collected involves verbatim accounts which need to be analysed to understand the meaning and essence of the phenomenon. Significant statements are extracted and categorised as per the themes identified in the data.

Other Research Designs

Case study

The case study method was first introduced into social science by Frederic Le Play in 1829. It was used by Glaser and Strauss in the development of a new theory. It is defined as a research strategy, an empirical inquiry that investigates a phenomenon within its real-life context.

Case study as a method of research involves an up-close, in-depth and detailed examination of the subject of the study (the case), as well as its related contextual conditions. It had a prominent place in many disciplines and professions such as psychology, anthropology, sociology, nursing and medicine. The 'case' being researched may be an individual, patient, rare disease patient, organisation, event or action, existing in a specific time and place.

According to Thomas, "Case studies are analyses of persons, events, decisions, periods, projects, policies, institutions, or other systems that are studied holistically by one or more methods. The case that is the *subject* of the inquiry will be an instance of a class of phenomena that provides an analytical frame, an *object* within which the study is conducted and which the case illuminates and explicates". According to Creswell, data collection in a case study occurs over a "sustained period of time". It can include quantitative evidence, rely on multiple sources of evidence, and benefit from the prior development of theoretical propositions. Therefore, it should not be confused with qualitative research as it can be based on any mix of quantitative and qualitative evidence.

Selection of case An average or typical case is often not the richest in information; therefore, is not suitable for case study research. It is more useful to select subjects that offer an interesting, unusual or particularly revealing set of circumstances. When selecting a subject for a case study, researchers will therefore use information-oriented sampling, as opposed to random sampling. Outlier cases (that is, those which are extreme, deviant or atypical) reveal more information than the potentially representative case.

Three types of cases may thus be a choice for selection in case study research:

- Key cases
- Outlier cases
- Local knowledge cases

Beyond decisions about case selection and the subject and object of the study, decisions need to be made about purpose, approach and process in the case study. Thomas proposes evaluative or exploratory typology for the case study, where the purposes are first identified, followed by delineation of the approaches (theory-testing, theory-building or illustrative), and then a decision is made about the processes to be used (whether the study is to be single or multiple; retrospective or snapshot).

Secondary data analysis

Secondary data analysis as a research design refers to the analysis of data collected by someone else to answer the research questions. Secondary data can include any data that is examined to answer a research question other than the question(s) for which the data were initially collected (Vartanian 2010). When the same individual/team of researchers designs, collects and analyses the data, it is referred to as primary data analysis. The sources of data for secondary analysis are many:

- Large government-funded datasets
- University/College records
- Authors websites
- Census of India
- Simple Online Data Archive for Population Studies (SodaPop) – http://sodapop.pop.psu.edu/data-collections
- National Family Health Survey
- Sample research survey

Advantages of secondary data analysis

- It saves a lot of time and energy as study design and data collection is already completed
- It provides access to international and cross-historical data that would otherwise take several years and millions of rupees to collect
- It may improve the quality of the data
- Research projects funded by the government usually involve larger samples that are more representative of the target population
- Oversampling of minority groups/behaviours allows for increased statistical precision
- Datasets often contain considerable breadth

Disadvantages of secondary data analysis

- Study design and data collection are already completed
- Data may not facilitate that particular research question
- Data may *potentially* lack depth
- It may require knowledge of survey statistics/methods which is not generally provided by basic graduate statistics courses

Meta-analysis

Meta-analysis is a research design that uses the data/results of studies on similar topics to answer the research question of interest. It is also known as 'conducting research about previous research'. It is a **statistical technique** for combining findings from independent studies. It should not be equated with review of literature as that is more subjective in nature and provides a biased description of the work which has been done on a topic of interest. Meta-analysis is objective in nature and the data of the previous research is again subjected to analysis to draw unbiased inferences about the phenomenon of interest. The purpose of a meta-analysis is to aggregate information in order to achieve a higher statistical power for the variable of interest, as opposed to a less precise measure derived from a single study. Meta-analysis is most often used to assess the **clinical effectiveness of healthcare interventions**, and it does this by combining data from two or more randomised control trials.

Meta-analysis is useful in evidence-based practice which aids in decision-making about whether a particular intervention is useful for practice by analysing the results of studies on similar topics. The advantages of meta-analysis are as follows:

- Generalisability of the findings is extended to a larger population.
- The precision and accuracy of estimates can be improved as more data is used. Inconsistency of results across studies can be quantified and analysed.
- The presence of publication bias can be investigated.

Steps in a meta-analysis

1. Formulate the research problem.
2. Search the literature.
3. Select relevant studies based on incorporation criteria, e.g., the requirement of randomisation and blinding in a clinical trial, decide whether unpublished studies are included to avoid publication bias.
4. Decide which dependent variables or summary measures are allowed. For instance, differences (discrete data) and means (continuous data).
5. Select a meta-regression statistical model. It is a tool used to examine the impact of moderator variables on study effect size using regression-based techniques.

Evaluation research

Evaluation research design is used when the researcher wants to evaluate the impact of a newly implemented program/policy. According to Weiss (1998), evaluation is, "The systematic assessment of the operation and/or the outcomes of a program or policy, compared to a set of explicit or implicit standards, as a means of contributing to the improvement of the program or policy". Outcomes refer to the results of the program. For example, the researcher may ask the question 'Has your attitude to HIV/AIDS changed as a result of your training program?'. Measuring group differences or pre/post-testing is used to measure outcomes. Process refers to the internal working/operation of the program/policy. Designing the evaluation of the process of the program requires thoughtful planning of what the researcher intends to investigate, for example, monitoring staff action during the program or collecting surveys from different levels of staff to explore problems with work efficiency.

Focus groups interviews

A focus group interview is a group discussion organised for research purposes on a particular topic. This discussion is moderated and guided by a researcher. It is useful in generating a rich understanding of the participant's experiences and beliefs. The composition of a focus group needs attention so as to get the best quality of discussion. The researcher should give due consideration to the impact of group mix (e.g., how the group may interact with each other) before the focus group proceeds. The venue for the focus group should be comfortable, quiet and free from distractions. Prior arrangement should be made to record the interview (audio or video tape). The researcher should acknowledge the presence of the audio recording equipment at the outset of the interview and provide assurance of confidentiality and opportunity to withdraw if any participant is uncomfortable about being taped.

The optimum size for a focus group is 6–8 participants, however, it can work successfully with as few as three and as many as 14 participants. The interview questions should move from the general to the specific and the order of the questions should be relative to the importance of issues in the research agenda. The researcher may also probe and expand on issues as and when required during the discussion. In the focus group, the researcher/moderator should ensure smooth progress of group discussion, keeping it focused without leading it and prevent the discussion being dominated by one member, and make sure that all participants have ample opportunity to contribute.

However, it is important to note that the analysis of focus group data is different from other qualitative data because of their interactive nature, and this needs to be taken into consideration during analysis.

CHAPTER SUMMARY

- Quantitative research involves the collection of data in the form of quanta/numbers which allows the researcher to undertake statistical operations for data analysis.
- Unlike quantitative research, qualitative research is focused on gaining a rich and complex understanding of people's lived experience, culture and behaviour.

- Pragmatic approach is a blend of both quantitative and qualitative approach. Pragmatic researchers use any of the methods, techniques and procedures typically associated with quantitative or qualitative research.
- Participatory research aims towards some kind of reform; therefore, it is important that they involve the study group in the research at all stages of the research process.
- Experimental research aims to test the effectiveness of an intervention in which control is exerted over all the factors that can affect the result of an intervention.
- The essential criteria for true experiments are experiment, randomisation and control.
- Randomisation is the process of random allocation of the study subjects to the experiment and control groups.
- Solomon four-group design is used to remove the effect of pretesting on the dependent variable as well, as it allows the researcher to understand the magnitude of the effect of pretesting on the dependent variable.
- In factorial design, all levels of each independent variable are combined with all levels of the other independent variables to produce all possible conditions.
- Cross-over design is used to assess the effectiveness of two or more interventions in a single study. They can be used to assess which intervention is superior to other, whether treatment X is better than treatment Y or vice versa.
- In randomisation block design, there are two independent variables, but the second one is not subjected to manipulation (it is a naturally occurring extraneous variable which is interwoven in the design as an independent variable).
- Quasi-experimental design lacks one of the essential requirements (either control or randomisation) for the true experiment.
- Non-equivalent control group design is useful when the researcher wants to assess the effectiveness of an intervention, but for some reason it is not possible to have either a control group or randomly assign the subjects to the experimental and control groups.
- Time series are useful in research design to assess the long-term effects of an intervention in which at a specified interval, intervention is withheld or intensified.
- Pre-experiments are the weakest form of experiments as they lack two essential characteristics of true experiments: randomisation and control.
- When the researcher identifies the *effect* first and looks back to identify the *cause,* it is termed a retrospective study.
- When the researcher identifies the *cause* first and looks forward to identify the *effect,* it is termed a prospective study.
- Cross-sectional studies are those in which there is one point of data collection. The phenomenon of interest is captured at a given point of time.
- Longitudinal study involves multiple points of data collection over an extended period of time.
- Descriptive studies involve the observation and description of the phenomenon and facts about how they are present in their natural setting.

- Historical research is the systematic study of past events to give an account of what has happened in the past.
- External criticism is the process of determining the validity, trustworthiness or authenticity of the source (to ascertain if the source is what it claims to be).
- Internal criticism is the process of determining the extent to which the information contained in the sources collected is reliable and authentic. This is done by positive and negative criticism.
- Historical researchers often use three techniques while handling evidence. These are corroboration, sourcing and contextualisation.
- According to Glaser and Strauss (1967), "Grounded theory investigates the actualities in the real world and analyses the data with no preconceived ideas or hypothesis". It is the discovery of theory from data systematically obtained from social research.
- Ethnography is a qualitative research design aimed at exploring cultural phenomena and at representing it graphically and in writing. It is a research tradition rooted in anthropology and sociology.
- The phenomenological researcher aims to provide a rich textured description of lived experience. The lived experience is a key concept and focus of investigation for phenomenology.
- The researcher aims to bracket or keep on hold previous assumptions or understanding in order to be open to the phenomenon as it appears.

EVALUATE YOURSELF

Long Answer Questions

Q1: Explain the following research deigns with suitable examples:
(a) Cross-over design (b) Randomised block design
(c) Factorial design

Q2: How will you control extraneous variables in an experimental study?

Q3: Explain the criteria for a true experiment.

Q4: What are the criteria to establish a cause and effect relationship?

Q5: Define phenomenology. What are the methods of data collection in grounded theory?

Q6: Define historical research. Explain the steps of historical research.

Q7: What are the advantages and disadvantages of experimental research?

Q8: How will you control extraneous variables in your study? Explain in detail.

Q9: Elaborate the threats to internal and external validity of a study?

Short Answer Questions

Q1: Define the following:
(a) Quantitative research (b) Experiment study
(c) Quasi-experiment (d) Control
(e) Randomisation

Q2: Write short notes on
1. External and internal criticism in historical research
2. Pre-experimental research design
3. Retrospective and prospective study
4. Cohort study
5. Trends studies
6. Secondary analysis
7. Meta analysis
8. Threats to external and internal validity
9. Phenomenology
10. Ethnography
11. Differentiate qualitative research from quantitative research

Multiple Choice Questions

Q1: Cross-over design is a:
(a) True experiment (b) Quasi-experiment
(c) Pre-experiment (d) Non-experiment

Q2: Factorial design is represented by:
(a) Each independent variable has two or more levels
(b) Each dependent variable has two or more levels
(c) Both a and b
(d) None of the above

Q3: Which of the following is/are essential requirement/s for a true experiment?
(a) Manipulation (b) Control
(c) Randomisation (d) All of the above

Q4: Solomon four-group design is used to:
(a) Study testing effect (b) Study systematic bias
(c) Describe a phenomenon (d) All of the above

Q5: Phenomenology is
(a) Study of culture (b) Study of lived experience
(c) Study of social process (d) All of the above

Q6: Ethnography is
(a) Study of culture (b) Study of lived experience
(c) Study of social process (d) All of the above

Q7: Grounded theory is
(a) Study of culture (b) Study of lived experience
(c) Study of social process (d) All of the above

Q8: Which of the following is a threat to internal validity?
(a) Hawthorne effect (b) Novelty effect
(c) Instrumentation (d) Experimenter effect

Q9: Which of the following is a threat to external validity?
(a) External events (b) Instrumentation
(c) Novelty effect (d) Maturation

Q10: Identify the control mechanism for extraneous variables in a quasi-experimental study:
(a) Randomised block (b) Cross-over
(c) Statistical control (d) All of the above

Answers

1. a	**2.** a	**3.** d	**4.** a	**5.** b
6. a	**7.** c	**8.** c	**9.** c	**10.** c

FURTHER READING

Ashworth PD. 2003. An approach to phenomenological psychology: The contingencies of the life world. *Journal of Phenomenological Psychology* 34(6):145–156.

Borgatti S. 2013. *Introduction to grounded theory.* (http://www.analytictech.com/mb870/introtogt.htm), accessed on 23/02/2013.

Burns N, Grove SK. 2007. *Understanding Nursing Research, Building an Evidence- based Practice. 4th ed.* Elsevier Publications, New Delhi p. 66–69.

Garza G. 2007. Varieties of phenomenological research at the University of Dallas, *Qualitative Research in Psychology* 4(4):313–342.

Glaser B. 1992. *Basics of Grounded Theory Analysis.* Sociology Press, Mill Valley, California.

Glaser BG, Strauss AL. 1967. *The Discovery of Grounded Theory. Strategies for Qualitative Research.* Aldine Transaction, Inc., accessed on 23/02/2013.

Grounded theory. (http://www.analytictech.com/mb870/introtogt.htm), accessed on 23/02/2013.

Husserl E. 1931. *Ideas: General Introduction to Pure Phenomenology*. B Gibson and WR Trans (eds). George Allen and Unwin, London. (Originally published 1913).

Husserl E. 1970. *The Crisis of European Sciences and Transcendental Phenomenology*. Ill Evanston (ed.). Northwestern University Press. (Originally published in 1936).

Jing K, Wenglensky S. 2010. Course Title: *Research Method,* accessed on 23/02/2013.

Langdridge D. 2007. *Phenomenological Psychology: Theory, Research and Method*. Pearson Prentice Hall, Harlow, England.

Moran D. 2000. *Introduction to Phenomenology*. Routledge, London.

Polit DF, Tatano BC. 2008. *Nursing Research, 8th ed.* Lippincott Williams and Wilkins Publications, p. 250–256.

Sharma SK. 2011. *Nursing Research and Statistics*, Elsevier Publication, New Delhi, p. 132–135.

Smith JA, Osborn M. 2003. Interpretative phenomenological analysis. In: *Qualitative Psychology: A Practical Guide to Research Methods*. JA Smith (ed.). Sage Publications, London.

Thomas G, James D. 2006. Reinventing grounded theory: Some questions about theory, ground and discovery, *British Educational Research Journal* 32(6):767–795, accessed on 23/02/2013.

Thomas G. 2011. Sonia is typing..... A typology for the a case study in social science following a review of definition, discourse and structure. *Qualitative Inquiry* 17(6):511–521.

Thornberg R. 2012. Informed grounded theory. *Scandinavian Journal of Educational Research* 56: 243–259, accessed on 23/02/2013.

William MK, Trochin WMK. 2010. (http://www.socialresearchmethods.net/kb/expsimp.phpental designs).

Theoretical/ Conceptual Framework

Chapter overview

- Introduction and definition of terms
- Theories: definition, characteristics, significance, common concepts and classification
- Conceptual model/framework/schemes
- Selecting the appropriate conceptual framework
- Criteria for evaluating conceptual models/frameworks
- Criticism of nursing theories

INTRODUCTION TO THEORETICAL/CONCEPTUAL FRAMEWORK

Qualitative research involves studying a phenomenon in-depth, leaving no stone unturned, and leading to the development of a theory. A theory can also be developed through intuition, systematic observation and experience. A theory may include a group of concepts, the relationship among the concepts, proposition statements and assumptions that provide a systematic view of the phenomenon and proposes actions that guide the practice of nursing. Kerlinger has defined theories as, "A set of interrelated concepts that give a systematic view of a phenomenon that is explanatory and predictive in nature". Qualitative research gives birth to theories through the inductive approach, whereas quantitative researchers derive their hypothesis deductively from nursing theories and test it using empirical data. Therefore, integration of theory in research not only helps generate hypotheses but also paves the way for application of the results of a research study in nursing practice through a theoretical framework. Nursing philosophers and scientists have developed many nursing theories and conceptual models to develop the scientific base of the nursing profession. Unfortunately, nursing practice is still largely based on tradition, and nurse practitioners often fail to integrate nursing theories into practice. Similarly, nurse researchers are also reluctant to integrate or fit the key study variables in a conceptual model or theoretical framework. This results in findings that are not integrated into practice. This isolation of theory, practice and research is a grave situation for the nursing profession as it can diminish its scientific status.

Definition of Terms

Before exploring the details of nursing theory, conceptual models and how to utilise them in nursing research, some key terms need to be defined.

Concept The basic building blocks of a theory (Fig. 5.1). These are vehicles of thought that involve images and words that portray objects, properties or events. For example, anxiety is a concept portrayed as a person looking tense, with grim facial expressions and increased pulse rate.

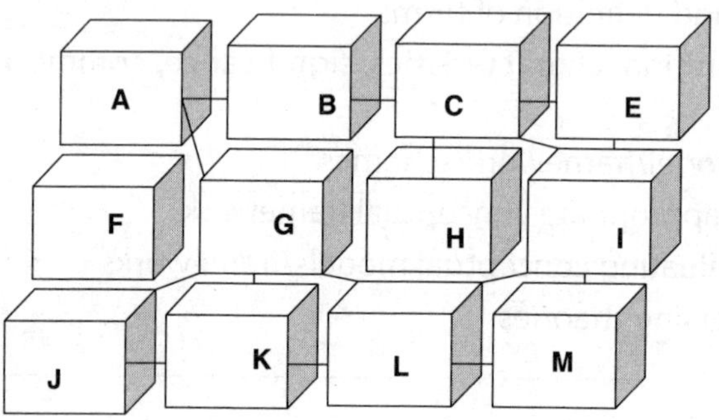

Figure 5.1 Concepts knitted together to shape a theory

Construct Deliberately invented/created and defined by the researcher for scientific purposes in a research project. For example, quality of life, medication adherence behaviour.

Conceptual models/framework/schemes The visual portrayal of interaction among concepts which brings to the surface some common themes relevant to the interrelatedness of the concepts. It shows the pathway to how a theory can be applied in nursing practice. A conceptual model simplifies the perception of a theory by providing a tangible picture that encompasses the basic components and the relationship/interactions among them. Concepts are assembled by virtue of their relevance to a common theme. It is more loosely structured than a theory. For example, Betty Neuman's system model and Roy's adaptation models are conceptual models used in nursing. Their concreteness makes them easy to remember and apply; on the other hand, a theory is more abstract and difficult to understand, thereby reducing its applicability. Conceptual model has been described as a less formal attempt to organise the phenomenon of interest.

Framework refers to the conceptual underpinnings of a study. Every study is necessarily based on a framework but may not necessarily be based on a theory or conceptual model.

If a study is based on a theory, the framework of the study is referred to as a theoretical framework and when it is based on a conceptual model, it is known as a conceptual framework. Sometimes, the study framework is implicit. This means it is not based on any explicit theory or conceptual model. The researcher formulates conceptual definitions of the study variable to explain the framework of the study based on the world view of the phenomenon.

A schematic model uses boxes, arrows and symbols to graphically represent the concepts and relationships among them.

Proposition Closed sentences that are distinguished from what is expressed by an open sentence. The proposition in classical theories indicates the relationship among the concepts. These are considered statements that speak the truth. For example, Imogene King's theory of goal attainment involves the concepts of perception, communication, interaction, transaction, role, stress, coping and goal attainment. The relationships among these concepts are further explained by the propositions:

- If role conflict is felt by a nurse or patient or both, it will lead to stress in the nurse–patient interaction.
- Perceptual accuracy in the nurse–patient interaction leads to transaction.

Theory Abstract generalisation that provides an explanation of a relationship about how concepts are inter-related. This classical definition of theory requires that theory must embody at least two concepts in a manner that can explain the phenomenon of interest.

Another school of thought believes that theory is a broad characterisation of a phenomenon of interest. This type is termed descriptive theory as it describes the features of a phenomenon of interest. Grounded theory researchers strive to develop a conceptualisation of a phenomenon that is grounded in empirical data.

Theory has been defined as a set of inter-related concepts, propositions and relationships arranged in such a way that they provide a different perspective to a phenomenon of interest. It describes, explains, predicts and elaborates the phenomenon central to nursing practice.

Characteristics of Theories

- Theories inter-relate concepts in such a way as to create a different way of looking at a particular phenomenon.
- Theories are logical in nature.
- Theories are generalisable.
- Theories are bases for hypotheses that can be tested.
- Theories increase the general body of knowledge within a discipline through the research implemented to validate them.

- Theories are used by practitioners to guide and improve their practice.
- Theories are consistent with other validated theories, laws and principles but will leave open unanswered questions that need to be investigated.

Significance of Theory

Nursing theory aims to describe, predict and explain the phenomenon of nursing (Chinn and Jacobs 1978). It serves as a springboard for nursing practice through the explanation of phenomenon of interest and describing nursing explicitly. It facilitates the advancement of knowledge and points towards the direction in which nursing should develop in the future (Brown 1964). According to Pearson (1949), theory is important because it helps nurses decide what is known and what it is necessary to know. This can be seen as an attempt by the nursing profession to maintain its professional boundaries and identities. For example, Betty Neuman's system model appreciates primary, secondary and tertiary prevention as nursing intervention.

Common Concepts in Nursing Theory

Nursing theories help distinguish nursing from other related disciplines such as medicine, surgery and paramedical by providing a sound basis for the practice of nursing, which is different from that of other related professions. The phenomenons of interest that influence and determine nursing practice are depicted in Fig. 5.2.

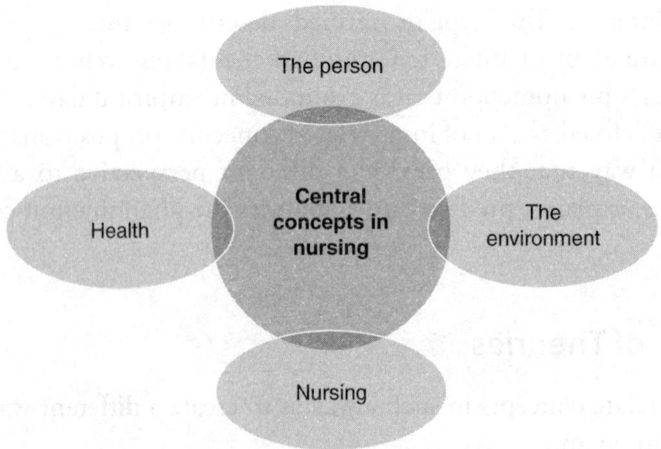

Figure 5.2 Central concepts in nursing

Each of these concepts is defined differently and uniquely by various nursing theorists. For example, Sister Callista Roy proposed Roy's adaptation model in which she defined the concept of health as, "A state and a process of being and becoming integrated and whole".

Theory, Research and Practice Relationship

Nursing theories and research are complementary to each other. Theories and models are developed inductively through empirical observations and in-depth interviews in qualitative research. The concepts and inter-relationship among these concepts, which are the building blocks of a theory, are subjects for validation enquiry, which can be achieved through deductive hypothesis formulation and testing in quantitative research. Thus, the role of research is dual as it helps in building a theory and also provides avenues for testing and validation of the theory. Theory provides thrust for scientific investigation and research findings shape the development of theory.

However, it is noteworthy that research in nursing can be conducted without a guiding theory and later on the results can be linked to theory to guide nursing practice (Fig. 5.3).

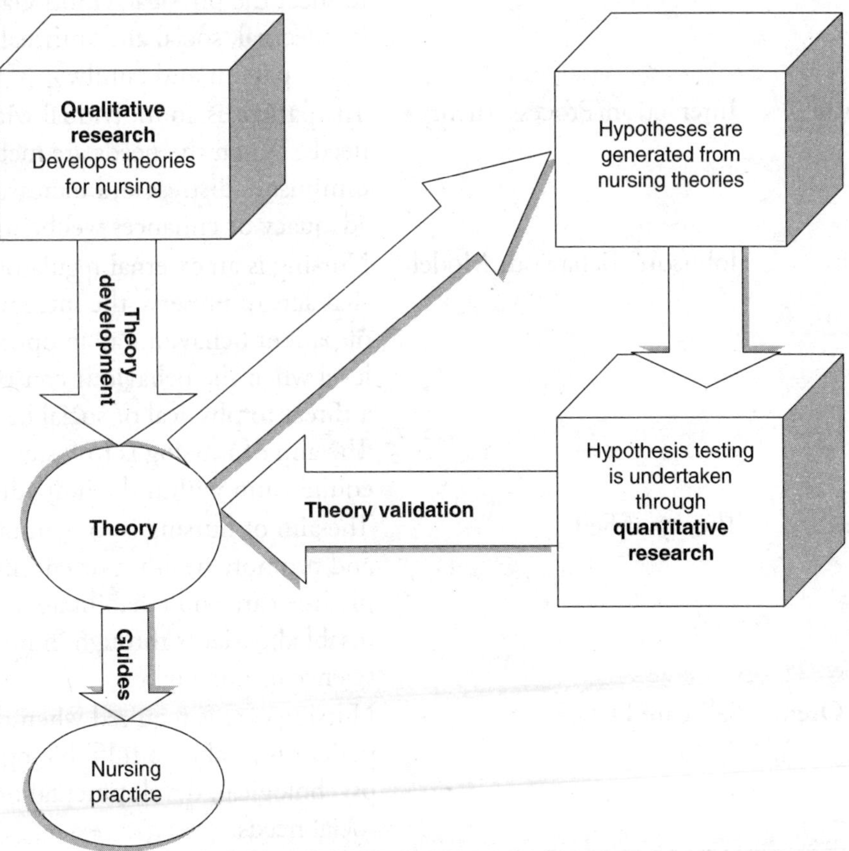

Figure 5.3 Theory development and validation

Table 5.1 Summary of nursing theories

Theorist	Theory/Model	Key concepts
Florence Nightingale	*Notes on Nursing: What it is, What it is not* (1860)/ Environmental Theory	Manipulation of the patient's environment facilitates the body's reparative process
Hildegard E Peplau	Theory of Interpersonal Relations	Nursing is a therapeutic interpersonal process
Virginia Henderson	Need Theory	Fourteen basic needs of human beings.
Faye Abdellah	Need Theory	■ 21 nursing problems ■ 10 steps to identify the patient's problems ■ 11 nursing skills to develop a treatment typology Nursing care should be comprehensive to meet the physical, emotional, intellectual, social and spiritual needs of the patient and family.
Ida Orlando	Interaction/Process Theory	The patient is an individual with needs. When the needs are met, it diminishes distress and increases adequacy or enhances wellbeing.
Dorothy E Johnson	Johnson's Behaviour Model	Nursing is an external regulatory force that acts to preserve the integration of patient behaviour at an optimum level when the behaviour constitutes a threat to physical or social health. The aim of nursing is to foster equilibrium within the individual.
Carl Rogers	Theory of Self	The aim of nursing is to maintain and promote health, prevent illness, provide care and rehabilitate ill and disabled patients through 'humanistic science of nursing'.
Dorothea Orem	Self-care Deficit	Nursing care is required when the patient is unable to fulfil biological, psychological, developmental or social needs.

(*continued*)

Table 5.1 Continued

Theorist	Theory/Model	Key concepts
Sr. Callista Roy	Adaptation Model	Promoting adaptation for individuals and groups in the four adaptive modes, thus contributing to health, quality of life and dying with dignity by assessing behaviours and factors that influence adaptation.
Imogene King	Goal Attainment Theory	The theory describes a dynamic, interpersonal relationship in which a person grows and develops to attain certain life goals. Factors that affect the attainment of goal are roles, stress, space and time. Use communication to help the patient re-establish positive adaptation to the environment.
Betty Neuman	System Model	Stress reduction is the goal of the system model of nursing practice.
Jean Watson	Theory of Caring	Caring is inclusive, circular and expansive. It is for the self, for each other, for patients/families, and for the universe. Caring changes self, others and the culture of groups/ environments. The theory attempts to define the outcome of nursing activity as regards the humanistic aspects of life.
Myra Estrine Levine	Conservation Theory/Model	Conservation model is focused on promoting adaptation and maintaining wholeness using the principles of conservation. The nurse should focus on the conservation of energy, structure and personal and social integrity.
Madeleine Leininger	Theory of Culture Care Diversity and Universality	Care and culture are inextricably linked. All cultures have practices related to caring. Culture should determine the way that individuals receive care, based on the different ways their cultures meet their basic needs.

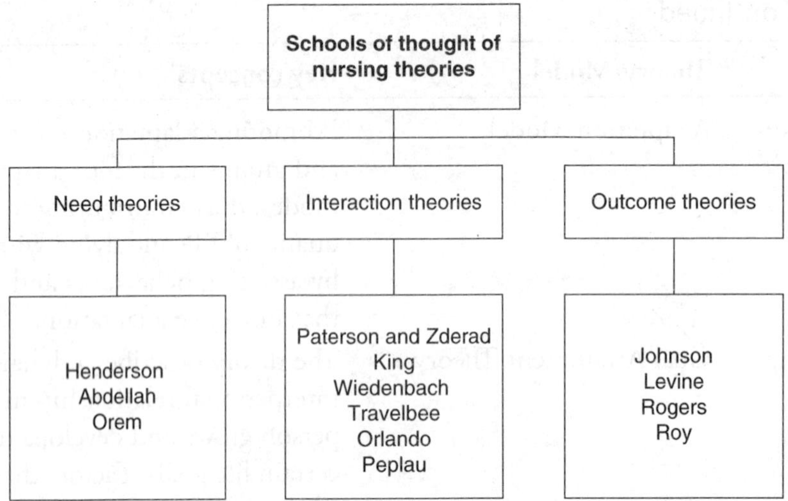

Figure 5.4 Schools of thought of nursing theories

Classification of Theories (Fig. 5.5)

- **Meta theory:** It is the theory of theory. Meta theory utilises abstract concepts to identify the phenomenon. A higher level of abstraction is difficult to understand and utilise in nursing practice.
- **Grand nursing theories**: These theories are broadest in scope and present abstract general concepts and propositions. They are intended to be applicable to all instances of nursing. They define broad perspectives for practice and ways of appreciating the nursing phenomena. However, grand nursing theories reflect and provide insights that are useful for practice but are not designed for empirical testing. Therefore, the use of these theories for directing, explaining and predicting nursing in specific situations is limited. They provide a broad conceptual framework that helps identify the key concepts and principles of the discipline.
- **Middle-range nursing theories**: These theories are more precise and narrower in scope than grand nursing theories. They serve as an effective bridge between grand nursing theories and nursing practice. The concepts and propositions are presented at a lower level of abstraction and thus provide an opportunity for theory-based research and nursing practice strategies.
- **Nursing practice theories**: These are theories that have utility and applicability to enhance nursing practice within a specific range of nursing situations. They have the most limited level of abstraction and provide frameworks for nursing interventions, and predict the outcome of the same. They identify explicit goals of nursing care and provide details on how these goals will be achieved (Polit et al. 2001).

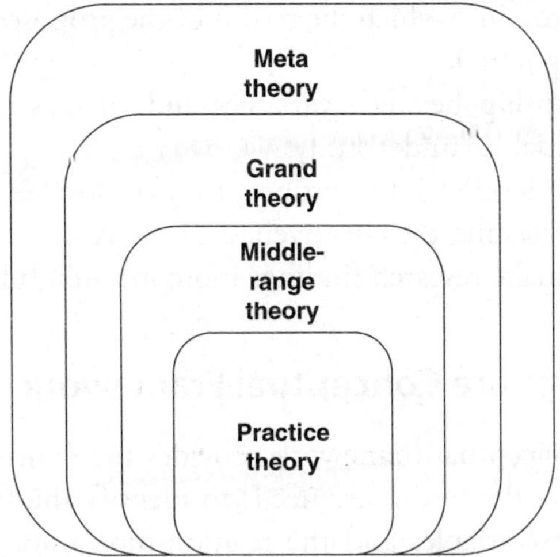

Figure 5.5 Types of theories

Conceptual Model/Framework/Schemes

Most research studies have explicit or implicit theoretical underpinnings, which describe, explain or predict the phenomenon under study. Descriptive study uses descriptive theory as its framework; similarly, experimental study is based on predictive theory. According to Burns and Groves (2001), theories are linked to conceptual models and frameworks whereas a conceptual model is more abstract than a theory and a theory may be derived from a model. A model, as an abstraction of reality, provides a way to visualise reality to simplify thinking. A conceptual model shows concretely and in simplified ways how various concepts are inter-related in a theory. According to Fawcett (2000), the conceptual model, "Gives direction to the search for relevant questions about the phenomena of central interest to a discipline and suggests solutions to practical problems". It is used to make conceptual distinctions and organise ideas in a systematic way. Strong conceptual frameworks capture something real and do so in a way that is easy to remember and apply. The purposes of a conceptual/theoretical framework can be explained as follows:

- It provides a theoretical context to a research problem. It serves as a pilot that helps in the overall study process.
- Theoretical framework provides a theoretical rationale for the development of hypothesis.
- It provides background information for the development of operational definitions of variables.
- It offers a guideline about how the variables under study can be inter-related with each other.

- It puts forward a skeleton into which the results of the proposed study can be fitted and integrated into nursing practice.
- It predicts the relationship between variables and enables the researcher to clearly identify the various variables under study.
- It helps the researcher develop intervention protocols for the experimental study and provides guidelines for testing the effectiveness of the same.
- Theories and models make research findings more meaningful and generalisable.

Selecting the Appropriate Conceptual Framework

As mentioned above, a conceptual framework provides the conceptual underpinnings of a research study. Therefore, the researcher needs to identify the framework that can best explain the study concepts/variables and the relationships among them. The researcher needs to have an understanding of different theories or frameworks available within the area of interest. A comprehensive review of literature may assist the investigator in making an informed choice while selecting the conceptual model.

- Descriptive nursing theories can be used to guide a descriptive study.
- Predictive nursing theories can guide an experimental study.

The issue of concern with the use of conceptual models is that most Indian nurse scientists use them as the organisational structure of their study. They rarely use it to select research problems, design or data collection instruments. Therefore, the results of the study are interpreted in isolation and not integrated with the theory, contributing to widening of the theory–practice gap. Integrating the result with the chosen model can help validate it and offer guidelines about how the results can be utilised to improve nursing practice.

In an ideal situation, the conceptual framework of interest should be the founding stone of a research study which can later include the formulation of a problem statement, hypothesis, interventional protocols and selection of research design, sample and data collection tools. However, in practice, researchers select a research problem and later try to explore conceptual models that can provide an organisational structure to the problem. This practice is not useful as the study finding will be less meaningful in the context of the selected theory; it will also offer no suggestions about the validity of the selected theory. Further, the research results will not be useful in increasing the scientific evidence base of the nursing profession. Fabrication of research problem onto a theory is of little use; nurse scholars are required to plan research projects derived directly from a theory/model to widen the scientific status of the profession at large. Silvia (1986) has identified three ways used by researchers to incorporate theory into research:

- **Minimal use of theory:** It refers to the use of theory to provide an organisation structure to the study. Theory is not used to develop and test hypothesis; thereby the study results cannot be integrated with the theory.

- **Moderate use of theory:** In this instance, concepts from theories are used to organise the research process; however, testing of the theory is not undertaken. Rather, the researcher provides an overview of the linkage between theoretical concepts and research variables.
- In the third type of theory use, as described by Silvia, the researcher uses the theory not only to explain the theoretical underpinnings of the study but also to **test the hypothesis** generated from it. The results of the study either support or reject the theory and are integrated with the theoretical framework which offers a solution about how the findings can be utilised in practice.

Criteria for Evaluating Conceptual Models/Frameworks

Fawcett (1995) has given criteria for evaluating a conceptual model/framework:

Comprehensiveness of content: This is appraised in terms of its depth and breadth (Fawcett 1995). When a conceptual model incorporates sufficient descriptions of the constructs and provides details about how the constructs are related with the propositions, it ensures that adequate depth is present in the conceptual model. Breadth of the model is related to its scope to provide guidance in various clinical nursing situations and serve as a basis for practice, research, education and administration.

Logical congruence: Fawcett mentioned that logical congruence is linked with the logic of the internal structure of the model, which is evaluated through critical reasoning. Through critical reasoning, the evaluator is required to judge the world's views and the type of nursing knowledge reflected by the model. In order to be logically congruent, a conceptual model should merge different perspectives and redefine concepts from different schools of thought before using them in the model.

Conceptual clarity: This appraises whether the concepts are clearly identified and described explicitly, whether the relational statements, which show association among concepts, have been identified clearly. Fawcett pointed out that the developer of the model should state the assumptions and basis on which the model or framework was built, i.e., observation, experience, middle range or grand theory.

Level of abstraction: This criterion examines the extent and intensity of abstraction for the concepts incorporated in the model. Level of abstraction can range from concrete to very abstract. Olszewski and Avant (1995) defined abstract concepts as those that are not limited by time or space and are not directly measurable. Similarly, concrete concepts are those that are directly measurable. By looking at the level of abstraction, an analyst can find out the concretisation or abstractness of the theory.

Clinical utility: Clinical utility of the model refers to the applicability and relevance of the model to the real world of practice (Sidani 2000); whether the model is significant to the nurse practitioners to guide their practice. The two main issues to be considered are the setting where the model can be applied and the clinical situations which can be tackled by the model by influencing nursing practice.

The researcher must critically appraise the selected conceptual model in order to determine which model is the most appropriate to guide the development of an intervention and overall process for a research study.

The nurse researcher typically uses a variety of conceptual models to guide her study; here some of the models that have been extensively used in nursing research as the organisational structure of the study are discussed.

Systems Theory as a Framework

Systems theory is concerned with changes caused by interactions among all the factors that constitute the system. Systems theory was proposed in 1936 by the biologist Ludwig von Bertalanffy, and it was further developed by Ross Ashby. Von Bertalanffy emphasised that real systems are open to, and interact with, their environments, and that they can acquire qualitatively new properties through emergence, resulting in continual evolution. A system is defined as, "A whole with interrelated parts in which the parts have a function and the system as a totality has a function" (Auger 1976). A human being can be considered as a system where the human being as a whole has a function and the various organ systems which constitute the human being have their own functions which are inter-related and which interact with each other and as a whole; they provide integrity to the human being. A system is said to be closed if no material enters or leaves it; it is considered open if there is import and export of material. The important components of a system are input, throughput, output and feedback. The system framework has been used extensively in nursing research. An example of a research study which uses system framework is given as: A study to evaluate the effectiveness of a training programme on the knowledge, attitudes and practice of Basic Life Support techniques among Class 9 students from selected schools in Punjab (Fig. 5.6).

In the current study, input includes the (learners') characteristics of Class 9 students such as age, gender, height, weight, attitude, knowledge and skill to perform BLS. These characteristics will be processed with structured BLS training which will include delivery of knowledge and demonstration of the steps of BLS. The students will be provided a pretest before the administration of BLS training to assess their knowledge, attitudes and practice to perform BLS. After the intervention, students will again be assessed on the same parameters. As a result of BLS training, students will have increased knowledge about Basic Life Support, enhanced practice to perform it and develop a favourable attitude towards it. In this study, as per systems theory, the student is envisioned as an open system that is in constant interaction with the environment which influences his/her knowledge, attitudes and practice of BLS. When the input variables (Fig. 5.6) are processed while conducting BLS training, it would enable students to achieve the desired output, i.e., in

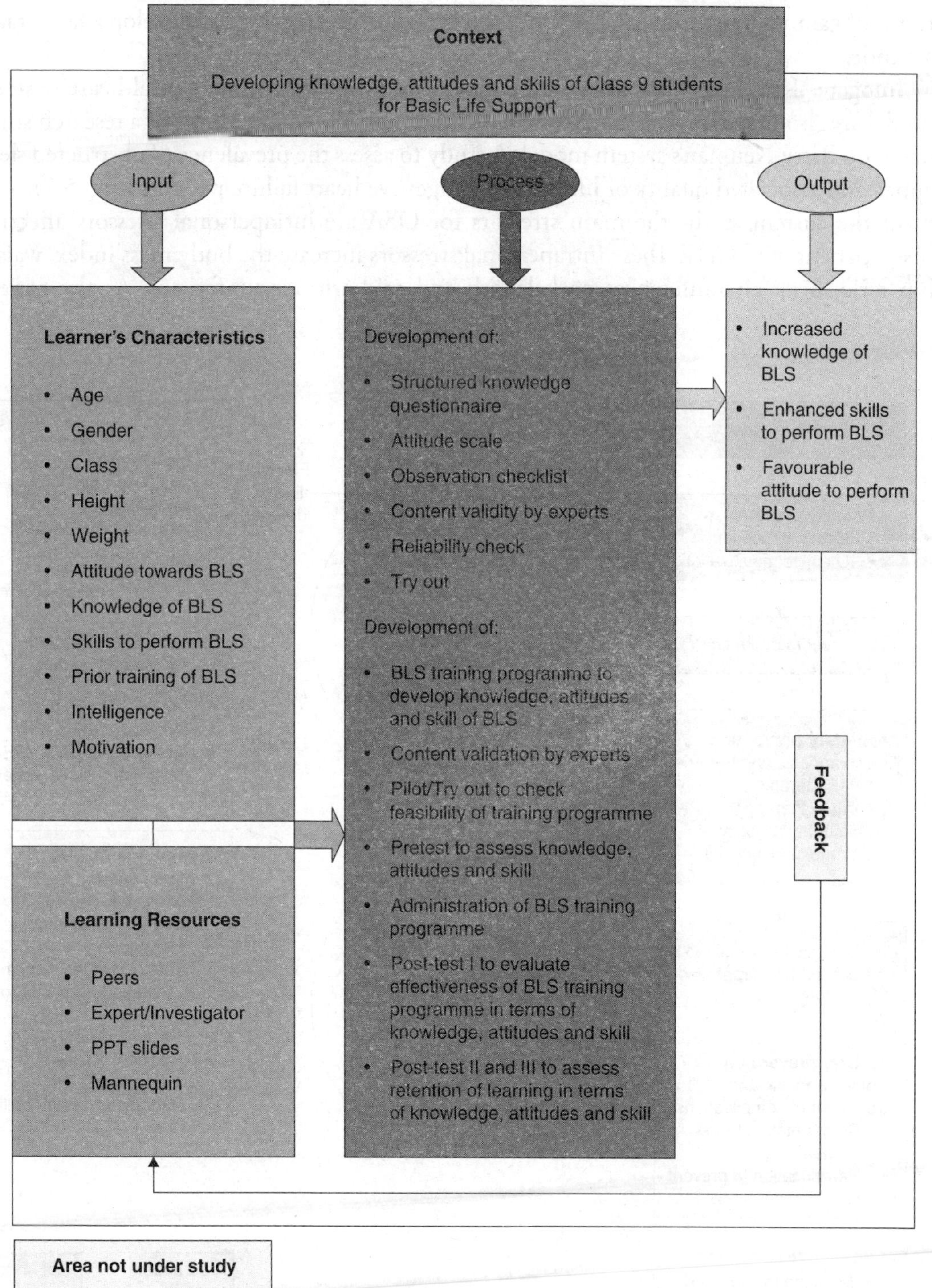

Figure 5.6 Conceptual framework of the study based on Ludwig von Bertalanffy's systems theory

terms of gaining knowledge and practice to perform BLS and thereby develop a favourable attitude.

Imogene King's systems interaction model and Betty Neuman's healthcare systems model are also based on systems theory. Consider the following example of a research study based on Betty Neuman's system model: A study to assess the prevalence of obstructed sleep apnea and associated quality of life among congestive heart failure patients (Fig. 5.7).

In the current study, the main stressors for OSA are intrapersonal stressors affecting obese patient with CHF. These intrapersonal stressors increase the body mass index, waist–hip ratio, neck circumference, neck length and mid-arm circumference. As the patient

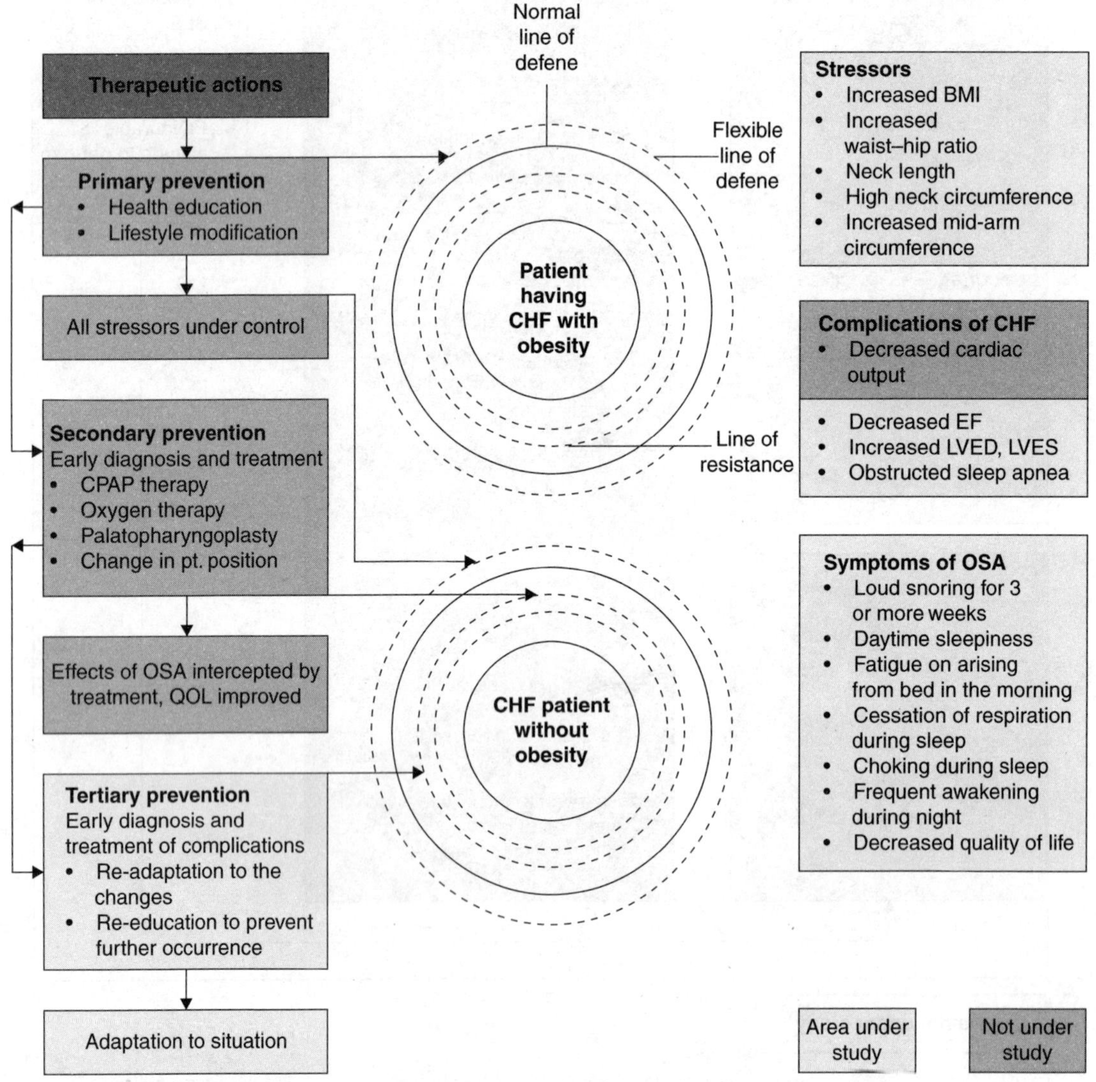

Figure 5.7 Conceptual framework of a study based on Neuman's system model

is already diagnosed with CHF, it can be assumed that the normal line of defence and resistance is already broken and the patient is more susceptible to the invasion of stressors. Due to this, there is a response pattern exhibited by the individual, which includes various signs and symptoms of obstructed sleep apnea.

The symptoms of OSA include snoring for three or more weeks, daytime sleepiness, feeling of fatigue on awakening in the morning, choking during sleep and decreased quality of life. This study is done to assess the prevalence of obstructed sleep apnea in congestive heart failure patients and associated quality of life.

Neuman has stated the nursing actions as primary, secondary, tertiary and prevention. In the current study, primary prevention includes prevention of encounters with stressors in order to prevent these stressors from invading the flexible LOD; so in primary prevention, the nurse's responsibilities are to prevent the occurrence of increase in body mass index and waist–hip ratio among CHF patients. Primary prevention is applicable for patients with congestive heart failure without obesity, where all stressors are under control.

Secondary prevention according to Neuman includes early diagnosis and treatment. In the current study, secondary prevention focuses on physical examination to diagnose obstructed sleep apnea at an early stage. In order to assess the disease, the nurse should be able to assess various anthropometric parameters and symptoms of obstructed sleep apnea. The treatment of obstructed sleep apnea includes continuous positive pressure ventilation, continuous nasal oxygen and palatopharyngoplasty.

The goal of tertiary prevention is to maintain this adaptability by strengthening the line of resistance, thus preventing future occurrence. This goal is primarily accomplished by the use of re-educative measures and by optimum use of the system's resources, including the external and internal environment. In the current study, as shown in Fig. 5.7, tertiary prevention is applicable because the patient is encountered in a situation where he/she has already developed obstructed sleep apnea.

Criticisms of Nursing Theories

In India and globally, there is a wide theory–practice gap despite theory and practice being viewed as inseparable. Most practicing nurses do not apply relevant nursing theories in their routine practice. The reason for this may be because the majority of nursing theory is developed by and for nursing academics (Lathlean 1994); therefore, it is far from the reach of clinical nurses. Another aspect of the problem is that traditionally nurses are used to 'speaking with their hands' (Levine 1995). Therefore, many nurses have not had the training or experience to deal with the abstract concepts presented by nursing theory. This makes it difficult for the majority of nurses to understand and apply theory in practice (Miller 1985). The situation calls for the necessity of the 'dual role' of nurses so that the communication gap between the nurse academician and nurse practitioner can be minimised; this can provide a road map for the application of nursing theories in clinical nursing practice. Secondly, nurse scientists should generate research problems from existing nursing theories so that findings can be easily integrated in practice.

CHAPTER SUMMARY

- A theory includes a group of concepts, the relationship among the concepts, propositions statements and assumptions that provides a systematic view of phenomenon and proposes actions that guide the practice of nursing.
- Qualitative research gives birth to theories through the inductive approach, whereas quantitative researchers derive hypotheses deductively from nursing theories and test it through empirical data.
- Concepts are the basic building blocks of a theory. These are the vehicles of thought that involve images and words that portray objects, properties or events.
- A construct is deliberately invented/created and defined by the researcher for scientific purposes in a research project.
- A conceptual model simplifies the perception of a theory by providing a tangible picture that encompasses the basic components and the relationship/interactions among them.
- If a study is based on a theory, the framework of the study is referred to as theoretical framework, and when it is based on a conceptual model, it is known as conceptual framework.
- Schematic model uses boxes, arrows and symbols to graphically represent the concepts and relationships under study.
- Propositions refer to closed sentences to distinguish them from what is expressed by an open sentence. The proposition in classical theories indicates the relationship among concepts. These are considered as statements which bear truth.
- Theory has been defined as abstract generalisations which provide an explanation of how concepts are inter-related. It has also has been defined as a set of inter-related concepts, propositions and relationships arranged in such a way that it provides a different perspective of a phenomenon of interest.
- Theory serves as a springboard for nursing practice through the explanation of the phenomenon of interest and describing nursing explicitly.
- The person, environment, health and nursing are the four main concepts of nursing theories.
- The relationship of theory and research is mutually beneficial. Research helps in building a theory; it also provides avenues for testing and validation of the theory. Theory provides thrust for scientific investigations, and research findings shape the development of theory.
- Nursing theories are classified as grand nursing theory, middle-range theory and practice theory.
- A conceptual model shows concretely and in a simplified way how various concepts are inter-related in a theory.
- In an ideal situation, the conceptual framework of interest should be the founding stone of a research study which later can include the formulation of the problem statement,

hypothesis, interventional protocols and selection of research design, sample and data collection tools.

- Fawcett (1995) has given criteria for evaluating a conceptual model/framework, which includes comprehensiveness of content, logical congruence, conceptual clarity and level of abstraction.
- The theory–practice gap may exist because most nursing theory is developed by and for nursing academics (Lathlean 1994) and is therefore far from the reach of clinical nurses.

EVALUATE YOURSELF

Long Answer Questions

Q1: How do you develop, use and test a conceptual framework?

Q2: Explain the criteria for the evaluation of a conceptual framework.

Q3: Explain the role of theory in research.

Q4: Write a short note on conceptual framework.

Q5: Elaborate the relationship between theory and research.

Q6: Explain the characteristics of a theory.

Q7: Define nursing theory. What are the components of a theory? Explain the four major concepts used in nursing theories.

Q8: Prepare a conceptual/theoretical conceptual framework for the following study: "A descriptive study to assess the patient's satisfaction with nursing services in selected hospitals of Kolkata, India".

Q9: Elaborate the classification of nursing theories.

Short Answer Questions

Write short notes on:

1. Concept
2. Construct
3. Proposition
4. Characteristics of a theory
5. Theory–practice–research relationship
6. Purpose of conceptual framework
7. Criteria for evaluation of a conceptual framework

Multiple Choice Questions

Q1: If a study is based on a theory, the framework of the study is referred to as:
(a) A theoretical framework (b) A conceptual framework
(c) A framework of utility (d) A framework of judgement

Q2: Which of the following are considered as statements that speak the truth?
(a) Proposition (b) Concepts
(c) Constructs (d) None of the above

Q3: Which of the following is not a common concept in nursing theory?
(a) Person (b) Health
(c) Environment (d) Place

Q4: Qualitative research is concerned with:
(a) Development of nursing theory
(b) Testing and validating theory through hypothesis testing
(c) Collection of numerical data
(d) Use of highly structured instruments of data collection

Q5: Theory of interpersonal relationship was proposed by:
(a) Handerson (b) Paplau
(c) Orlando (d) Orem

Q6: Which of the following is an outcome theory?
(a) Orem's theory of self care (b) Levine's conservation theory
(c) Kings's theory of goal attainment (d) Paplau theory of interaction

Q7: Which of the following is termed a theory of theory?
(a) Grand theory (b) Middle range theory
(c) Practice theory (d) Meta theory

Q8: Theory of culture care diversity and universality was proposed by:
(a) Jean Watson (b) Myra Estrine Levine
(c) Both a and b (d) Madeleine Leininger

Answers

1. a **2.** a **3.** d **4.** a **5.** b
6. b **7.** d **8.** d

FURTHER READING

Brathwaite A. 2002. *Selection of a Conceptual Model/Framework for Guiding Research Interventions. The Internet Journal of Advanced Nursing Practice.* 6:1.

Burns N, Groves S. 2001. *The Practice of Nursing Research, Conduct, Critique, and Utilization, 4th ed.* WB Saunders Company, Toronto, Ontario.

Fawcett J. 1995 *Analysis and Evaluation of Conceptual Models of Nursing, 3rd ed.* FA Davis Company, Philadelphia.

Olszewski Walker L, Coalson Avant K. 1995. *Strategies for Theory Construction in Nursing, 3rd ed.* Appleton & Lange, Norwalk, CT.

Polit DF, Beck CT. 2008. *Nursing Research. 8th ed.* Lippincott Williams and Wilkins Publications.

Bertalanffy L Von. 1969. *General System Theory*. George Braziller Inc. New York.

Chinn PL, Jacobs MK. 1991. *Theory and Nursing, 4th ed.* CV Mosby, St. Louis.

Fawcett Downs F. 1986. *The Relationship of Theory and Research*. Appleton-Century-Crofts, Norwalk, Connecticut.

Barnum BJS. 1990. *Nursing Theory, Analysis, Application, Evaluation, 3rd ed.* Scott, Forman/Little, Brown, Glenview, Illinois.

Neuman B. 1989. *The Neuman Systems Model, 2nd ed.* Appleton & Lange, Norwalk, CT.

Silvia MC. 1976. Research testing nursing theory: State of the art. *Advances in Nursing Sciences* 9(1):1–11.

Young A, Taylor SG, Renpenning KM. 2001. *Connections: Nursing Research, Theory and Practices.* CV Mosby, St. Louis.

6 Sampling Techniques

Chapter overview

- Need for and characteristics of a sample
- Definition of key terms
- Factors influencing the sampling process
- Types of sampling techniques
- Determination of sample size
- Sampling errors

NEED FOR A SAMPLE

Studying the entire population for a given problem situation is almost impossible. For example, if a researcher wants to discover the attitude of healthcare professionals towards HIV/AIDS, she has to collect data from all the healthcare professionals in the country—an impossible task. Secondly, it is not cost-effective or time-efficient to conduct research for the whole country. Therefore, the researcher must either drop the study project or proceed using a sample. Most healthcare research cannot be conducted for the entire population. Therefore, the researcher must select a subset of the population—known as the sample—that represents the entire population. Sampling is necessary for the following reasons:

- Cost effectiveness
- Less time consuming
- Less labour intensive
- Feasibility to conduct research
- Quality of data gathered

CHARACTERISTICS OF A GOOD SAMPLE

- It should be representative of the entire population.

- It should be unbiased—provide equal opportunity to all subjects to be recruited to the study.
- The sample size should be large enough to provide sufficient precision.
- The sample should be selected randomly

DEFINITION OF KEY TERMS

Population The aggregate of the subjects/elements/objects for which a researcher is interested to explore or describe some phenomenon or to test an intervention. It is the large group of individuals, items or elements from which individuals are selected to participate in a study. In research methodology, population can be of two types:

- **Target population**: The aggregate of the subjects/elements/objects for which the researcher wants to generalise the findings of the research study; in other words, it is population that is targetted for generalising the findings of a research study.
- **Accessible population**: The aggregate of the subjects/elements/objects that are accessible to the researcher as a pool of subjects from which she can recruit the study sample.

> **For example**: A researcher is undertaking a research project titled 'A descriptive study to assess the prevalence of obstructed sleep apnea and associated quality of life among congestive heart failure patients seeking treatment in selected hospitals of New Delhi, India'. In this study, the researcher wants to generalise her findings to all congestive heart failure patients in India. Therefore, the target population is Indian CHF patients, and the accessible population is patients with congestive heart failure who attend the outpatient department of selected hospitals in New Delhi, India.

Sample The selected **subset of the (accessible) population** on which the research study is conducted and data collected to answer the research question. In the example given above, the researcher will recruit the study sample from the accessible population, that is, patients with congestive heart failure who seek treatment at the outpatient department of selected hospitals in New Delhi.

Sampling error The difference between sample statistics and population parameters. Research studies are usually conducted on a selected sample rather than the entire population. This is done for practical reasons, as it is not feasible to study the entire population every time. Therefore, the population parameters are estimated based on the data collected from the sample. However, the population parameters cannot be estimated accurately using data from only one sample. Different samples drawn from the same population may lead to different results, which are scattered around the population parameters. This difference in the data is called sampling error. Sampling error cannot be avoided entirely but its magnitude can be calculated and minimised by taking steps such as increasing the sample size and ensuring that the sample adequately represents the entire population.

Sampling criteria The list of characteristics of elements that the researcher has determined beforehand and which serves as eligibility criteria for a subject to become part of the sample.

For example, these criteria may include:

- Age (between 18 and 60 years)
- Gender (male/female)
- Marital status
- Ethnicity
- Ability to understand English, Urdu, German, etc.

Sampling frame The list of all subjects of the given population from which a random sample is drawn. A researcher who wants to draw a random sample will require a sampling frame. Sometimes, she may use an existing listing of the subjects, for example, a telephone directory, voter list, attendance register of a school, and so on. However, in such situations she may need to define the population as individuals who are listed in the telephone directory or voter list. If such a preformed list of subjects is not available, then the researcher must prepare it herself.

Sampling bias It refers to the bias in the study results due to under or over representation of the population's key attributes in the sample, which are relevant to the research question. When the population is homogeneous, there are very few chances of sampling bias. However, with increase in population variability in terms of key characteristics of interest, the chances of sampling bias increase. The researcher can minimise sampling bias by increasing the sample size.

FACTORS INFLUENCING THE SAMPLING PROCESS

The sampling process is the process of recruiting subjects for the study. The researcher must make various decisions about the sample, taking into account a number of factors:

- Experience of the researcher
- Characteristics of the study subject
- Sample size
- Sampling technique to be used
- Time available for the study
- Geographical location of the population

Experience of the researcher

A novice researcher may find it difficult to handle and recruit a large sample. However, an expert researcher could probably do so with ease. Similarly, the time available to conduct the study, academic workload and researcher's interest may influence the sampling process as well as the sample size.

Characteristics of the study subject The nature of the subjects to be recruited for the sample play a very important role in the sampling process. These characteristics may include diagnosis, gender, employment status, geographical location and educational status of the patient. Sometimes, it may be difficult for the researcher to identify and locate the study subjects. This makes the sampling process time consuming.

Sample size Recruiting a large study sample can only be accomplished with sufficient resources and time. Therefore, it may not be suitable for a novice researcher or a non-funded project. Secondly, sampling by convenience may require a large study sample as compared to simple random sampling in order to obtain a sample that is representative of the population. The sample size is also influenced by many other factors, which in turn influence the process of sampling. These factors are listed below:

- Sampling method
- Cost
- Administrative concerns (e.g., research deadlines, administrative permission)
- Minimum acceptable level of precision
- Confidence level
- Variability within the population (e.g., stratum) of interest

Sampling technique This may be a critical factor influencing the sampling process. Sampling by convenience is the simplest to execute, and therefore the researcher can recruit a large study sample if time and other factors permit. On the other hand, simple random sampling or other forms of random sampling may require expenditure of time and effort, and it may be quite difficult to execute the sampling process.

Time available for the study Time is another critical factor. Postgraduate students who must complete the research project within a specified time period cannot recruit a large study sample dispersed over a wide geographical area. However, seasoned researchers can do so.

Geographical location of the population If the population is distributed over a large geographical area, it may be very difficult for the researcher to collect data, even from a very small randomly selected sample. However, if the population is limited within a small geographical boundary, the researcher will easily be able to recruit the study sample.

Process of Sampling

Recruitment of study sample is an important task for a researcher. A number of factors influence the researcher's decision on how to select a representative sample for the study. The process of sampling includes the following steps:

1. **Identify and define the target population:** As defined earlier, the target population is the aggregate of elements/subjects/object which meets the designated criteria set by the researcher. The researcher is intended to generalise the study results to the target population.
2. **Identify the accessible population:** Here, the researcher must identify the portion of target population that is accessible to her as a pool of subjects that can be recruited to collect data for answering the research questions.
3. **Determine the inclusion and exclusion criteria:** Inclusion criteria specify the conditions that make a person eligible to be included in the study. It may be specified age, diagnosis, willingness of the subject, ability to read and write and so on. Exclusion criteria are those that exclude a subject from the study sample. For example, unconscious patient, serious illness or other associated conditions. These criteria are the sole determinant for whether a person is eligible to be included in the study or not.
4. **Specify the sampling method and technique:** Probability and non-probability sampling are two methods which include various techniques for sample selection. The researcher must consider the influencing factors for a sample before finalising the appropriate technique for sampling. These factors has already discussed in this chapter.
5. **Decide on the sampling frame:** It is the list of all elements/subjects of a population. It is required for probability sampling techniques only. The researcher is required to identify the sampling frame or prepare it if it is not available. Preparing the sampling frame is a labour-intensive task which may sometimes force the researcher to opt for non-probability sampling. Sometimes, the researcher may define the population in terms of the available list of subjects. For example, a study to assess the prevalence of anemia among mothers registered at the antenatal clinic of a selected hospital in Chennai. It may solve the problem of unavailability of sampling frame as the researcher has defined the population as mothers who are already registered at the antenatal clinic of the selected hospital.
6. **Determine the sample size:** For sample size determination, the rule of thumb is that it should be as large as possible. However, power analysis is used for the same to compute the exact number of participants required for a study.
7. **Select the sample** by implementing the appropriate technique and sampling plan.

TYPES OF SAMPLING TECHNIQUES

Sampling techniques can be broadly classified as **probability sampling** and **non-probability sampling**.

Probability sampling is further classified as:

- Simple random sampling
- Stratified random sampling
- Systematic random sampling
- Cluster/Multistage random sampling

Non-probability sampling is further classified as:

- Convenience sampling
- Purposive sampling
- Quota sampling
- Snowball sampling
- Sequential sampling
- Consecutive sampling

Probability Sampling Techniques

These techniques are based on the theory of probability and ensure equal probability for every subject to be recruited into the sample. Research scholars consider probability sampling techniques to be scientific and superior to non-probability methods as they result in samples that are representative of the entire population (*although they cannot guarantee the same*). There are several techniques of probability sampling, explained in detail below.

Simple random sampling

This technique provides equal chance to each individual in the population to be selected for the study sample. This is not as easy or simple in practice as it appears to be in theory. However, the greatest advantage of simple random sampling is that it yields a sample that can be considered as representative of the population (though there is no guarantee of this). This technique commands great respect from research scholars.

Steps in simple random sampling

1. Identify the accessible population of the study (the population from which you intend to select the sample).
2. Determine the sample size.
3. Prepare a list of all the subjects or individuals or elements of the population (called the sampling frame) or use an existing list, if available.
4. Select the sample by using the lottery method or a table of random numbers.

A table of random numbers can be generated online. The researcher must specify the maximum and minimum number to be generated, depending on the number of subjects listed in the sampling frame. For example, if 1000 subjects are listed in the sampling frame, the minimum number must be set as 1 and the maximum number as 1000. The output will be a table of random numbers ranging from 1 to 1000.

The researcher must then place a finger on the table after closing her eyes. The person listed with that number in the list of subjects (sampling frame) is the first participant.

Table 6.1 Sample table of random numbers generated from www.graphpad.com

60	65	136	91	134	149	84	102	31	142
111	97	151	13	158	20	167	93	113	119
158	104	195	151	14	70	82	74	176	78
21	106	117	125	173	46	129	187	79	178
30	54	36	28	54	93	151	183	101	1
187	111	91	3	161	109	144	174	200	171
105	84	127	157	5	173	150	44	15	38
24	127	175	23	100	9	29	92	37	176
125	89	21	26	73	155	90	33	113	35
138	86	198	103	128	168	158	91	139	117
193	32	33	52	173	112	130	133	22	177
101	194	37	2	27	41	107	192	43	108
47	70	138	179	112	67	196	81	111	69
76	16	114	72	148	178	189	122	195	108
7	102	167	164	99	111	52	167	194	108
175	99	142	169	138	75	184	27	145	2
112	126	15	67	39	141	35	124	152	67
181	35	91	89	151	170	113	22	124	104
153	151	134	5	178	186	120	104	196	187
44	159	36	134	66	67	170	200	17	97
195	33	27	34	180	106	57	62	168	10
135	169	12	180	36	94	92	141	51	98
113	10	3	30	198	49	75	111	198	164
35	172	110	103	171	114	66	164	71	176
37	7	22	126	133	71	91	11	56	4
13	161	122	163	156	8	21	66	31	162
117	107	146	39	157	139	130	165	55	124
52	195	81	154	11	113	31	22	127	152
94	180	63	197	186	181	73	86	180	148
126	180	124	176	174	107	45	17	131	47

Moving horizontally right in the table, the researcher must find the next number and recruit the subject listed with that number in the sampling frame. This process is continued until the desired numbers of participants is recruited for the study.

Advantages

- It is highly representative, if all the selected subjects participate in the study.

- A little advance knowledge about the population is all that is required to recruit the sample.
- Sampling errors can be computed easily.

Disadvantages

- This is not possible without a sampling frame (complete list of population members)
- The time frame may be too long—the data/sample could change over time.
- It may be uneconomical and time consuming.

Stratified random sampling

This is a probability sampling technique in which the researcher divides the entire population into different subgroups or strata, and then **randomly** selects the final subjects, either proportionally or disproportionally, from the different strata (Fig. 6.1). This type of sampling is used when the researcher has advance knowledge of the population and can divide it into strata based on some key factors to ensure adequate representation of specific subgroups in the final sample. Some of the common strata used are age, gender, religion, educational attainment, socio-economic status and nationality. Stratified random sampling can be of two types: proportionate and disproportionate.

Proportionate stratified random sampling The proportion of each stratum in the sample is the same as is present in the population from which the sample is drawn. For example, a population of 4500 nursing students in Punjab can be divided into the

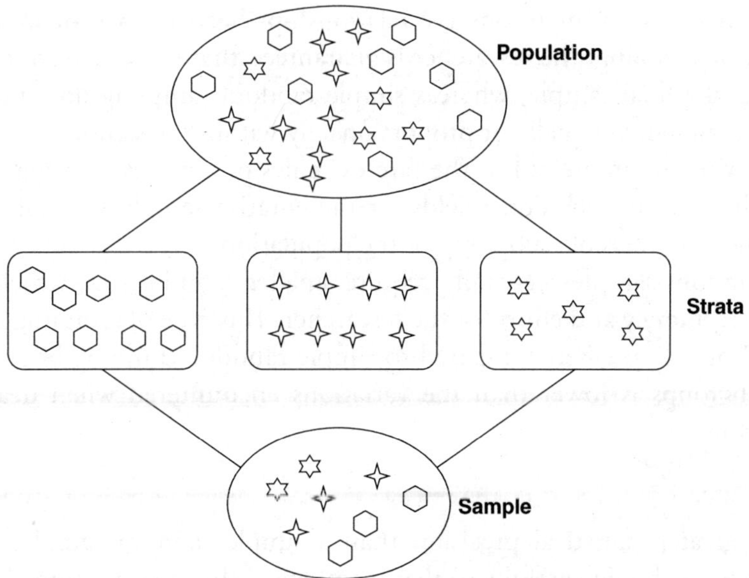

Figure 6.1 Stratified random sampling

following four strata on the basis of the type of nursing education programme in which they are enrolled:

- GNM – 1000
- Post-basic BSc (N) – 1000
- Basic BSc (N) – 2000
- MSc Nursing – 500

The proportion of the strata in the population is: 1000:1000:2000:500 that is 2:2:4:1. Now if the researcher wants a sample of 900 subjects, then she must randomly select 200 GNM students, 200 Post-basic BSc (N) students, 400 Basic BSc (N) students and 100 MSc Nursing students (as per the proportion). This will ensure the same proportion of each stratum in the sample as it exists in the given population, that is, 200:200:400:100 = 2:2:4:1.

Disproportionate stratified random sampling In this case, an equal number of subjects from each stratum is selected randomly. For example, if the researcher wants a sample of 400 subjects, then she can select 100 subjects from the each stratum. This is disproportionate stratified random sampling as it does not take into consideration the proportion of each stratum in the population. The limitation of this methoid is that it may under-/over-represent subgroups in a population.

Need for stratified sampling There are many situations in which researchers would prefer stratified random sampling to other types of sampling. It may be used when the researcher wants to highlight a specific subgroup within the population. Stratified sampling ensures the presence of key subgroups within the sample.

Researchers may also want to observe relationships between two or more subgroups. With this type of sampling, the researcher is guaranteed that subjects from each subgroup are included in the final sample, whereas simple random sampling does not ensure that subgroups are represented equally or proportionately within the sample.

Researchers who are interested in the rare extremes of a population may use stratified random sampling as this technique yields a representative sample that contains even the smallest and most inaccessible subgroup of the population.

Stratified random samples generally require smaller sample sizes, which in turn can save a lot of time, money and effort for the researcher. This type of sampling technique has high statistical precision when compared to simple random sampling because variability within the subgroups is lower than the variations encountered when dealing with an entire population.

Advantages

- It ensures greater statistical precision than a simple random sample, provided the strata have been chosen carefully so that members of the same stratum are as similar as possible in terms of the characteristic of interest (homogeneous stratum).

- It is often more convenient to recruit a stratified sample than a simple random sample.
- It guarantees better coverage of the population than a simple random sample.

Disadvantages

- It can be difficult to identify appropriate strata for a study.
- Advance knowledge about the population is required to divide it into mutually exclusive strata.

Cluster random sampling

This is also known as multistage sampling and is used when researchers want to generate evidence that is generalisable across a population distributed over a large geographic area. In this situation, if the researcher uses a non-probability technique, it is likely to yield an unrepresentative sample, thereby compromising the purpose of the study. Alternatively, the researcher can opt for simple random sampling, which might fulfil the underlying purpose of the study as it generates a representative sample. However, there are practical concerns in this situation that make simple random sampling unsuitable. Cluster sampling is a practical choice to fulfil the study purpose as it yields a representative sample from a population distributed across a large geographic area. In this type of probability sampling, a cluster (i.e., a group of population elements constituting the sampling unit) instead of a single element of the population is selected randomly across the large area.

Consider that a researcher wants to estimate the pulse polio immunisation coverage in Bhopal. She could take a random sample of 500 households. This would require a sampling frame of Bhopal households. If such a list is not available, then the researcher would have to prepare it by conducting a census of the households in Bhopal—an expensive and labour-intensive task.

Alternatively, she could select 10 blocks randomly (say, the city is divided into 200 blocks), and in each block, she could select 10 households randomly. Now, she needs to construct the household listing frame only for 10 blocks, which requires must less time and cost compared to a complete listing of all households in Bhopal. In this example, the blocks are the **primary sampling units** (PSUs) or clusters. The households are **secondary sampling units** (SSUs).

Advantages

- This is a less expensive method.
- It is less time consuming.
- A large geographical area can be covered.

Disadvantages

- The chance of error exists.
- This may be less accurate than a simple random sample.

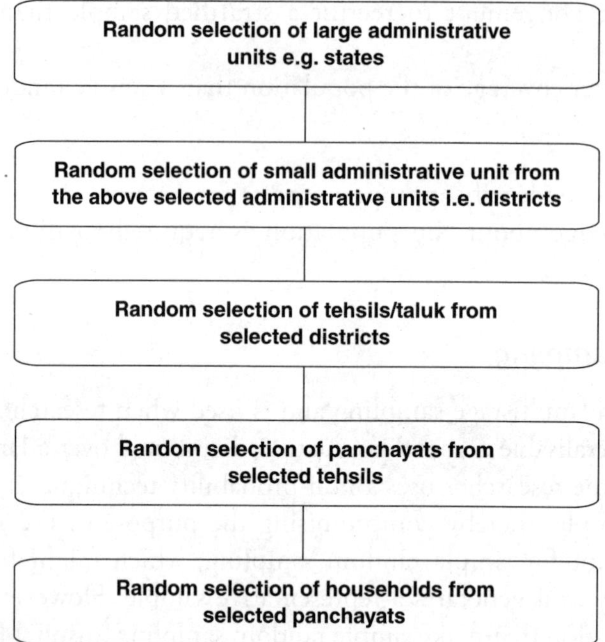

Figure 6.2 Process of cluster random sampling

Systematic random sampling

This is a method of selecting subjects from a larger population in which the first subject is selected randomly from the sampling list; thereafter, a fixed periodic interval (sampling fraction) is chosen and subjects listed at the chosen interval are picked up for the sample. Typically, every k^{th} member is selected from the total population for inclusion in the sample. Systematic random sampling yields a sample that is representative of the population unless certain characteristics of the population are repeated for every k^{th} individual. In order to identify the sampling interval k, the researcher calculates the sample size required. Then, the total number of subjects in the population is divided by the desired sample size to obtain the sampling fraction. The sampling fraction is then used as the constant difference between subjects.

$$\text{Sampling fraction or sampling interval } (k) = \frac{\text{Size of population}}{\text{Sample size}}$$

Steps in systematic random sampling

1. Determine the sample size required for the study.
2. Identify the population size and obtain a sampling frame.
3. Calculate k using the formula given above.

4. Select the first subject from the population list randomly (just place your finger on a table of random numbers).
5. Select every k^{th} person from the list of the population or sampling frame.
6. Move throughout the list in a circular fashion if desired till a sample of the desired size is selected.

For example, if a researcher want to select a random group of 1000 people from a population of 50,000 using systematic sampling, she could simply select every 50th person after selecting the first subject randomly, as here k is 50,000/1000 = 50.

Advantage

- More likely than consecutive sampling to produce a representative sample, if done correctly

Disadvantages

- It is more difficult to execute the sampling plan correctly
- More attention is required for procedural details of the sampling process
- Non-random selection of the first patient will make the sample non-random

Non-probability Sampling Techniques

Non-probability sampling refers to techniques where the sample is assembled in a process that does not give all the individuals in the population an equal chance of being selected. Random sampling is not possible in all settings as most researchers are bound by constraints such as time, money and resources. Hence, it becomes necessary to use other sampling techniques. Non-probability sampling techniques serve as an appropriate alternative when random sampling is not feasible.

Subjects in a non-probability sample are usually selected on the basis of their accessibility or by the personal judgment of the researcher. The drawback of non-probability sampling is that the sample *may or may not* represent the entire population accurately. Therefore, the generalisability of results of the research is compromised.

Non-probability sampling is often used in nursing research because the sampling procedure is much easier, quicker and cheaper than in probability sampling. For undergraduate and postgraduate students, such practicalities often lead to the use of non-probability sampling techniques. However, they are often viewed as inferior to probability sampling because the sampling units are not selected randomly.

Quantitative researchers resort to non-probability sampling techniques only when they are unable to use probability sampling due to some constraints, such as lack of sampling frame. For qualitative researchers, however, non-probability sampling techniques can provide strong theoretical reasons for their choice of units (or cases) to be included in their sample. Here, the goal is not to achieve objectivity in the selection of samples or to make generalisations, but to discover the intricacies of the sample being studied.

The types of non-probability sampling are examined in detail below.

Convenience sampling

Convenience sampling is probably the most common of all sampling techniques used by nurse researchers. Here, the subjects are selected as per the convenience of the researcher or their easy accessibility to the researcher. Subjects are chosen mostly because they are easy to recruit. This technique is considered the easiest, cheapest and least time-consuming. It is, however, least acceptable to serious researchers because the resulting sample may not be representative.

Advantages

- It is easy to recruit the study sample.
- It is cost effective.
- It is less time consuming

Disadvantages

- It may not be representative of the entire population.
- The results are less reliable.
- Generalisability of the study results is limited (low external validity of study results).

Consecutive sampling

It is a strict version of convenience sampling, when the complete accessible population is selected as a study sample. This non-probability sampling technique can be considered as the best of all non-probability samples because it includes all the available subjects; this makes the sample a better representative of the entire population.

Advantage

- It is relatively easy to use

Disadvantage

- Variations in who is selected at different times of the year are possible (for example, in the rainy season, a patient from a rural area may find it difficult to visit the OPD/clinic)

Quota sampling

This is a non-probability sampling technique where the population is first divided into subgroups or quotas, just as the population is divided into strata in stratified sampling. The criteria for dividing the population are pre-decided by the researcher based on the purpose of the study to ensure equal or proportionate representation of subjects. This basis may be gender, occupation, educational status, age, and so on. Subjects are selected **conveniently** (not randomly) from the strata, either proportionally or disproportionally, depending on the study requirements.

Proportional quota sampling is useful when the researcher wants a sample that is the miniature of the entire population, where the main characteristics of interest have the same distribution as in the population. For example, if a population has 40% women and 60% men, and the researcher wants a sample of 100 subjects, using proportionate quota sampling, she should select 40% women and 60% men (same as the population proportion). The researcher must decide the specific characteristics on which she will base the quota. Will it be by gender, age, education race or religion? The advantage of quota sampling is that it provides a better representation of the attributes of interest in the sample.

Non-proportional quota sampling is typically used to ensure that smaller groups are adequately represented in the study sample. Here, the researcher selects an equal number of subjects from each quota to achieve the desired sample size. For example, a researcher wants to study the attitude of nursing students in Punjab towards the profession. The total population (5000 students in Punjab) is divided into two strata, namely, male (200) and female (4800). With proportionate quota sampling, the resulting study sample will not accurately depict an overall picture of the attitude of nursing students because of under-representation of male students. Therefore, in this situation, non-proportional sampling is preferred to ensure better representation of the minority subgroup (male).

Advantages

- Sophisticated skills are not required for sample selection.

Disadvantages

- It does not provide an equal chance to every individual, leading to bias in the sample.

Judgmental/Purposive sampling

Judgmental sampling is more commonly known as purposive sampling. In this type of sampling, subjects are chosen with a specific purpose in mind. The researcher may believe that some subjects are more suitable for research than others. She therefore chooses the sample based on who she thinks would be appropriate for the study. This technique is used primarily when only a limited number of people have expertise in the area being researched. Purposive sampling requires that the researcher have advance knowledge about the population so that she can choose subjects who are knowledgeable about the phenomenon of interest.

Purposive sampling techniques include homogeneous sampling, maximum variation sampling, extreme (or deviant) case sampling, typical case sampling, total population sampling and expert sampling. Each of these techniques has a specific goal, focusing on certain types of sampling elements.

Advantage

- Less field work is required to select the sample.

Disadvantages

- This requires advance knowledge about the population.
- The chance of bias is present.

Snowball/Network sampling In this technique, the initial study participants are asked to suggest someone else who can meet the study criteria and be willing to participate in the study. This is usually done when the population size is very small and the researcher is unable to locate study participants on her own. Therefore, she can ask the initial subjects to identify another potential subject who meets the sampling criteria. The disadvantage of using a snowball sample is that it may not be representative of the population. The first study subject refers a friend; the friend also refers another friend, and so on. Snowball sample is biased because it provides people with greater social connections a higher chance of selection (Berg 2006).

Types

- **Linear snowball sampling:** In this type, each selected subject is asked to provide the reference of one person who is similar to him (Fig. 6.3). This process is like a linear chain and hence is termed linear snowball sampling. This method is appropriate when the desired sample size is small. However, there is a chance that the sample may not be representative of the population as people usually refer those who are in a similar socio-economic status.

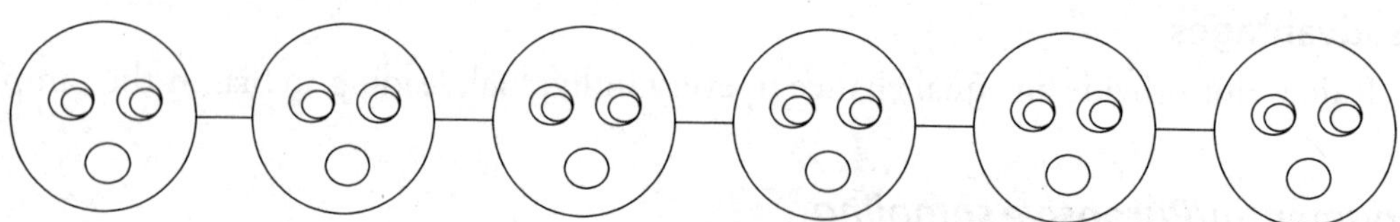

Figure 6.3 Linear snowball sampling

- **Exponential non-discriminative snowball sampling:** Here, the subject initially recruited is asked to provide a reference to at least two similar subjects, and each of them further provides references to two subjects (Fig. 6.4). It is appropriate when the desired sample size is large.
- **Exponential discriminative snowball sampling:** The subject initially recruited is asked to refer two subjects. From these two subjects, reference is sought from only one (Fig. 6.5). It may enhance the representativeness of the sample.

Advantages

- It makes studies in which members of the population are difficult to locate feasible.
- It is especially useful in cases where the subjects/population are hard to locate.

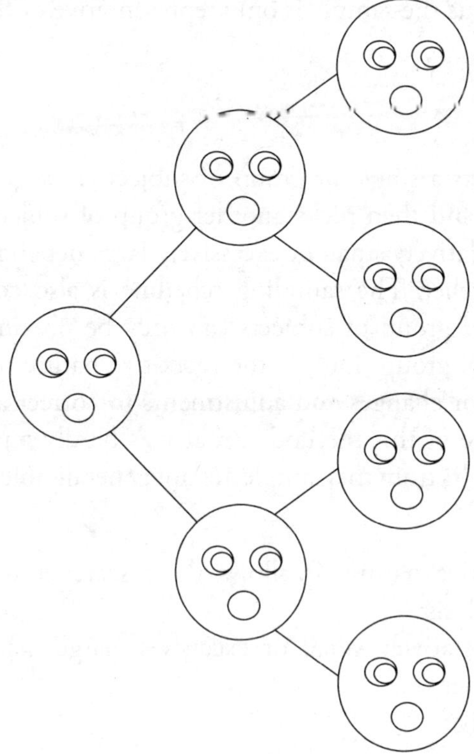

Figure 6.4 Exponential non-discriminative snowball sampling

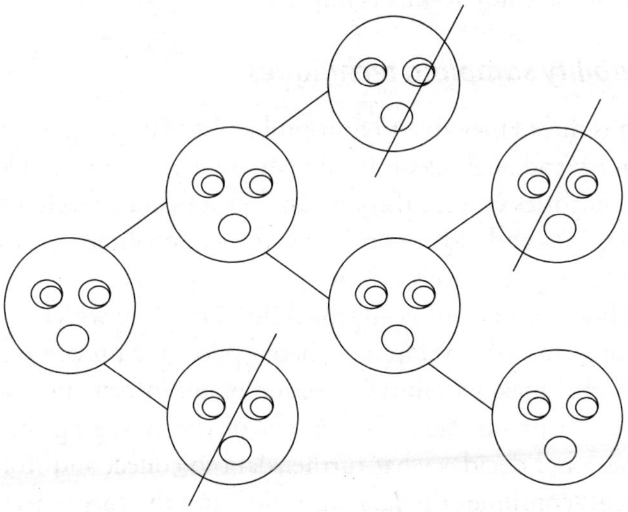

Figure 6.5 Exponential discriminative snowball sampling

Disadvantage

- It is highly prone to sampling bias as the initial subjects tend to nominate people they know well. Therefore, it is possible that the subjects share the same traits and characteristics, and thus the sample is only representative of the small subgroup of the entire population.

Sequential sampling

Here, the researcher selects a single or group of subjects in a given time period, collects data, analyses the results and then picks another group of subjects if needed, and so on. The sample size can be relatively small or excessively large depending on the requirements determined by the researcher. The sampling schedule is also completely dependent on the researcher as a second group of subjects can only be obtained after the experiment is conducted on the initial group. Due to the repetitive nature of this sampling method, it provides scope for minor changes and adjustments to correct and sharpen the research method. The disadvantage of this method is that it is hardly representative of the entire population; therefore, results from this sample are not generalisable to the entire population.

Advantages

- Because of its repetitive nature, it allows the researcher to fine-tune her research methodology and analysis
- Sample size can be relatively small or excessively large depending on the decision making of the researcher
- Not workforce extensive

Disadvantages

- Sequential sampling is hardly representative of the entire population
- Generalisability of the study results is limited

Use of non-probability sampling techniques

Qualitative research is most amenable to non-probability sampling techniques because it is concerned with inquiry and analysis of social phenomena, culture and lived experiences in which themes and categories emerge through analysis of data collected by such techniques as interviews, observations and videotapes. Therefore, in qualitative research, the sample is usually small and is often purposively selected.

Theoretical sampling is a form of non-probability sampling which is used in qualitative research. Here, the objective of developing a theory pilots the process of sampling and data collection. The researcher makes an initial selection of key informants; collects and analyses the data and produces a preliminary explanation of the emerging theory. Based on this explanation, the researcher decides what further data to collect and from whom, to refine the theory. The process continues till data saturation and the theory has evolved fully.

Sample size determination

Determination of sample size is a difficult task for novice researchers. The calculation of number of subjects required so as to obtain significant results involves careful planning and statistical operations. Some important factors that can affect the sample size are discussed in detail.

- **Availability of time**: Data collection time determines the amount of time a researcher has to collect data from the available subjects. If it is short, for example, one month or two months, the researcher must determine how many subjects can be visited for data collection in the given time frame.
- **Availability of resources**: Resources like availability of budget, travelling expenses, stationary and compensation may place restrictions on the sample size.
- **Geographical location**: The researcher must determine whether the study subjects are available in a limited geographic area or if they are distributed over a wide geographic area.
- **Administrative concerns**: Administrative concerns such as the complexity of the design, research deadlines and accessibility to participants can have an impact on the sample size.
- **Nature of the study**: Longitudinal studies may require a small sample size, but for extensive and cross-sectional one-time data collection studies, a larger sample size is expected.
- **Population**: For a homogeneous population, a small sample may suffice. However, with increase in variability in the population, a larger sample is required to represent the population.
- **Effect size**: If the relationship between the independent and dependent variables is strong, then a small sample size would be sufficient.
- **Attrition**: This refers to a condition where people who were initially willing to participate fail to continue participation and leave the study. If the data is collected from multiple points, the possibility of attrition exists. So, the sample size should be selected including the expected rate of attrition.
- **Minimum acceptable level of precision**: This is an important parameter that has a large impact on the sample size requirement. It is also known as margin of error (ME). It expresses the maximum expected difference between the true population parameter and a sample estimate of that parameter. For example, an opinion poll might report that 60% of voters will choose Candidate X. To indicate the quality of the survey result, the opinion poll agency should add that the margin of error is + 5%, with a confidence level of 90%. This means that if the same survey is repeated with different study samples, the true percentage of Candidate X would fall within the margin of error 90% of the time.
- **Sampling method**: This is another important determinant of sample size. Probability sampling usually requires a smaller sample size than convenience sampling.

For example, a researcher is conducting a survey. The sampling method is simple random sampling, without replacement. To choose the right sample size for a simple random sample, the following inputs need to be defined:

- The desired margin of error (also known as measure of precision)
- The level of significance (alpha)
  - In an experimental study for a hypothesis test, alpha is the significance level.
  - For an estimation problem, alpha is: 1 – Confidence level.
- The critical standard score z
  - For a two-tailed hypothesis test or an estimation problem, the critical standard score (z) is the value for which the cumulative probability is 1 – alpha/2. However, for one-tailed hypothesis testing, z is the value for which the cumulative probability is 1 – alpha.
- The size of the population (N). If the population size is very large, it need not be specified.

The smallest sample size can be calculated for mean and proportion sample statistics using the following formula that provides the desired level of precision.

Population size	Sample statistics	Sample size calculation formula
Known	Proportion	$n = [(z^2 * p * q) + \text{ME}^2]/[\text{ME}^2 + z^2 * p * q/N]$
Known	Mean	$n = \{z^2 * \sigma^2 * [N/(N-1)]\}/\{\text{ME}^2 + [z^2 * \sigma^2/(N-1)]\}$
Unknown	Proportion	$n = [(z^2 * p * q) + \text{ME}^2]/(\text{ME}^2)$
Unknown	Mean	$n = (z^2 * \sigma^2)/ME^2$

Sample size determination can be illustrated with the help of the following example.

At the end of every academic year, the State Nursing Council administers a test to a simple random sample from a population of 1000 nursing graduates. Over the past three years, students who took the test correctly answered 60% of the test questions. What sample size is required to achieve a margin of error equal to ±2%, with a confidence level of 95%?

To solve the sample size requirement, the researcher must proceed as follows:

- The specified margin of error is ±2% or 0.02.
- The specified confidence level is 95% or 0.95.
- Compute alpha (1– Confidence level) = 1 – 0.95 = 0.05.
- Determine the critical standard score (z). This is the value for which the cumulative probability is 1 – alpha/2 = 1 – 0.05/2 = 0.975 (this calculation is applicable for an estimation problem). To find the critical standard score, use the normal distribution table for the given cumulative probability. The table shows that the z value is 1.96 for a cumulative probability of 0.975.
- Now, assume that the population proportion p is equal to its past value over the previous three years. That value is 0.60.
- By putting these values in the formula (population known; sample statistics proportion), estimate the required sample size.

$$n = [(z^2 * p * q) + ME^2]/[ME^2 + z^2 * p * q/N]$$

$$n = [(1.96)^2 * 0.60 * 0.4 + 0.0004]/[0.0004 + (1.96)^2 * 0.60 * 0.40/1000]$$

$$n = (0.9219 + 0.0004)/(0.0004 + 0.0009219) = 697.707$$

Therefore, to achieve a margin of error of ±2%, the researcher must survey 698 students, using simple random sampling.

Sample size calculation techniques vary from study to study depending on the type, design, nature and sampling technique of the study. Therefore, novice nurse researchers should consult statistical experts for the same. Nowadays, online software can be used for sample size calculation:

- PS: Power and Sample Size Calculation software
- G* Power
- PASS
- STATA
- Splus
- DSTPLAN
- NQuery Advisor
- PC-Size
- Russ Lenth's Power and Sample Size
- UCLA Calculation Service

Some of these software are free. Interested readers are advised to log on the website of the software to know more about the same.

SAMPLING ERRORS

The use of samples instead of the entire population is necessary for practical reasons. However, with the use of samples, there is a chance that there may be some differences between the sample analysis results and the population analysis results. Sampling error is the difference between the sample statistics used to estimate a population parameter and the actual but unknown value of the parameter (Bunns and Grove 2009). As the sample does not include all the members of the population, sample statistics such as mean and percentage generally differ from parameters on the entire population. For example, if the researcher measures the weight of 1000 individuals from a state of 1 million, the average height of the 1000 people will typically not be the same as the average height of all 1 million. This difference is termed sampling error. If the researcher draws different samples of 1000 subjects from the given population, she will get a different mean height every time. Therefore, errors will exist when population mean is estimated based on the sample statistics. When plotting the mean of different samples on a graph, a normal distribution will emerge, also known as **sampling distribution of mean**. The standard deviation of the sampling distribution of mean is referred to as the **standard error of mean**. However, for practical reasons, it is not feasible to draw many samples from the population and then calculate the mean of each sample to construct the sampling distribution of mean. Statisticians have instead derived a formula for the estimation of the standard error of mean using data from one sample:

$$\text{Standard Error of Mean} = \frac{\text{Standard deviation of the sample}}{\text{Square root of the sample size}}$$

This formula gives an estimate of the standard deviation of the sampling distribution of mean, which is the quantitative measure of sampling error. Therefore, using a large study sample, the sampling error can be reduced. The more individuals or elements the sample includes, the smaller the sampling error.

CHAPTER SUMMARY

- A sample is defined as a subset of the (accessible) population on which the research study is conducted and data is collected.
- Sampling criteria are the list of characteristics of the elements that the researcher has determined beforehand and which serve as eligibility criteria for a subject to become part of the sample.
- Sampling frame is the list of all the subjects of the given population from which a random sample is drawn.
- Scholars consider probability sampling techniques as scientific and superior to non-probability methods as it results in a sample that is representative of the entire population (*although there no guarantee of the same*).
- Simple random sampling technique provides an equal chance to each individual in the population to be selected for the study sample.
- A stratified sample is a probability sampling technique in which the researcher divides the entire population into different subgroups or strata, and then randomly selects the final subjects, either proportionally or disproportionally, from the different strata.
- In proportionate stratified random sampling, the proportion of each stratum in the sample is the same as in the population from which the sample is drawn.
- In disproportionate stratified random sampling, an equal number of subjects is selected from each strata.
- In cluster random sampling, a group of population elements constitutes the sampling unit, instead of a single element of the population.
- Systematic random sampling is a method of selecting subjects from a larger population according to a random starting point and thereafter a fixed periodic interval (sampling

fraction). Typically, every k^{th} member is selected from the total population for inclusion in the sample.

- Non-probability sampling refers to sampling techniques where the sample is assembled in a process that does not give all the individuals in the population an equal chance of being selected.
- With convenience sampling, the subjects are selected as per the convenience of the researcher or their easy accessibility to the researcher.
- Sample size is predetermined in convenience sampling, before sample recruitment. However, in consecutive sampling, all accessible subjects are selected for the study sample.
- Quota sampling is a non-probability sampling technique wherein the population is first divided into subgroups or quotas, just as in stratified sampling. The subjects are selected conveniently (not randomly) from the strata, either proportionally or disproportionally, depending on the study requirements.
- In judgmental or purposive sampling, subjects are chosen by the researcher with a specific purpose in mind.
- Snowball or network sampling is a non-probability sampling process in which the initial study participants are asked to suggest someone else who might meet the study criteria and be willing to take part in the study.
- Sequential sampling is a non-probability sampling technique wherein the researcher selects a single or a group of subjects in a given time period, collects data, analyses the results and then picks another group of subjects if needed, and so on.

EVALUATE YOURSELF

Long Answer Questions

Q1: Define probability and non-probability sampling. List the probability sampling techniques and explain systematic random sampling in detail.

Q2: What are the characteristics of a good sample? Explain the factors influencing sampling.

Q3: Explain the need for a sample. Describe the characteristics of a good sample.

Q4: Describe the types of non-probability sampling techniques.

Q5: Elaborate the factors that affect sample size.

Q6: What inputs are required to calculate sample size for a study? Explain in detail with examples.

Short Answer Questions

Q1: Write short notes incorporating relevant examples on the following:

1. Accessible population
2. Target population
3. Sampling frame
4. Sequential sampling method
5. Consecutive sampling
6. Quota sampling
7. Stratified sampling
8. Simple random sampling
9. Snowball sampling
10. Systematic sampling
11. Sampling error

Q2: Suppose you are selecting every fourth person passing a subway; determine which type of sampling technique this is, if the population is defined as:
1. people passing the subway,
2. people residing near the subway.

Multiple Choice Questions

Q1: Which of the following is a probability sampling technique?
(a) Sequential sampling
(b) Consecutive sampling
(c) Purposive sampling
(d) Stratified random sampling

Q2: In systematic sampling, every k^{th} subject is selected from the sampling frame; however, the first subject is selected by:
(a) Convenience
(b) Reference
(c) Random
(d) Any of the above

Q3: Quota sampling is a type of:
(a) Simple random sampling
(b) Probability sampling
(c) Non-probability sampling
(d) Consecutive sampling

Q4: Sampling error is:
(a) Error in estimation of population parameters by sample data
(b) Error in estimation of sample statistics by population parameters
(c) Error in the sampling process
(d) None of the above

Q5: Snowball sampling is used when:
(a) Researcher is conducting a study in hilly areas
(b) Researcher is unable to locate participants
(c) Participants are distributed in large geographical areas
(d) Researcher has less experience in conducting study

Q6: Which of the following probability sampling methods is appropriate when the population is distributed over a large geographical area?
(a) Consecutive random sampling
(b) Cluster random sampling
(c) Stratified random sampling
(d) Sequential sampling

Q7: Which technique of snowball sampling is appropriate for recruiting a large sample?
(a) Simple linear sampling

(b) Exponential non-discriminative sampling
(c) Exponential discriminative sampling
(d) All of the above

Answers

1. d **2.** c **3.** c **4.** a **5.** b **6.** b **7.** b

FURTHER READING

Babbie E. 2001. *The Practice of Social Research, 9th ed.* Wadsworth Thomson, Belmont, CA.

Berg S. 2006. Snowball Sampling–I, pp 7817–7821. In: *Encyclopedia of Statistical Sciences*, S Kotz, C Read, N Balakrishnan, B Vidakovic (eds). John Wiley and Sons, Inc., Hoboken, NJ.

Castillo JJ. 2009. Stratified Sampling Method. Experiment Resources. (https://explorable.com/stratified-sampling), accessed in March 2012.

Determining Sample Size – University of Florida. (http://edis.ifas.ufl.edu/pd006), accessed on April 24, 2013.

Lunsford TR, Lunsford BR. 1995. Research Forum: The Research Sample, Part I: Sampling. *JPO* 7(3):105–112.

PASS – NCSS software. (http://www.ncss.com/pass.html), accessed on April 24, 2013.

Polit DF, Tatano BC. 2008. *Nursing Research, 8th ed.* Lippincott Williams and Wilkins Publications, pp 340–341, 348–353.

Sampling bias – Scholarpedia. (http://www.scholarpedia.org/article/Sampling_bias), accessed on April 26, 2013.

Sampling bias – Wikipedia. (http://en.wikipedia.org/wiki/Sampling_bias), accessed on April 24, 2013.

Sampling in Research – Schatz. (http://www.socialresearchmethods.net/tutorial/Mugo/tutorial.html), accessed on April 24, 2013.

7 Data Collection Tools and Techniques

Chapter overview

- Introduction to data collection
- Data—what, from whom, when and where to collect
- Data collection methods and instruments
  - Methods of data collection
  - Data collection process
  - Questionnaire
  - Interview
  - Observation
  - Rating scales
  - Likert scale
  - Guttmann scale
  - Visual analogue scale
  - Vignettes
  - Q-sorts
  - Bio-physiological methods
  - Validity and reliability of the instrument
  - Pilot study
  - Data collection procedure

INTRODUCTION TO DATA COLLECTION

Data collection is the process of gathering and measuring information on variables of interest in a systematic way to answer the research questions and test hypotheses. High-quality data is essential for maintaining the integrity of the research study. Therefore, reliable and valid data collection tools must be selected to reduce the chance of errors.

The data collection process is labour-intensive, involving longs hours of work in the research setting, interacting with study participants and gathering the required information from them. Therefore, the researcher should plan for systematic data collection by answering the following initial questions:

- What data is needed for the study?
- From whom should the data be collected?
- When should the data be collected?
- How should the data be collected?

Qualitative data collection, as compared to quantitative methods, is open-ended, with fewer structured protocols (open-ended interviews, unstructured observation). Regardless of the type of data involved, data collection in a qualitative study is more labour-intensive and takes a great deal of time.

DEVELOPING THE DATA COLLECTION PLAN

The data collection plan identifies the type of data needed for the study and helps the researcher select or develop the tools for data collection. If a standardised instrument is to be used, then permission must be sought from the author of the tool. The researcher must pilot-test the developed tools before administering them for final data collection. Data collection forms and procedures should be established before the researcher moves to the research setting for data collection. The researcher should also determine the sequence in which the tools should be administered.

Data collection tools may vary from one study to another. However, questionnaires, interviews, observations and bio-physiological methods are the common data collection tools used in quantitative nursing research.

Questionnaires

This is a paper-and-pencil instrument widely used for data collection in nursing research. A questionnaire is a list of questions used to gather the required information from the study subject. It is a pre-planned set of questions designed to yield specific information about the feelings, beliefs, attitudes and opinions of the study sample. It has been used extensively in nursing research to measure key variable of interest, for example, anxiety, quality of life, excessive daytime sleepiness and many others. It is easy to administer to a large number of people and saves the researcher time and money. The responses of the participants are kept anonymous; this gives them the liberty to be truthful while responding to questions about controversial issues. While developing questions, ambiguities should be reduced to the minimum. The layout of the questionnaire should also be planned according to the analysis plan of the study.

Characteristics of a good questionnaire

- A good questionnaire should be as brief as possible; however, it should be long enough to obtain the essential data.
- It should be attractive in appearance and neatly arranged.
- Instructions should be clear and complete.
- Each question should deal with a single idea.
- Questions should be clearly worded.
- There should not be suggestions for the desired response.
- Questions should be presented in psychological order—from the general to the specific.
- Questions of intimate nature should be placed at the end of the questionnaire.

Guidelines for constructing and administering questionnaires

- Identify the **construct/concept** to be captured using the questionnaire.
- Review the **pertinent literature** to identify the key areas about which questions should be developed.
- Frame **semi-structured/structured questions** involving a close choice for the participant.
- The stem of the question should be in **clear, simple language** and should not be unnecessarily lengthy.
- **Negative wording** should be clearly contrasted in the stem by using underline or bold italic fonts.
- **Double-negative statements** should be avoided in the stem of the question.
- All alternatives should be **grammatically consistent** with the stem of the test item.
- Carefully **avoid verbal clues** that might enable participants to select the correct answer or eliminate an incorrect alternative.
- **Avoid similarity of wording** in both the stem and the correct answer.
- Make the **distracters similar** to the correct answer in both length and complexity of wording.
- Avoid the use of **alternatives** such as 'All of the above' or 'None of the above'.
- Make sure that each question is **independent** of the other items and does not provide leading answers.
- The wording of the statement in true–false items should be **highly precise** so that it can be judged as unequivocally true or false.
- Avoid the following types of questions:
  - *The double question:* The wording of such questions makes them difficult to understand and answer accurately. The question may contain two or more unrelated parts, or the parts may be contradictory; for example, 'Would you agree that it is not unlikely that our next Chief Minister will not be a woman?'.
  - *The wrong choice question:* 'Is your eye yellow, purple or green?'. This type of question discourages the participants from attempting the next question.

- *The 'fuzzy word' question:* Fuzzy words like 'rarely', 'occasionally' and 'often' can result in meaningless answers.
- *Jargon questions:* Jargon refers to technical words that may have one meaning to the professionals in that field and another, or none, to the public. Therefore, it is always better to avoid jargon. For example, 'defibrillator' is a technical word that is not likely to be understood by a student of Class 10 in India; therefore, this should be replaced with '*electrical shock-producing machine*'.
- *Leading questions:* 'Why do you think nurses are good at maintaining ethical principles?'. This question leads the respondent to answer based on the assumption that nurses are ethical practitioners.

- The **covering letter** should explain the purpose of the study and the procedure to maintain the confidentiality of the responses. The due date by which the questionnaire should be returned must be mentioned.
- The **layout and design** should be attractive and appealing. Questions should be arranged in logical sequence. Instructions should be provided at the beginning of the questionnaire in bold font. Questions of an intimate nature should be presented towards the end of the questionnaire.
- Use a sample from the target population to **pilot-test** the questionnaire to know the reaction of the participants. Revise and retest the questionnaire if required.
- Prepare a **follow-up letter** and, with a copy of the questionnaire, send it to those who have not responded. Stress the importance of the study and the contribution the respondent can make.

Methods of questionnaire administration

Web-based questionnaire The researcher can send the questionnaire as a soft copy using the internet or by electronic mail to the potential study participant, along with instructions and other information related to the study. This is a method frequently used in market research. Nurses can also use this technique to reach participants around the world. The disadvantages of this method include the exclusion of people who do not have a computer or are unable to access one. Also, the validity of such a questionnaire survey is in doubt, as people may complete it in a hurry or may not give an accurate response.

Mail questionnaire Mail questionnaires are mailed in printed form to the respondents whose names and addresses have already been obtained by the researcher. A covering letter is attached to the questionnaire to explain the purpose of the study, emphasising how valuable the respondent's completion of the questionnaire is to the study. A self-addressed and stamped envelope for return of the questionnaire is also included. The advantage of mail questionnaire is that respondents may be more frank and honest on sensitive issues. Also, it is free from interviewer bias. Certain segments of the population may be reached more readily by mail. It provides enough time for the respondents to think about their responses.

The main disadvantages are:

- Low response rates—the subjects may not return the filled-in questionnaire.
- Sequence of questions cannot be controlled.
- Probing and clarification about any doubt is not possible.
- Proxy response—someone else may have responded to the questionnaire on behalf of the targetted participants.

Self-administered questionnaire This is presented to the respondents by the researcher or by someone in an official position. The purpose of the questionnaire is explained, and then the respondents are left alone to complete the questionnaire. This method assures a high response rate, accurate sampling and provision of explanations if required.

Advantages of questionnaires

- Less expensive
- Less time is involved in data collection
- Can be administered to large groups
- Respondents can attempt the questionnaire at their own pace and convenience
- Provides liberty to participants to answer questions out of order and in several sessions

Disadvantages of questionnaires

- The researcher cannot probe deeply into the beliefs and attitudes of the participants
- Modifications to questions cannot be made once the questionnaire has been distributed

Interviews

This is a conversation between two or more persons in which questions are asked by the interviewer to explore the views, experiences, beliefs and/or motivations of the interviewee. It is a direct face-to-face attempt to obtain reliable and valid data in the form of verbal responses from respondents. Channel and Kahn (1968) defined interview as, "A two-person conversation initiated by the interviewer for the specific purpose of obtaining research-relevant information, and focused by him on content specified by the research objectives of systematic description, prediction, or explanation".

In quantitative research, interviews are more structured—the researcher asks a standard set of questions and nothing more. Qualitative interviews, however, are unstructured, enabling the researcher to probe as and when required to fully understand the phenomena of interest. Unstructured interviews are therefore appropriate when little is known about the study phenomenon or when detailed insights are required from participants.

Types of interviews

Structured interview This refers to **verbally administered questionnaires** where the sequence and wording of the questions are pre-determined by means of a schedule and the interviewer is not allowed to make any changes. There is no scope for follow-up questions to responses that require further explanation. The questions and protocols are organised well in advance and, therefore, it is relatively quick and easy to administer. However, as mentioned earlier, it is of little use for seeking in-depth information about the phenomenon of interest. The drawback of the structured interview is that it rigidly follows procedures and does not allow the researcher to probe. However, this rigidity provides an opportunity for the researcher to execute it in different modes, for example, face-to-face, by telephone/videophone and over the internet.

Face-to-face interviews offer the distinct advantage of enabling the researcher to establish rapport with the potential participants and gain their cooperation. These interviews yield the highest response rates in survey research. It also allows the researcher to clarify ambiguous answers and seek follow-up information, if required. It offers control over the sequence of questions and there is no systematic exclusion of illiterate or physically handicapped people. However, structured interviews are expensive and time-consuming. The presence of the interviewer may lead to a biased response (social desirability bias) from the participant; similarly, the age, race or gender of the interviewer may introduce bias into the study.

Telephone interviews are less time-consuming and less expensive than to face-to-face interview. It offers an opportunity to access anyone who has a telephone and to avoid the interviewer bias. However, the response rate is not as high as in face-to-face interviews, but it is considerably higher than with the mailed questionnaire. Telephone interview can cause bias in sampling as people without phones are excluded from the study.

Semi-structured interview These, unlike structured interviews, consist of several key questions that help the interviewer define the areas to be explored. It also allows the interviewer or interviewee to diverge in order to pursue an idea or response in more detail. The interviewer can probe to yield meaningful information whenever it is required. This flexibility allows for the elaboration of information that is important to participants but which may not have been thought of as pertinent by the research team.

Unstructured interviews These are more flexible and provide the freedom to ask questions. The questions to be asked in the interview are derived from the research questions; however, the content, sequence and wording are left entirely to the interviewer. The interview may simply start with an opening general question such as 'Can you tell me about your experience of tsunami?' and then progress based on the initial response. The interviewer can probe the initial answers and follow up unexpected clues, and thus redirect the inquiry in a more fruitful way. This is usually time-consuming (often lasting several hours), but is a useful data collection strategy when significant depth is required in data or when virtually nothing or little is known about the phenomenon under investigation.

Unstructured interviews can, however, generate data that is difficult to quantify and so testing and verifying of hypotheses cannot be undertaken.

General instructions to conduct a successful research interview

- The **setting** for the interview should be calm and quiet. It should be free from distractions and mutually agreed upon by the interviewee and the interviewer. It may be a home, restaurant, etc.
- The **time** of the interview should be pre-decided by the interviewer and the interviewee.
- **Questions** are either developed in advance (structured interview) or during the interview (unstructured interview). An interviewer needs to be able to think fast on her feet to conduct an unstructured interview.
- The interviewer should list the **material required** for the interview and keep it in a carry bag. It may include the interview schedule (questionnaire), pen, pencil, stationery items (for structured interview) and pictures, newspaper cuttings, artefacts for the unstructured interview. A tape-recorder, if required, should be checked to ensure that it is in proper working condition.
- The interview schedule should be **pilot-tested** on several respondents prior to data collection to check if the schedule is clear and understandable to the participants, if it will yield reasonably unbiased data and if any changes to the schedule are required. Sometimes, after pilot-testing, questions may need to be rephrased or procedures revised. Opening statements and methods of recording responses need to be evaluated to ensure that rapport is maintained with the interviewee.
- Some rules should be observed while **conducting the interview.** Dress properly, greet the interviewee and introduce yourself to establish an appropriate level of rapport and gain trust when sensitive topics are being discussed. Switch on the tape-recorder. Explain the purpose of the study and present questions in the pre-decided order (structured interview) in language that can be understood by the interviewee or start with broad general questions (unstructured interview) and probe as the interview advances. Be an active listener, observe the non-verbal cues, and do not interrupt the respondent unnecessarily. Clarify if the response appears to be vague; clarify and probe if required (unstructured interview). Tape-recording provides a more accurate record of the interview. However, it may inhibit the response. Computer software can also be used to record responses.

Conducting a research interview

Arrival process: Introductions, background noise checks, greetings and getting to know each other, setting up of audiotape/recording equipment and settling down.

Introducing the study

- Explain the purpose of the interview/study.

- Explain why the interviewee has been chosen for the study.
- State the time duration of the interview.

Informed consent

- Use the subject/patient information sheet to explain about the study.
- Explain how the information will be kept confidential and the responses anonymous.
- Explain why a tape-recorder is required.
- Obtain written/documented oral consent.

Conducting the interview: The interview should be gradual, unhurried and relaxing. The protocols for conducting structured, semi-structured and unstructured interview are as follows:

- **Structured interview:** Ask the pre-planned questions in the predefined order.
- **Semi-structured interview:** Ensure that you have pre-planned questions to ask; however, also allow questions to flow naturally based on the response provided. Do not be rigid about asking specific questions in the specific order. In fact, the flow of the conversation dictates the questions to be asked/omitted and the order of the questions.
- **Unstructured interview:** This requires preplanning of general questions to be asked at the outset of the interview. Thereafter, as the conversation advances, questions are put up by the interviewer as per the situation in order to obtain in-depth information. The interviewer must be competent to frame relevant questions while listening to the participant.

During the interview process, the interviewer should

- Make the interviewee comfortable
- Appear interested in what the interviewee is saying
- Use appropriate non-verbal behaviour and keep personal feelings and opinions on hold
- Observe body and facial gestures, pauses, silence and laughter
- Use probing questions as and when required; for example, 'Could you explain it further?'
- Seek clarity and a deeper understanding from the respondent throughout the interview (unstructured interview)
- Not push the pace unnecessarily, or 'put words into the participant's mouth'
- Transit smoothly from one topic to the other
- Close the interview with thanks

Advantages of interviews

- Opportunity to clarify questions whenever required
- Data can be collected from young children and from illiterate persons
- The verbal and non-verbal behaviour of the participant can be observed

- Sequence and pace of the questions can be controlled
- Opportunity to probe

Disadvantages of interviews

- More expensive than the questionnaire method
- Time-consuming
- Cannot provide anonymity for the respondent

Interviews v/s Questionnaires

- **Cost:** Interviews are more expensive to conduct than questionnaires. Travelling and existence expenses are also incurred for interviews.
- **Time:** Interviews require a great deal of time for information collection. However, questionnaires require less than 30 minutes, preferably 15–20 minutes, to complete.
- **Bias:** Interviews are prone to more bias than questionnaires because of the interviewer factor. Studies have also shown that race, religion, age and social class can be potential sources of bias in an interview.
- **Anonymity:** Anonymity is one of the features sought in questionnaires. The anonymous mailed questionnaires provide a greater portion of socially unacceptable responses than face-to-face interviews.
- **Response rate:** The mailed questionnaire tends to have a considerably lower response rate than the face-to-face interview. The refusal rate for personal interviews is typically much smaller than the non-response rate for postal questionnaires.

Observations

Whenever it is not possible to collect data using paper-and-pencil instruments or through interviews, the researcher must look for other ways to collect the information required for the study. Observation is a method of data collection that comprises observing/watching behaviour, events or physical characteristics in their natural setting. Some events/behaviour can be observed directly; however, sometimes it is also possible to observe them indirectly. When interactions, processes or behaviour are watched as they occur, it is **direct observation**. When the results of interactions, processes or behaviour are watched, it is **indirect observation**. For example, to study whether a new food is acceptable to students or not, the researcher can observe the amount of food left on the plate by the students.

Observations can also be overt or covert. **Overt observation** is when study participants know that they are being observed by the researcher; in **covert observation**, on the other hand, the study participants are not aware that they are being observed by the researcher. The researcher/observer is concealed and observes the participants without informing them. Covert observation is required when it is expected that the subjects will not behave naturally if they know that they are being observed (Hawthorne effect). The benefit is that people are more likely to behave naturally if they do not know they are being observed.

Research situations where observation can be used as an important data collection instrument are given below:

- **To study an ongoing process or situation**, for example, how the nurses communicate with the patients in the Emergency Room in the morning shift.
- **To study individual behaviour or interactions between people**, for example, to study how people living in a slum area interact on health-related issues.
- **To study a physical setting**, for example, whether a classroom or training facility is conducive to learning.
- **When the study subjects cannot provide data through questionnaires or interviews**

Planning for observation

This is essential for the success of an observation. The researcher must make decisions about the following:

- **What is to be observed?**: The researcher must determine the focus for observation. For example, she may want to know how well BLS skills training is being implemented in the nursing college. Here, her focus area may be BLS skills observation among students.
- **Who is to be observed?**: The researcher must determine the individual/groups she intends to observe and also whether the study subjects will be observed individually or in groups.
- **When to observe?**: The researcher must determine the time when the event/process/ interaction will be observed and also the frequency with which the event/process/ interaction happens in the population.
- **Where to observe?**: The researcher must decide the location/setting where the participants will be observed to collect the required information; for example, in the ward, ICU or classroom. It is the place where the desired behaviour/event/process takes place naturally.
- **How to observe?**: The researcher must determine the nature of the observation, whether it will be direct or indirect, overt or covert. They must also decide the number of observers required for the study. It is critical that the observers are well trained in data collection to ensure high-quality and consistent data. The researcher must also consider whether a camera will be used to record the event/process or if she will observe through the senses.
- **How to collect data?**: Observation data can be collected in three ways. Recording sheet and checklist are the most standardised ways. The observation guide lists the interactions, processes or behaviour to be observed with space to record open-ended narrative data. Field notes are open-ended narrative data that can be written or dictated to a tape-recorder.

Advantages of observation

- Observation does not rely on people's willingness or ability to provide information.
- It permits the researcher to directly see what people do rather than relying on what they say.

Disadvantages of observation

- Observer bias may affect the quality of data collected.
- It is susceptible to the Hawthorne effect (people usually perform better when they know they are being observed) and therefore the data collected may not depict the truth.
- It is expensive and time-consuming.

Participation observation

This is an important data collection strategy in phenomenology, ground theory, ethnography and other qualitative designs. It is a labour-intensive task in which the researcher is immersed in a variety of activities over an extended period of time. This enables her to observe cultural members in their daily lives, to participate in their activities as a full-time resident/member and to fully grasp the cultural behaviour and activities. Living in the context facilitates prolonged engagement and is one of the activities listed by Lincoln and Guba (1994) to establish trustworthiness. Bernard (1994) defines participant observation as, "The process of establishing rapport within a community and learning to act in such a way as to blend into the community so that its members will act naturally, then removing oneself from the setting or community to immerse oneself in the data to understand what is going on and be able to write about it". It enables the researcher to describe existing situations using the five senses, providing a 'written photograph' of the situation under study. Researchers can observe events/processes/interactions that informants may be unable or unwilling to share and observe situations that informants have described in unstructured interviews (data triangulation) to identify and clarify the inaccuracies in description. Therefore, it is a way to increase the validity of the study as it helps the researcher obtain a better understanding of the context and phenomenon under study. As the researcher serves as the instrument for data collection, she must understand how her gender, ethnicity, class and theoretical approach may affect observation, analysis and interpretation.

The novice researcher is required to practice reflexivity at the beginning of research to understand the biases she has that may interfere with the correct interpretation of what is observed. Gold (1958) has provided a description of observer stances in qualitative research:

- **Complete participant**: The researcher conceals her role from the group to avoid disrupting normal activity.
- **Participant as observer**: The researcher is a member of the group being studied, and the group is aware of the research activity.
- **The observer as participant**: The researcher participates in group activities as desired, yet the main role is to collect data, and the group being studied is aware of the researcher's observation activities.
- **Complete observer**: The researcher is completely hidden from view while observing and the participants being studied are unaware of being observed.

Participating observation is undertaken using the following process:

Gaining entry and establishing rapport This determines the success of data collection in any qualitative study using unstructured interview or observation. To assist in gaining permission from the community to conduct the study, the researcher may bring letters of introduction, utilise her affiliation and funding sources or request the gatekeepers, i.e., Sarpanch, Mukhiya, Headmaster, Principal. Personal contacts with key informants can be used to ease entry into the research field. Agar (1980) suggests that the researcher be cautious about accepting the first people she encounters in the research setting as key informants, as these people may be 'professional stranger handlers'. Key informants must be people who are respected by other participants and who are viewed as neutral.

'Hanging out' is the process by which the researcher gains trust and establishes rapport with participants (Bernard 1994). It involves meeting and conversing with people to develop relationships over an extended period of time. The researcher must speak the language of the people under study. Fluency in the native language helps gain access to sensitive information and increases rapport with participants. In an ethnography study, it is common for the researcher to live in the culture under study for extended periods of time and to return home for short breaks, and then return to the research setting for more data collection. When the researcher lives in a culture that is different from her own, she will constantly be bombarded by new stimuli, which may result in culture shock. Therefore, the researcher must take a break from the constant observation.

Once the researcher has gained entry into the field, she must decide what she should observe to fulfil the study purpose. Dewalt and Dewalt (2002) suggest that the researcher first study what is happening and why it is happening; sort out the regular from the irregular activities and search for variations to view the event in its entirety from a variety of viewpoints. She should check for negative cases and when behaviour matches the theoretical purpose of the observation, seek similar opportunities and plan systematic observations of those events/behaviour.

Taylor et al. and Merriam and Dewalt et al. have provided several tips for conducting observations:

- Be low profile in dress and actions.
- Become familiar with the research field/setting.
- Initially focus on a single activity/interaction and then return to a view of the overall situation.
- Explore the keywords in people's conversations.
- During breaks, mentally replay remarks and scenes that have been observed.
- Actively observe the interactions—who talks to whom, whose opinions are respected, how decisions are made. Try to remember as many verbatim conversations, non-verbal expressions and gestures as possible.
- Note-taking and writing-up practices are the critical part of fieldwork; therefore, make it part of the daily routine to keep the entries up to date.
- Field notes should include specifics such as day, date and time, along with a simple coding system for keeping track of entries. Field notes may include records of what is

observed, including informal conversations with participants, records of activities and journal notes kept on a daily basis.

Observation checklist/structured observation

This is a two-dimensional tool used to assess and record the presence or absence of behaviour or traits or activities when some incident has occurred. Development of a checklist requires a category system that involves listing the behaviour that the observer is intended to observe and record. A decision has to be made by the evaluator regarding the exhaustiveness of the phenomenon and the number of categories to be included in the checklist. The checklist does not rate the frequency or extent of the behaviour or trait.

Advantages of checklists

- Adaptable to most subject matter that is observable
- Can evaluate learning activities in relation to procedure, process, personal trait or characteristics

Limitations of checklists

- Determines only presence or absence of an action, behaviour or trait
- Provides no means of determining the extent to which a behaviour or trait is possessed by the student

The following is an example of a checklist.

Table 7.1 Checklist for oral medications

Steps	Yes	No
Wash hands		
Recall safety measures		
Locate the drug, read the label on the bottle and see that it is the right medicine and shake the bottle		
Collect medicine in the container		
Measure liquids accurately with a minim glass and read the lower level of the meniscus		
Pour liquid from side opposite the label, wipe the mouth of the bottle, recap the bottle.		
Take the tablet/capsule in a spoon or medicine cup		
Identify the patient with the patient chart		
Explain the procedure		
Place patient's towel under the chin		
Position the patient comfortably in upright sitting position		

(*continued*)

Continued

Steps	Yes	No
Administer each drug separately followed by water		
Record the drug given, details of the dose, route, date, time, signature, omissions, etc.		
Clean and replace the articles		

Note: Please tick (✓) the appropriate column for each step

Rating scale

As mentioned above, checklists cannot quantify the extent or frequency of observed behaviour. Here, a rating scale is a useful tool which eliminates this limitation of the checklist. It is a device that facilitates the appraisal of a number of traits or characteristics in reference to a common qualitative scale of values. It provides the scope of quantification of the judgment in relation to an observed behaviour of the subject. A rating scale may have 5–7 points of rating in the form of abstract labels (quantitative) along with their description. For example A, B, C, D, E or 5, 4, 3, 2, 1.

Qualitative form:
Superior – 5
Above average – 4
Average – 3
Poor – 2
Very poor – 1

Sometime, frequency labels like Always, Usually, Frequently, Sometimes and Never can be used depending on the trait to be rated. These abstract labels are assigned a numerical value to quantify the frequency and extent of the observed behaviour.

Bondy (1983) developed a criterion reference rating scale in which there were five levels of competency:

- Independent
- Supervised
- Assisted
- Marginal
- Dependent

Types of rating scales

Descriptive rating scale: This provides a list of descriptive phrases for each trait. The rater selects the one most applicable to the student and records her selection, usually by means of a (✓) mark.

Sample of descriptive rating scale

Rating item	3 Dependent	2 Independent	1 Partly independent
Behaviour			
Problem-solving skill			
Physical examination			
History taking			

Independent: Student is able to handle it on her own; *Partly independent:* Student is able to solve simple problems; *Dependent:* Student needs help in solving complex problems. Withdraws from it and needs counselling and guidance. Total score range = 4–12

Interpretation of the score obtained by a particular student: 10–12: Superior; 7–9: Above average; 4–6: Average, needs improvement

Numeric rating scale: The rater assigns a code number (which refers to a descriptive phrase) to each trait of the person being rated. Code numbers are assigned to the descriptive phrases, arranged in order of degree or level with which they indicate possession or lack of occurrence of each trait.

Sample of numerical rating scale

Behaviour	Excellent	Very good	Fair	Poor	Very poor
	5	4	3	2	1
1. Able to identify the priority needs of patients.					
2. Communication with the patient.					
3. Evaluation of interventions.					

Total score range: 3–15

Interpretation of the total score obtained by the student: 13–15 Excellent; 10–12 Very good; 9–11 Fair; 6–8 Poor; 3–5 Very poor

Graphic rating scale: This has descriptive phrases printed horizontally at various points (underneath as a straight line across the page). The rater indicates the performer's standing for each trait by placing a check mark at an appropriate point along the line.

Sample graphic rating scale for assessment of workshop

Instructions: Place a tick mark (✓) on the line at the point which best describes the person.

Sloppy worker	Frequently makes mistakes	Occasionally does fine work	Excellent worker
1	2	3	4
Careless about use of equipment.	Careless in use and handling of equipment.	Needs help looking after equipment at times.	Takes cares of equipment in a professional manner. Ensures patient's safety and comfort.

1 and 2 – Needs constant supervision; 3 – Needs guidance; 4 – No need for supervision

Likert scale

Named after its inventor, Rensis Likert (1932), this is a psychometric scale commonly used in survey research and to evaluate the attitude of nursing students towards a controversial issue or phenomenon of interest. It is a bipolar scaling method measuring either positive or negative response to a statement. It consists of Likert items that are statements about which the respondent is asked to rate their level of agreement or disagreement. An individual's score on a particular scale is the sum of her ratings on all the items. This score reflects the respondent's overall attitude towards the issue in question. Dividing the total score by the number of items, the mean attitude score is calculated.

Usually, a Likert scale is a symmetric scale because there are equal numbers of positive and negative statements. Often five ordered response levels are used, though many psychometricians advocate using seven or nine levels because the former may produce slightly higher mean scores relative to the highest possible attainable.

The format of a typical five-point Likert scale is:

1. Strongly disagree
2. Disagree
3. Neither agree nor disagree
4. Agree
5. Strongly agree

Likert scales may be subject to distortion from several causes. There may be *central tendency bias* in which respondents may avoid using extreme response categories (strongly agree or strongly disagree), *social desirability bias* in which respondent try to portray themselves as socially desired and *acquiescence bias* which includes selecting items as they are presented. Designing a scale with balanced keying (an equal number of positive and negative statements) can obviate the problem of acquiescence bias, as acquiescence on positively keyed items will balance acquiescence on negatively keyed items, but central tendency and social desirability are somewhat more problematic issues associated with the Likert scale.

Constructing items for the Likert scale A large pool of potential items on the particular topic is prepared with the help of experts in the field.

Guidelines for writing statements

- The statements should be brief.
- Each statement should convey one complete thought.
- The statement should belong to the attitude variable that is to be measured.
- The statements should cover the entire range of the affective scale of interest.
- Statements should be such that they can be endorsed or rejected (agree/disagree).
- Acceptance and rejection should indicate something about the attitude measured.
- Care should be taken about the language of the statements:
  - Avoid double negatives
  - Avoid All, Always, None and Never
  - Use with care – Only, Just, Merely
  - Avoid words with more than one meaning

How to improve the Likert scale A group of judges is asked to score the statements. The item scores given by the judges are summed. Inter-correlations between the paired items are calculated. Those items that have low correlation with the summed scores are eliminated. The average score is calculated based on the top quarter and lowest quarter provided by the judges and a t-test is carried out on the mean between the two. Questions with low t-values, which indicate that they have low discriminating power, are eliminated.

Given below is an example of a five-point Likert scale to measure the attitude of high school students towards BLS techniques.

Item	Response					Score
	SA	A	?	SD	D	
Basic Life Support should be learnt voluntarily by every citizen of the country.						
If you encounter a person lying unresponsive, you will immediately start Basic Life Support.						
It is harmful to administer mouth-to-mouth breathing with barrier devices.						

(continued)

Continued

Item	Response					Score
	SA	A	?	SD	D	
It is better to start chest compression, instead of no cardiopulmonary resuscitation, if you don't have barrier devices with you for mouth-to-mouth ventilation.						
The government should install automatic external defibrillators at all public places so that the number of out-of-hospital deaths due to cardiac arrest can be prevented.						
Basic Life Support should be included in school curricula of secondary school students.						
Learning Basic Life Support is not useful until we have a nationwide uniform emergency medical service (EMS) number.						
Fear from legal actions can hinder your performing Basic Life Support.						
Basic Life Support should be given by a professional only.						
Basic Life Support training for school children should be adequate to prepare them for providing Basic Life Support.						

SA = Strongly Agree; A = Agree; SD = Strongly disagree; D = Disagree; ? = Uncertain

Reliability of the Likert scale The Likert scale measures are at the ordinal level of measurement because responses indicate a ranking only. As the numbers of scaling points are increased from 2 to 20, there is rapid increase in reliability but it tends to level off at about 7, and after 11 points there is little gain in the reliability of the scale (Nunally 1978).

Guttman scale

Guttman scaling is a method of scale construction developed by Louis Guttman in 1940. A typical Guttman scale includes a series of items or statements tapping progressively higher levels of a single attribute. In this attitude scale, the items are ordered from low to high according to their difficulty level so that approval of any specific item in the list implies approval of all items prior to that item.

Visual analog scale

This is a widely used psychometric response scale to measure subjective characteristics (sensations/feelings) or attitudes along a continuum that cannot be easily measured directly. For example, the amount of pain that a person feels ranges across a continuum from none to very severe. From the patient's perspective, this scale appears continuous and their pain does not take discrete categories such as none, mild, moderate and severe. Participants are required to specify their level of agreement to a statement by indicating a position along a continuous line between two end-points. It consists of 100-mm-long lines, the starting point and the end of which is marked, with the extreme of the dimension being measured; for example, best–worst. Between these two extreme ends, the respondent provides her response for the phenomenon measured, which is later measured using a ruler from the left side. The continuous (or analogue) aspect of the scale differentiates it from discrete scales such as the Likert scale, allowing a wider range of statistical methods for data analysis. It is used to measure the intensity of certain subjective sensations and feelings such as pain, anxiety, discomfort, quality of sleep, level of alertness, functional ability and attitude towards certain issues. There is evidence that visual analogue scales have superior metrical characteristics than discrete scales; thus a wider range of statistical methods can be applied to these measurements.

The patient marks on the line the point that they feel represents their feelings/perception of their current situation. The VAS score is determined by measuring in millimetres from the left-hand end of the line to the point that the patient marks.

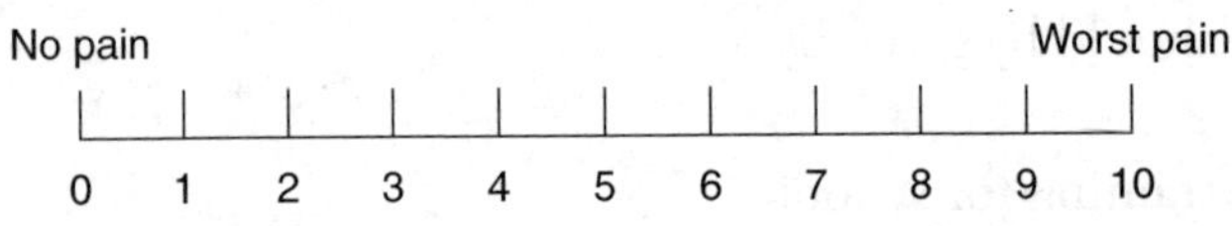

Figure 7.1 Visual analogue scale

Advantages of VAS

- Highly subjective sensations and feelings can be measured reliably through VAS.
- The quantitative assessment of highly subjective phenomenon is possible by this scale.

Disadvantages VAS

- This scale cannot be used for making comparisons across a group of individuals at the same time.
- In measuring pain, the scale does not afford the patient opportunity to record increases in pain, thereby creating bias in the study in favour of treatment.

Osgood's semantic differential scale

This is another scale used to measure attitude. This scale has bipolar adjectives used to measure the reaction of participants to the issue in question. The overall attitude score is obtained by summing across the individual items in the questionnaire submitted by each respondent. Dividing the total score by the number of adjectives, the mean score is obtained.

Sample of semantic differential scale

Assessment of final year students regarding their attitude towards patients

Positive adjectives	7	6	5	4	3	2	1	Negative adjectives
Communicative								Non-communicative
Polite								Rude
Considerate								Callous
Pleasant								Unpleasant
Respectful								Disrespecting
Friendly								Insincere

Vignettes

Vignettes have been used quantitatively to study attitudes, perceptions and beliefs. Vignettes are simulations of real events that can be used in research studies to elicit the subject's knowledge, attitudes or opinions based on their statements about how they would behave in the hypothetical situation depicted. Participants are presented with a hypothetical scenario and characters. Enough context and information is also provided for participants to have an understanding of the scenario being depicted, but needs to be vague in ways that compel participants to 'fill in' details. They can be asked about how a character should ideally act and/or how they would realistically act. 'Should' questions focus participants' attention on the moral dimensions of situations and 'would' questions on the pragmatic. Use of vignettes enables the researcher to collect information simultaneously from a large numbers of subjects, to manipulate a number of variables at once in a manner that would not be possible in observation studies. Vignettes are useful for studying potentially sensitive topics as it is less threatening for participants to respond to a hypothetical scenario than being directly asked about their experiences or views. It can also be useful if participants lack direct personal experience and knowledge about a topic.

Designing a vignette

The process of designing a vignette is very similar to that of designing a story completion task. However, vignettes are more directive than story completion tasks.

- The scenario and characters should be meaningful to the participant group. Contextual detail along with character names using authentic language makes a vignette vivid.
- Write the scenario from the point of view of characters.
- Decide to what extent you want to direct participants to focus on particular issues and how much freedom you want to allow them while 'filling in' the details. This will determine the information you provide in the vignette, and the questions you ask.
- You can use a single vignette or one presented in stages. A stage usually involves a major plot for character development. However, using more than four stages has the potential to confuse participants.

- Determine whether you want to direct participants to focus on the moral aspects of a situation and/or the pragmatic. This affects your use of 'should' versus 'would' questions.

In quantitative vignette research, the gap between vignettes and 'reality' is of great concern, because vignettes are used to measure and predict people's responses to real-life situations (Hughes 1998). However, qualitative vignette research explores people's perceptions and understanding around the issue.

Vignette data can be analysed through thematic analysis, grounded theory and pattern-based discourse analysis.

Projective Techniques

Projective techniques are the use of vague, ambiguous, unstructured stimulus objects or situations in which the subject 'projects' his or her personality, attitude and opinions to give the situation some structure. Instead of questioning them directly about a third party or an object, the subjects project their covert feelings on to the third party or object. It is a useful method of research to unearth feelings, beliefs, attitudes and motivation which many subjects find difficult to articulate and to 'break the ice' in focus-group discussions.

Design and structure of projective technique

The more ambiguous the stimulus, the more the subjects will project their emotions, motives, attitudes and values. The Thematic Apperception Test is an interesting projective technique which requires the participant to view a photograph or drawn picture. The participant must then explain what the person in the photo is feeling or thinking. The projective techniques can be categorised into the following types as per the response required by the subjects.

- *Association:* The subjects are presented with a stimulus and they are asked to respond by speaking out the first word or thought elicited by the stimulus. It helps determine what underlying thoughts occur when someone reflects on an image, figure or idea.
- *Construction:* The subject is given a stimulus concept and asked to construct a story or a picture. It presents the opinions of other people's actions, feelings or attitudes.
- *Completion:* It requires the participant to finish an incomplete sentence, story or conversation. The response of the participant provides insight into the thoughts of the participant.
- *Expressive:* A subject is asked to role-play, act, draw or paint a specific concept or situation. The researcher should focus on the manner in which the subject constructs something rather than on what it represents.
- *Choice ordering:* The subjects are asked to rank order or categorise the given product or services on the basis of certain factors.

Data analysis in quantitative projective research involves the classification of the content/ data into categories that are then given numerical values. Thus, data is tabulated in quantitative form. Whereas in qualitative projective technique, the description and explanation of the projections by the subjects form the database, which then requires ordering and interpretation.

Q Sorts

Q sort research aims to systematically study subjectivity, for example, a person's view point, opinion, beliefs and attitude. *Q-set* is the set of statements about the topic of interest presented to the participants (also known as *P-set*). They are asked to rank-order the statements about some topic according to some preference or feeling about them. These rankings are then subject to factor analysis. If significant clusters of correlation exist, they could be factorised and described as common view points. Q sort is a small sample study of human subjectivity based on sorting of the Q-set of unknown reliability. Results from Q methodological studies have often been criticised for their validity and hence the possibility for generalisation.

Brown (1993) has outlined the following steps for performing a Q methodological study:

Definition of the concourse: This is the raw material for the Q sort. According to Brown (1993), concourse is referred to as the flow of communicability surrounding any topic in ordinary conversation. All possible statements that the respondents can make about the subject at hand are collected. It may consist of self-referential statements through interviewing people, statements derived through participant observation, newspapers, magazines, research papers, etc.

Development of the Q-set: A subset of statements is selected from the concourse, called the Q-set. It often consists of 40–50 statements. The selected statements should be widely different from one another to enhance the representativeness of Q sort. The statements are edited wherever necessary and are randomly assigned a number. The statement and the corresponding number are printed on a separate card known as the Q deck.

Selection of the P-set: This is a non-random small sample of participants who are believed to be theoretically relevant to the problem under consideration.

Q sorting: The participants are asked to rank order the Q deck as per their point of view regarding the topic. The respondent is instructed to sort the statements into three piles:

- Statements he generally agrees with
- Statements he generally disagrees with
- Statements he is generally neutral or doubtful about

Thereafter, the respondent is asked to rank-order the statements and place them in the score sheet provided. The score sheet is a continuum ranging from 'Most disagree' at one end to 'Most agree' at the other end; in between is a distribution that usually takes the form of a quasi-normal distribution.

Bio-physiological Methods

Bio-physiological data collection measures can be used alone or in combination with other methods. They involve the collection of data related to the bio-physiological mechanism of a person with or without using a specialised instrument. Specific technical instruments and equipment may be required to measure the physiological and biological/physical variables such as temperature, blood pressure and oxygen saturation. However, physiological activity or dysfunction can be observed directly. For example, phenomena such pallor, redness, vomiting, cyanosis, edema and wound status can be observed directly without any equipment.

Nursing research typically involves testing of nursing interventions to improve the clinical outcomes of patients in terms of physiological variables such as blood pressure, edema, oxygen saturation, pulse and cyanosis. Also, the nurse, as a part of the healthcare team, is in a good position to easily access the equipment used to record these measures, such as sphygmomanometer, thermometer and pulse oxymeter. Therefore, bio-physiological measures have a distinct place in healthcare research and study the basic physiological process, physiological outcome of nursing care and effect of nursing interventions.

Bio-physiological measures can be classified into two categories: in vivo methods and in vitro methods. **In vivo methods** are performed directly on the subject. For example, temperature, pulse and respiration are in vivo methods. Whereas, measurements performed outside the subject, such as serum sodium level, blood urea nitrogen and blood sugar level are known as **in vitro bio-physiological measures**. The collection of in vivo measures requires a technical set-up that has six components, as shown in Fig. 7.2.

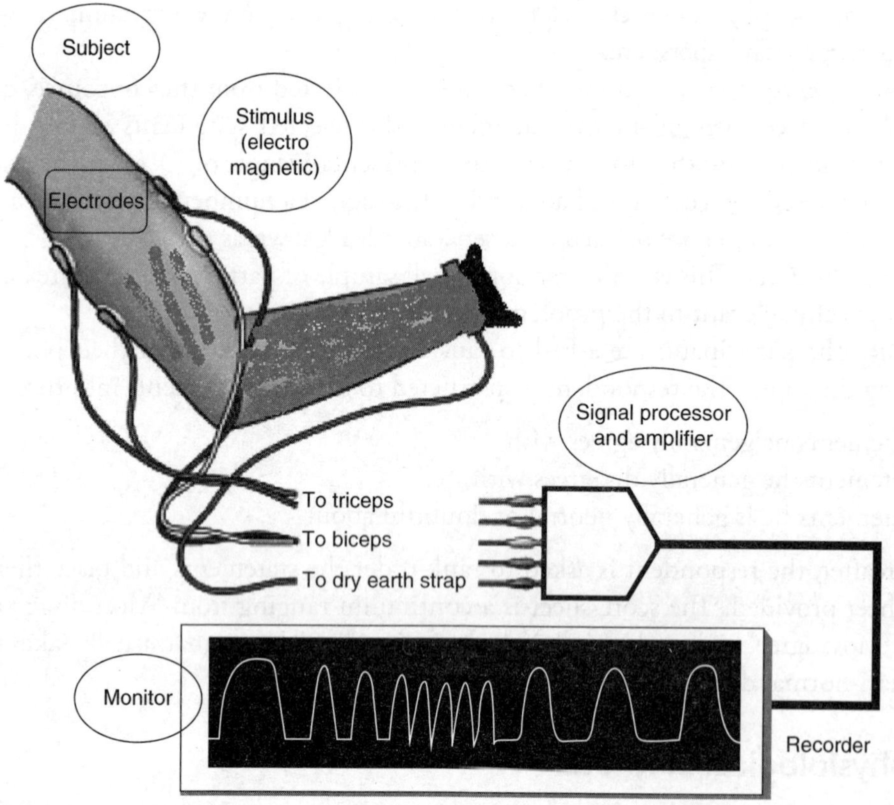

Figure. 7.2 Components used for the collection of in vivo measures

Similarly, various techniques are used to collect in vitro measures:

- Radiological: CT scan, X ray, magnetic resonance imaging (MRI), PET scan
- Biochemical: Blood sugar, blood urea, serum sodium, serum calcium
- Microbiological: Culture test, sensitivity test
- Cytological: Fine needle aspiration cytology, exfoliative cytology

Advantages of bio-physiological methods

- Provides more reliable and valid data
- More objective in nature—no subjective bias

Disadvantages of bio-physiological methods

- Some of the bio-physiological measures may have harmful effects on the subjects, such as X ray, and therefore may pose an ethical dilemma about whether to use them
- Instruments used to measure bio-physiological data may be expensive, such as PET scan and MRI
- Use of instrument/equipment may require training of operators
- Environmental interference in the measurement system may cause error in the data produced

Validity and reliability of the instrument

Validity Validity refers to how well a test measures what it supposed to measure. For example, if an anxiety test measures anxiety and not other closely related concepts, then it can be said to be a valid tool for anxiety measurement. However, how can it be determined whether a particular test measures the concept of interest? For this, the types of validity and how to ascertain the validity of a test must be studied.

- *Face validity* refers to whether the test appears to be assessing the intended construct. Experts ascertain the face validity of a test by looking at the overall appearance of the test items. It is noteworthy that it is not a scientific type of validity; however, it is an important indicator of the validity of a test. For example, the researcher may be able to determine if a person is stressed/ happy just by looking at the face of the individual.
- *Construct validity* is one of the main types of validity along with content and criterion validity. It is used to ensure that the test actually measures the intended construct of interest and not any other. Construct is deliberately invented by the researcher to conceptualise a variable under study. A panel of experts familiar with the construct is given the test to assess the construct validity. The experts can examine the items and decide what that specific item is intended to measure.

  Multi-trait multi-method matrix (MTMM) as described by Campbell and Fiske is an important method to ascertain construct validity. Here, the newly designed test's score is correlated with other tests that are known to be closely related to the intended construct. Construct validity cannot be determined in a single study. Rather, it is a continuous process that involves evaluation, re-evaluation, refinement and development. It checks for convergence and discriminability of the intended test with the other methods of measurement of the same construct. Convergence refers to whether the test to measure the intended construct yields similar results with other methods of measurement of the same construct. Discriminability refers to the ability to differentiate the construct from other related but conceptually distinct constructs.

- *Criterion-related validity* is used to predict the future or concurrent performance of a test. It is further classified in two subtypes: concurrent and predictive validity. The test results are correlated with another concurrent or future criterion of interest. For example, if a nursing program designed a test to assess cumulative student learning throughout the four-year BSc Nursing degree course. The new test/measure could be correlated with a standardised future measure of ability in this discipline, such as an NCLEX-RN test. The higher the correlation between the established measure (NCLEX-RN) and the new test, the more predictive validity the new tool will have to assess cumulative student learning.
- *Content validity* ensures that the designed measure covers a broad range of content within the concept under study. As it is not possible to cover everything, selected items need to be sampled from all the domains of the topic. A panel of experts will then judge whether the sample items represent the entire domain on a particular topic of interest. For example, when designing an assessment of knowledge on Basic Life Support, it will not be useful to include only chest compression and respiration-related items. Other areas such as airway, choking and drowning should be included So that the assessment should reflect the content area in its entirety.

Reliability The reliability of a data collection instrument refers to the degree to which it produces stable and consistent results. Many ways can be used to determine the reliability of the measures.

- *Test–retest reliability* is a type of reliability used to evaluate a test for the stability of its scores over a period of time. If the variable measured by the instrument is liable to change over a period of time (time effect), then this method cannot be used to determine the reliability of the test. It is ascertained by administering the same test twice over a period of time to a group of individuals. The test scores at Time 1 and Time 2 are correlated to evaluate the test for stability over time. The greater the correlation coefficient, the more reliable the test. However, a correlation coefficient of 0.7 or more is considered acceptable for most tests. For example, reliability of the BLS knowledge questionnaire can be established by the test–retest method as follows:

Subject no.	Test score X	Retest score Y
1	6	7
2	7	7
3	8	9

(*Continued*)

Continued

Subject no.	Test score X	Retest score Y
4	5	6
5	7	7
6	10	10
7	9	8
8	8	8
9	6	6
10	5	6
	$r = 0.92$	

Formula for calculating correlation coefficient:

$$r_{xy} = \frac{\Sigma(X - \bar{X})(Y - \bar{Y})}{\sqrt{[\Sigma(X - \bar{X})^2][\Sigma(Y - \bar{Y})^2]}}$$

where r_{xy} = Correlation coefficient for variables x and y

X and Y = Individual score on variables x and y

$\bar{X}$ and $\bar{Y}$ = Mean score for variables x and y

- *Internal consistency reliability* is the measure of reliability used to assess the degree to which different test items that investigate the same construct of interest produce similar results. Split-half is one way to assess internal consistency reliability. Here, the test items intended to probe the same area of knowledge are split into two sets (odd number items and even number items). The test is then administered to a group of subjects and the total score for each set is computed. Split-half reliability is obtained by determining the correlation between the two scores of the two sets of test items. Thereafter, the Spearman–Brown prophecy formula is applied to calculate the split-half reliability coefficient.

  For example, the split-half reliability of 25 items in the BLS Knowledge Questionnaire is given below.

Subject number	Total score	Odd number items total score	Even number items total score
1	9	4	5
2	6	3	3
3	9	5	4

(*Continued*)

Continued

Subject number	Total score	Odd number items total score	Even number items total score
4	8	4	4
5	4	2	2
6	3	1	2
7	11	6	5
8	8	4	4
9	7	3	4
10	9	5	4
		$r = 0.849$	

Spearman–Brown prophecy formula

$$r^* = \frac{2r}{1} + r$$

$$= \frac{(2) \times (0.849)}{1} + 0.849$$

$$= \frac{1.698}{1.849}$$

$$= 0.918$$

The Spearman–Brown prophecy formula provides an estimate of the internal consistency of a test. It does this by splitting the test items into two halves. However, it underestimates the reliability as there are so many ways of dividing the test items into two halves. Cronbach's alpha is a measure that calculates the correlation coefficient for all possible half-splits of test items. Therefore, it is considered superior to the split-half method for estimation of internal consistency of a test. Coefficient alpha or Cronbach's alpha is calculated using the following formula:

$$r = \frac{k}{k-1}\left[1 - \frac{\Sigma\sigma_1^2}{\sigma_y^2}\right]$$

where:

r = Estimated reliability

k = Total number of test items

$\Sigma\sigma_1^2$ = Sum of variance of individual test item

σ_γ^2 = Variance of total test scores

Inter-rater reliability is a measure of the reliability of an observation checklist. Observer bias is an important concern when using checklist as a data collection tool. Therefore, the inter-rater reliability of the checklist must be assessed where two or more observers watch the event simultaneously and record their observation on the checklist as per the instructions. It is used to assess the degree to which different observers agree in their observation decisions. It is especially useful when judgments can be considered relatively subjective. The formula to calculate inter-rater reliability (index of equivalence) for a checklist is given below.

Index of equivalence = Number of agreement/number of agreements + Disagreements

$$= \frac{9}{10} = 0.9$$

The other methods to estimate inter-rater reliability are Cohen's Kappa, Fleiss's Kappa ANOVA, Pearson product–moment correlation coefficient, Spearman's rank correlation coefficient, intraclass correlation and Krippendorff's Alpha.

Inter-rater reliability is another measure of reliability for observation checklist. It is useful to examine the degree to which the single observer agrees in his observation decision by observing the same event twice. The formula to calculate index of equivalence for intra-rater reliability is the same as given above.

Specificity and sensitivity are two important measures for diagnostic tests. For the estimation of sensitivity and specificity, the test result is compared with the gold standard test. A gold standard test is one which is 100% accurate in identifying a disease.

Sensitivity refers to the extent to which the test diagnoses the condition positively. It can be calculated using this simple formula:

$$\text{Sensitivity of a test} = \frac{\text{Number of cases identified positive by the test}}{\text{Total number of cases in the population}}$$

For example, **Modified Berlin Questionnaire** is a sleep questionnaire to identify patients with obstructed sleep apnea. It consists of three categories and 12 items. The original Berlin Questionnaire was modified by Dr SK Sharma et al. at AIIMS, New Delhi, India for the Indian setting. Its sensitivity is 86%; this means that if it is administered to 100 patients diagnosed with obstructed sleep apnea, the questionnaire will declare only 86 patients to be positive for the condition.

Specificity refers to the ability of a test measure to exclude the condition when it is not present. In other words, it is the ability to exclude those who are negative for the condition/disease. It can be calculated using the formula

$$\text{Specificity} = \frac{\text{Total number of negative cases identified by the test}}{\text{Total number of healthy people in the population}}$$

For example, the specificity of the Modified Berlin Questionnaire is 95%. This means that if it is administered to 100 healthy individuals, it will diagnose 95 of them as negative for obstructed sleep apnea.

A false positive case is one that has been identified as positive by the test measure, but which is actually negative for the disease. It is termed a type I error in diagnostics tests. Similarly, a false negative case is one that has been identified as negative for the disease but is in fact positive for the given disease. It is termed a type II error in diagnostics tests.

A test measure with high sensitivity has low type II error; similarly, a test measure with high specificity has low type I error. Therefore, the researcher must find a balance between sensitivity and specificity.

Pilot Study

A pilot study is a small-scale trial run undertaken before embarking on the main study to identify unforeseen obstacles in the execution of the actual study plan. The purpose of the pilot study is to test intervention protocols, data collection strategies and sample recruitment procedures in order to be prepared for the main trial. It is also known as a feasibility study as it assesses the overall feasibility of the trial. Expensive interventions or experiments can be tested through pilot study to determine whether they are promising and acceptable to the participants. It can provide useful data for sample size determination and the modifications required in the overall plan of the main study (sampling strategy, intervention protocols, data collection instruments, data collection plan, plan of data analysis). It will not test the hypothesis; however, the term pilot study has been misused by scholars as a reason for not using a larger sample for their study.

Data Collection Procedure

It is a standardised plan that is followed consistently with every study subject to collect empirical data to fulfil the study purpose. For example, an experimental study to assess the effectiveness of BLS training among school children in selected schools of Ludhiana, Punjab, specified the data collection procedure as follows:

1. Written permission for data collection was obtained from Principal, DMCH College of Nursing and the principals of the selected schools.
2. The school selection was randomised by tossing a coin for the control and experiment groups.
3. Students of Class 9, who fulfilled the inclusion criteria and were willing to participate in the study, were included.
4. Written informed assent was obtained from the students after explaining the nature, aims and purpose of the study to them.
5. The students were administered the English version of the assessment tools in the following order:
   (a) *In the experiment group:* Before intervention, the students were given a structured knowledge questionnaire and the attitude scale. The investigator filled the observation checklist by observing the student's performance on the dummy. Post-intervention, after seven days, the students were given Part II of the knowledge questionnaire and the investigator filled the observation checklist by observing the student's performance on the dummy. Post-intervention, after 30 days, the students were again given Part II of the knowledge questionnaire and the investigator filled the observation checklist by observing the student's performance on the dummy. Post-intervention, after 60 days, the students were given Part II of the knowledge questionnaire and attitude scale. The investigator filled the observation checklist by observing the student's performance on the dummy.
   (b) *In the control group:* The same protocol was followed but the students in this group were not given intervention.
6. Students filled the structured knowledge questionnaire and attitude scale in the classroom in the presence of the investigator. During this, they were called one by one for height and weight measurement. Height was measured using a non-elastic inch tape mounted on the wall. Similarly, weight was measured by a spring balance weighing machine. The same machine was used throughout the study. Skill was assessed in a separate room using the dummy. The students were asked to perform two cycles of cardiopulmonary resuscitation. The investigator observed the student's performance and filled the observation checklist.

CHAPTER SUMMARY

- Data collection is the process of gathering and measuring information on selected variables of interest, in a systematic way to answer the research questions and test hypotheses.
- Data collection plan identifies the type of data requried for the study and selects or develops the tools for data collection.
- Questionnaire is a list of questions used to gather the required information from the study subjects.

- The researcher can send the questionnaire as a soft copy using the internet or by electronic mail to the potential study participant.
- Mail questionnaires are mailed in printed form to the respondents whose names and addresses have already obtained by the researcher.
- Interview is a direct face-to-face attempt to obtain reliable and valid data in the form of verbal responses from respondents.
- Structured interview refers to verbally administered questionnaires in which the sequence and wording of the questions are pre-determined by means of a schedule and the interviewer is not allowed to make any changes.
- Semi-structured interviews consist of several key questions that help the interviewer define the areas to be explored.
- Unstructured interviews are more flexible and provide the freedom to ask questions.
- The interview schedule should be pilot-tested on several respondents prior to data collection to ensure that the schedule is clear and can be understood by the participants.
- Mail survey (questionnaire) tends to have a considerably lower response rate than the face-to-face interview.
- Observation is a method of data collection through observing/watching behaviour, events or physical characteristics in their natural setting.
- When interactions, processes or behaviour are watched as they occur, it is direct observation. When the results of interactions, processes or behaviour are watched, it is indirect observation.
- Overt observation is when study participants know that they are being observed by the researcher; in covert observation, the study participants are not aware that they are under observation by the researcher.
- Bernard (1994) defines participant observation as, "The process of establishing rapport within a community and learning to act in such a way as to blend into the community so that its members will act naturally, then removing oneself from the setting or community to immerse oneself in the data to understand what is going on and be able to write about it".
- Gaining entry and establishing rapport determine the success of data collection in any qualitative study using unstructured interview or observation.
- Hanging out is the process of meeting and conversing with people to develop relationships over an extended period of time.
- Observation checklist is a two-dimensional tool used to assess and record the presence or absence of a behaviour, trait or activity when the incident occurred.
- Rating scale is a device that facilitates appraisal of a number of traits or characteristics in reference to a common qualitative scale of values. It enables quantification of the judgment in relation to an observed behaviour of the subject.
- Likert scale is a psychometric scale commonly used in survey research. It is a bipolar scaling method that measures either a positive or a negative response to a statement.
- Likert scales may be subject to distortion from several causes, i.e., central tendency bias, social desirability bias and acquiescence bias.

- Guttman scale includes a series of items or statements tapping progressively higher levels of a single attribute.
- Visual analogue scale is a psychometric response scale widely used to measure subjective characteristics (sensations/feelings) or attitude along a continuum that cannot be easily measured directly.
- Osgood's semantic differential scale has bipolar adjectives used to measure the reaction of participants to the issue in question.
- Vignettes are simulations of real events that can be used in research studies to elicit the subject's knowledge, attitudes or opinions according to how they state they would behave in the hypothetical situation depicted.
- Projective techniques are the use of vague, ambiguous, unstructured stimulus objects or situations in which the subject projects his or her personality, attitude and opinions to give the situation some structure.
- Bio-physiological measures involve the collection of data related to the bio-physiological mechanism of a person with or without using a specialised instrument.
- Validity refers to how well a test measures what it is supposed to measure.
- Reliability of a data collection instrument refers to the degree to which it produces stable and consistent results.

EVALUATE YOURSELF

Long Answer Questions

Q1: How will you proceed for data collection in a qualitative study? Explain in detail.

Q2: How will you validate a structured interview?

Q3: How will you establish the reliability of a checklist?

Q4: What are projective techniques? Explain with examples.

Q5: How will prepare a questionnaire for data collection? Explain various techniques of administration of questionnaires.

Q6: Define observation. What are the types of observations? Explain in detail.

Q7: What are the types of research interviews used for data collection? How will you proceed for a structured interview? Discuss in detail.

Q8: Define validity. Explain the types of validity of a data collection instrument with examples.

Q9: What do you mean by reliability? Explain split-half reliability with a suitable example.

Q10: What is sensitivity and specificity? Discuss with relevant examples.

Short Answer Questions

Write short notes on:

1. Questionnaire method of data collection
2. Reliability
3. Validity
4. Participant observation
5. Likert scale
6. Q sort
7. Vignette
8. Unstructured interview
9. Structured Interview
10. Advantages of self-administered questionnaire
11. Bio-physiologic method of data collection
12. Criterion validity
13. Construct validity

Multiple Choice Questions

Q1: The validity of a data collection tool refers to the:
(a) Extent to which it measures what it is supposed to measure
(b) Stability of scores over a period of time
(c) Validity of the source of the tool
(d) All of the above

Q2: The reliability of an instrument refers to:
(a) Validity of the scores yielded by the instrument in relation to other similar measures
(b) The degree to which it produces stable and consistent results
(c) Both a and b
(d) None of the above

Q3: The scores of nursing undergraduates for a final college test is highly correlated with scores on the all-India postgraduate entrance examination. Which type of validity does the college test possess?
(a) Content validity (b) Construct validity
(c) Criterion validity (d) All of the above

Q4:
(a) The extent to which the test diagnoses the condition positively
(b) The extent to which the test diagnoses the condition negatively
(c) The extent to which the test diagnoses the condition neutrally
(d) None of the above

Q5:

(a) The extent to which the test diagnoses the condition positively
(b) The extent to which the test diagnoses the condition negatively
(c) The extent to which the test diagnoses the condition neutrally
(d) None of the above

Q6: Predictive validity is a type of:

(a) Content validity (b) Construct validity
(c) Criterion validity (d) Concurrent validity

Q7: Test retest reliability is not used for a test when

(a) Test scores are liable to change over a period of time
(b) Test scores are not liable to change over a period of time
(c) It is administered to literate participants
(d) It is administered to illiterate participants

Q8: Method to estimate inter-rater reliability is:

(a) Cohen's kappa (b) Fleiss's kappa
(c) Krippendorff's alpha (d) All of the above

Q9: The appropriate method/s of assessing the reliability of the Likert scale is/are:

(a) Test retest method (b) Split-half method
(c) Inter-rater method (d) Both a and b

Q10: The appropriate method(s) of assessing the reliability of a knowledge questionnaire is (are):

(a) Test retest method (b) Split-half method
(c) Inter-rater method (d) Both a and b

Answers

1. a **2.** b **3.** c **4.** a **5.** b
6. c **7.** a **8.** d **9.** d **10.** d

FURTHER READING

Adler PA, Adler P. 1994. Observation techniques. In: *Handbook of qualitative research,* NK Denzin, YS Lincoln (eds). Sage Publications, Thousand Oaks, CA. pp. 377–392.
Barchak LJ. 2003. Who performs the Q sort? *Operant Subjectivity* 26(2): 72–122.
Barter C, Renold E. 2000. 'I wanna tell you a story': Exploring the application of vignettes in qualitative research with children and young people. *International Journal of Social Research Methodology* 3(4): 307–323.

Britten N. 2999. Qualitative interviews in healthcare. In: *Qualitative research in health care, 2nd ed,* Pope C, Mays N (eds). BMJ Books, London. pp. 11–19.

Brown SR. 1978. The importance of factors in Q methodology: Statistical and theoretical considerations. *Operant Subjectivity* 1(4): 117–124.

Brown SR. 1986. Q technique and method: Principles and procedures. In: *New tools for social scientists,* Berry WD, Lewis-Beck MS (eds), Sage Publications, Beverly Hills.

Brown SR. 2002. Q technique and questionnaires. *Operant Subjectivity* 26(2): 117–126.

Campbell DT. 1959. Convergent and discriminant validation by the multitrait-multimethod matrix. *Psychological Bulletin* 56: 81–105.

DeWalt KM, DeWalt BR. 2002. *Participant observation: A guide for fieldworkers.* AltaMira Press, Walnut Creek, CA.

Diliman DA, Sinclair MD, Clark JR. 1993. Effects of Questionnaire Length, Respondent-Friendly Design, and Difficult Question on Response Rates for Occupant-Addressed Census Mail Surveys, *Public Opinion Quarterly* 57: 289–304.

Fine GA. 2003. Towards a peopled ethnography developing theory from group life. *Ethnography* 4(1): 41–60.

Foddy W. 1994. Constructing Questions for Interviews and Questionnaires *Public Opinion Quarterly* 58: 639–642.

Fontana A, Frey JH. 1994. Interviewing: The Art of Science. In: *Handbook of Qualitative Research,* NK Denzin, YS Lincoln (eds), Sage Publications, London.

Gans HJ. 1999. Participant observation in the era of ethnography. *Journal of Contemporary Ethnography* 28(5): 540–548.

Hammersley M, Atkinson P. 1995. *Ethnography: Principles in practice, 2nd ed.* Routledge, London.

Kaldenberg DO, Koenig HF, Becker BW. 1994. Mail Survey Response Rate Patterns in Population of the Elderly, *Public Opinion Quarterly* 58: 68–76.

Kitzinger J. 1994. The methodology of focus groups: The importance of interaction between research participants. *Sociol Health Illn* 16: 103–121.

Kottak CP. 1994. *Cultural anthropology, 6th ed.* McGraw-Hill, New York.

Krysan M, Schuman H, Scott LJ, Beatty P. 1994. Response Rates and Response Content in Mail Versus Face-to-Face Surveys, *Public Opinion Quarterly* 58: 381–439.

Legard R, Keegan J, Ward K. 2003. In-depth interviews. In: *Qualitative research practice: A guide for social science students and researchers.* Ritchie J, Lewis J (eds). Sage Publications, London. pp. 139–169.

Lincoln YS, Guba EG. 1985. *Naturalistic inquiry.* Sage Publications, Beverly Hills, CA.

May KM. 1991. Interview techniques in qualitative research: Concerns and challenges. In: *Qualitative nursing research.* Morse JM (ed.). Sage Publications, Newbury Park. pp. 187–201.

Morgan DL. 1998. *The focus group guide book.* Sage Publications, London.

Oppenheim AN. 1972. *Questionnaire Design and Attitude Measurement,* Heinemann Educational Books Ltd., London.

Oppenheim AN. 1992. *Questionnaire Design, Interviewing and Attitude Measurement,* Pinter Publishers, London.

Pike KL. 1966. Emic and etic standpoints for the description of behavior. In: *Communication and culture,* AG Smith (ed.), Holt, Reinhart and Winston, New York. pp. 52–163.

Polit DF. Beck CT. 2012. *Nursing Research: Generating and Assessing Evidence for Nursing Practice, 9th ed.* Wolters Klower Health, Lippincott Williams & Wilkins, Philadelphia, USA.

Russell BH. 1998. *Handbook of methods in cultural anthropology.* AltaMira Press, Walnut Creek, CA.

Scott C. 1961. Research on Mail Surveys *Journal of the Royal Statistical Society, Series A* 124: 143–205.

Spradley JP. 1979. *The ethnographic interview.* Harcourt Brace Jovanovich College Publishers, Fort Worth.

Spradley JP. 1980. *Participant observation.* Holt, Rinehart and Winston, New York.

Stephenson W. 1953. *The study of behavior: Q-technique and its methodology.* University of Chicago Press, Chicago.

Stephenson W. 1993. Introduction to Q-methodology. *Operant Subjectivity* 17(1): 1–13.

Thomas DB, Baas LR. 1992. The issue of generelization in Q methodology: Reliable schematics revisited. *Operant Subjectivity* 16(1): 18–36.

Westen D, Rosenthal R. 2003. Quantifying construct validity: Two simple measures. *Journal of Personality and Social Psychology* 84(3): 608–618.

Wilks T. 2004. The use of vignettes in qualitative research into social work values. *Qualitative Social Work* 3: 78–87.

8 Analysis of Data

Chapter overview

- Introduction to data analysis
- Classification of data
- Tabulation of data
- Presentation of data
- Interpretation of data

INTRODUCTION TO DATA ANALYSIS

Data collection is the most time-consuming and labour-intensive task in any research project. It involves a great deal of field work, contacting of subjects, providing them the necessary tools and collection of data using techniques such as interviewing, observation and self-report. Data is thus collected on paper and this needs to be classified and coded in order to make it amenable to analysis and finally to answer the research questions. The coded data is entered in a spreadsheet to enable execution of statistical software for analysis.

CLASSIFICATION OF DATA

Classification is the process of arranging data in groups/classes on the basis of certain characteristics/properties. Classification of statistical data condenses the raw data into a form that can be used for statistical analysis. It removes complexities and arranges the data set into homogeneous groups of similarity and dissimilarity. The basis for data classification is determined by the types of variables included in a study. Given below are examples of data classification.

- **Geographical classification**: Data can be classified on the basis of geographical distribution such as cities, districts or villages, rural or urban. The following is an example of a geographical distribution.

District:	Indore	Gwalior	Bhopal
Number of nursing colleges:	0	204	123

- **Chronological classification**: When data is listed in chronological order, starting with the earliest year, it is known as chronological classification.

Year	2002	2003	2004	2005	2006	2007
Number of nursing colleges in India	125	250	300	1300	1900	4000

- **Qualitative classification**: Data can be classified on the basis of descriptive qualitative attributes such as gender, occupation, religion, caste or education, which cannot be quantified. Qualitative data classification can be of two types:
  - **Simple classification**: Each class of data is divided into two subclasses; for example, place of stay: rural and urban, literacy: literate and illiterate, and so on.
  - **Manifold classification**: Each class is divided into more than two subclasses which may be further subdivided (Fig. 8.1).

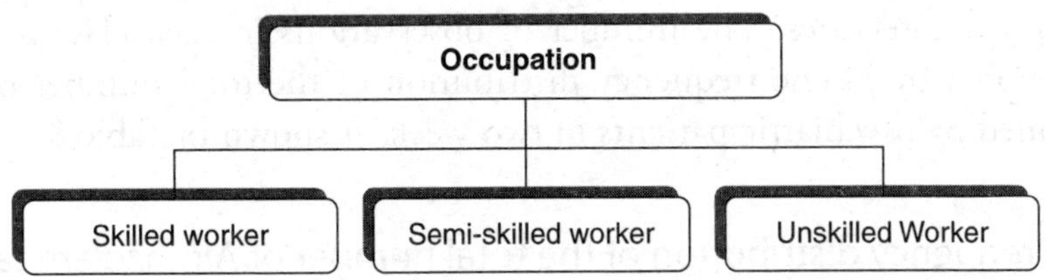

Figure 8.1 Manifold classification of occupation

- **Quantitative classification**: In this, data is classified on the basis of characteristics that can be measured quantitatively, such as height, weight and income.

Data can also be classified on the basis of the level of measurement used to measure a variable, such as nominal level, ordinal level, continuous level and ratio level. This is explained in more detail in Chapter 12.

ORGANISATION OF DATA

Data arrays are used to organise the research data. Collected data is presented in raw form and is not arranged in any particular order or sequence. For example, Table 8.1 depicts the total number of Alprazolam tablets consumed by psychiatric patients in two weeks.

Arranging data in data arrays enables the researcher to quickly check some of the characteristics of the data. When a raw data array is reorganised in rank order (smallest to largest) sequence, it is called an ordered array. Table 8.2 reorganises the data given in Table 8.1.

Table 8.1 Alprazolam tablets consumed by psychiatric patients in two weeks (raw data)

120	104	108	102	100
125	110	130	107	103
121	112	136	111	108

Table 8.2 Alprazolam tablets consumed by psychiatric patients in two weeks (rank order)

100	102	103	104	107
108	108	110	111	112
120	121	125	130	136

Frequency Distribution

Frequency distribution is used to divide a data set into conveniently established numerically ordered groups or categories. The number of observations in each class is referred to as frequency, denoted by *f*. The frequency distribution of the total number of Alprazolam tablets consumed by psychiatric patients in two weeks is shown in Table 8.3.

Table 8.3 Frequency distribution of the total number of Alprazolam tablets consumed by psychiatric patients in two weeks

Number of alprazolam tablets	Tally	Frequency
100	I	1
102	I	1
103	I	1
104	I	1
107	I	1
108	II	2
110	I	1
111	I	1
112	I	1
120	I	1
121	I	1
125	I	1
130	I	1
136	I	1

As the number of observations obtained becomes larger, frequency distribution as a way of condensing the data becomes quite difficult and time-consuming. Therefore, to condense larger data sets into a frequency distribution table, non-overlapping class intervals are constructed (steps are given below):

1. Determine the number of class intervals required as per the range of the data.
2. Determine the width of the class intervals.
3. Determine the class limits for each class interval to avoid overlap.

For the number of class intervals, the general rule is that there should be at least five class intervals, but not more than 15. However, the researcher is required to judge this requirement based on the data range. The width of each class interval can be decided by considering the difference between the largest and smallest numerical values in the data set and then dividing it by the number of class intervals desired.

$$\text{Class interval width} = \frac{\text{Range (Largest data value} - \text{Smallest data value)}}{\text{Desired number of class intervals}}$$

From Table 8.3, the data range can be calculated as 136 – 100 = 36 tablets. If the desired number of class intervals is 6, the width of the class intervals can be calculated as follows:

$$\text{Width of class interval} = \frac{36}{6} = 6$$

Once the class interval has been calculated, class limits (upper and lower limits) must be clearly defined so that each observation in the given data set belongs to one and only one class.

The lower limit of the first class should be a number slightly below or equal to the lowest value in the data set. The upper limit should be such that data can be condensed to the required number of class intervals. The width of the class interval should, as far as possible, be equal for all classes. The class midpoint is the point halfway between the upper and lower class limits of each class and is representative of all the observations contained in that class.

Observations in the data set can be classified exclusively or inclusively. When the upper limit of a class interval is the lower limit of the succeeding class interval, it is exclusive; whereas, when both the lower and upper limits of a class interval are included in the interval itself, it is known as the inclusive method of classifying data. To ensure continuity in distribution in the exclusive method, the correction factor must be calculated and then subtracted from the lower limits of all the classes and added to the upper limits of all the classes. A particular observation may be included in a class interval after giving due consideration to the correction factor. Given below is the formula to calculate the correction factor.

$$x = \frac{\text{Upper limit of a class} - \text{Lower limit of the next higher class}}{2}$$

Sometimes the investigator may decide to present data in a cumulative frequency (cf) distribution. This may be of two types (Table 8.4):

- In the **more than cumulative frequency distribution**, the frequencies of each class interval are added successively from bottom to top and represent the cumulative number of observations more than or equal to the class frequency to which it relates.
- In the **less than cumulative frequency distribution**, the frequencies of each class interval are added successively from top to bottom and represent the cumulative number of observations less than or equal to the class frequency to which it relates.

Table 8.4 Cumulative frequency distribution

Number of weeks	Number of patients	Cumulative frequency less than	Cumulative frequency more than
0–5	5	5	48
5–10	14	19	43
10–15	17	36	29
15–20	8	44	12
20–25	4	48	4

The **relative frequency of a class** is the frequency of that class divided by the total number of observations.

When the relative frequency of a class is multiplied by 100, it yields the **percentage frequency distribution** of the corresponding class (Table 8.5).

Table 8.5 Relative and percentage frequency distribution

Number of weeks	Number of patients	Relative frequency	Percentage frequency
0–5	5	0.10	10
5–10	14	0.29	29
10–15	17	0.35	35
15–20	8	0.16	16
20–25	4	0.08	8

TABULATION OF DATA

Tabulation is another way of summarising and presenting the given data in the form of rows and columns. It helps in statistical analysis and interpretation by bringing related information close to each other in rows and columns.

Constructing a Table

Table number Each table should be given a number for easy identification and reference. The table number should be placed above the title or along with the title of the table.

Table title The title of the table should be brief, self-explanatory and complete. It must indicate the nature of the data presented in the table. If required, a prefatory note may be provided just below the title for further clarification. It is usually enclosed in brackets and is about the unit of measurement.

Number of subjects *N* is placed at the top-right corner of the table and depicts the total number of subjects from whom the data was collected.

Captions and stubs Caption (headings of columns) and stubs (headings of rows) should be clear and concise. The body of the table should contain the numerical information arranged in columns and rows.

Footnotes Footnotes are provided below the table (if required) to clarify the captions and stubs. For example, if a table depicts data related to profits earned by an institute, the footnote may describe whether the profit is before tax or after tax computation.

Source note It defines the source of the data presented in the table. This may be given after the footnote.

Given below is an example of a table with the various elements depicted.

Table

N=

Stub heading	Caption				Total (Rows)
	Subhead		Subhead		
	Column head	Column head	Column head	Column head	
Stub Entries					
Total (Columns)					

Footnote:

Source Note:

Example of a table with data

Table 1.0 Comparison between the experimental and control group's mean knowledge scores from pretest to post-test I, II and III

N = 281

Knowledge score		Experimental group (n_1 = 191)	Control group (n_2 = 90)	*P* value
Pretest	Mean ± SD	9.76 ± 2.89	9.23 ± 2.45	$t = -1.564$
	95% CI	9.37 – 10.15	8.72 – 9.74	$P = 0.118$
				$df = 279$

(*Continued*)

Table 1.0 Continued

Knowledge score		Experimental group ($n_1 = 191$)	Control group ($n_2 = 90$)	P value
Post-test I	Mean	21.35 ± 2.71	9.38 ± 2.35	$t = 34.21$
	95% CI	20.93 – 21.76	8.89 – 9.87	$P < 0.0001$*
				$df = 279$
Post-test II	Mean	21.15 ± 3.04	9.57 ± 2.37	$t = -31.912$
	95% CI	20.72 – 21.59	9.07 – 10.06	$P < 0.0001$*
				$df = 279$
Post-test III	Mean	20.98 ± 3.29	9.48 ± 2.46	$t = 29.47$
	95% CI	19.89 – 20.76	8.96 – 9.99	$P < 0.0001$*
				$df = 279$

**p value significant at 0.05 level*

Classification of Tables

Tables may be classified as simple or complex. A simple table, also known as a one-way table, is one in which data based on only one characteristic is presented. A complex table, also known as a manifold table, is one in which data for two or more characteristics is presented. Complex tables are two-way or three-way tables according to whether two or three characteristics are presented simultaneously. When the variable under study is further subdivided into two groups, a two-way table is used. Similarly, a three-way table is used to present a variable that is further divided into three groups (Table 8.6). Manifold tables provide information about a large number of inter-related characteristics in the data set.

Table 8.6 Number of patients who visited the outpatient department in a week

Patient profile	Number of patients		Total
	Male	Female	
Cardiac	10	12	22
Oncology	09	11	20
Total	19	23	42

GRAPHICAL PRESENTATION OF DATA

Figures and graphs can be used to present data in pictorial form. This may provide a clearer understanding of the data at a glance. Figures and graphs provide a platform for quick and easy comparison of two or more frequency distributions. Also, any value that is extreme can be observed easily by looking at the graph. The size and shape of the graph give an exact illustration of the variations in the distribution trends. Figures and graphs should be prepared in such a way that they can be understood easily. For a large data set, it is advisable to prepare more than one figure or graph by splitting the data set into two or more categories.

Constructing a Graph

Microsoft Excel, a utility that forms part of the Microsoft Office suite, provides a platform for creating graphs of the desired type, such as bar graph, pie chart, line graph and scatter diagram. The user must select the data set and the type of graph required. The following guidelines can be used when presenting graphs in the research report.

Title Each figure or graph should have a clear and concise title. It is usually given below the figure. The title conveys the main theme that the graph intends to portray.

Size of the components of the graph The diagram should neither be too small nor too large. The size of each component of a diagram should be such that all the relevant characteristics of the data are properly displayed and easily understood. An appropriate proportion between the length and breadth of the diagram should be maintained.

Scale of data The scale used to depict data should specify the size of the unit and the nature of data it represents; for example, in centimetres, in kilogram, 1 large square on graph paper is equal to 100 cm. The scale adopted should be placed on the corresponding axes.

Footnotes Footnotes are given at the bottom of the diagram to clarify any points that need further explanation.

N *N* is the number of subjects for whom data is presented in the graph. It can be placed at the top-right corner of the graph.

Types of Figure and Graphs

Various types of graphs can be used to display data in pictorial form. Some important types of graphs used extensively by nurse researchers are given below.

- Histograms
- Frequency polygons
- Cumulative frequency distributions (Ogive)
- Pie diagrams
- Frequency curves
- Scatter diagram

- **Histograms** are used for both ungrouped and grouped data. For ungrouped data, values of the variable are scaled along the horizontal axis and the number of observations (or frequencies) along the vertical axis of the graph. The points are then connected by straight lines to enhance the shape of the distribution. The height of the boxes indicates the number of observations in each class. The bars are of the same width and only the length varies; therefore, the relationship among them can be easily established (Fig. 8.2).

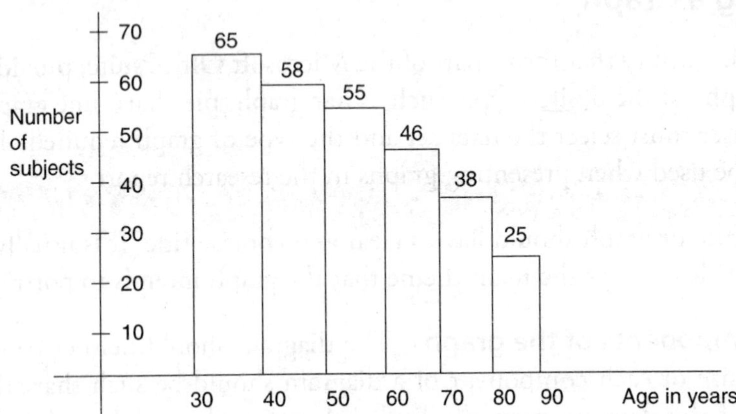

Figure 8.2 Histogram for age distribution in the study sample

Simple bar charts are used to represent only one characteristic of data. This means that there will be as many bars as the number of observations. For example, data obtained on the number of patients who attended antenatal clinic in a hospital over 10 years can be represented by such bars. Each bar would represent the number of patients who attended antenatal clinic in that year. As the bars are of the same width and only the length varies, the relationship among them can be easily established (Fig. 8.3).

It is the general rule that the bars be constructed vertically to depict observations that are the outcome of a numerical variable. However, when the observations are the outcome of a categorical variable, the bars can be constructed horizontally.

A **multiple bar** (also known as grouped or compound) **chart** is useful for direct comparison between two or more sets of data. Each set of data is represented in different shades or colours on the same scale. However, an index to explain the shades or colours must be given. Fig. 8.5 shows the number of male (series 2) and female patients (series 3) who attended OPD over 10 years.

Subdivided bar charts are suitable for expressing information in terms of ratios or percentages. While constructing these charts the components in each bar should be in the same order to avoid confusion. Different shades must be used to represent various ratio values but the shade of each component should remain the same in all the bars. An index of the shades should be given with the diagram. For example, Fig. 8.5 presents information on the percentage of male and female patients who attended OPD over 11 years (series 1 = male; series 2 = female).

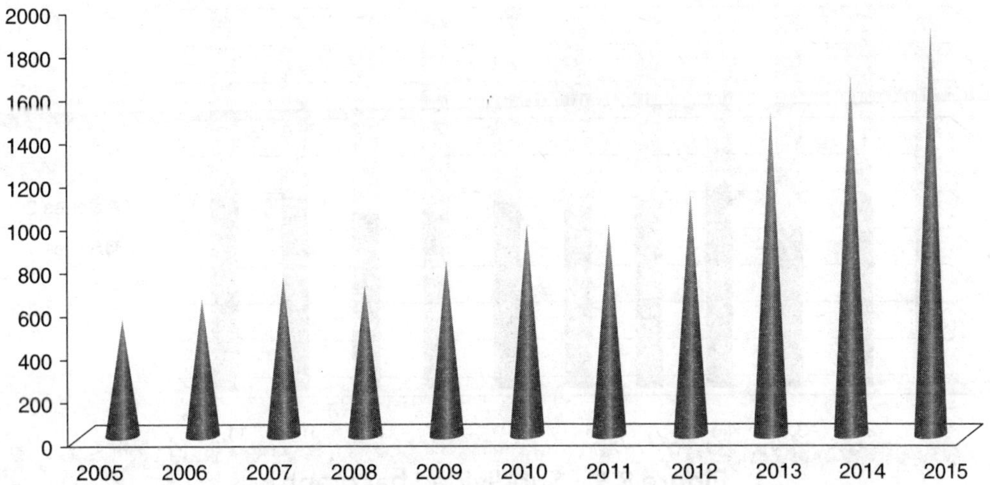

Figure 8.3 Bar graph depicting patients who attended antenatal clinic over a period of 10 years

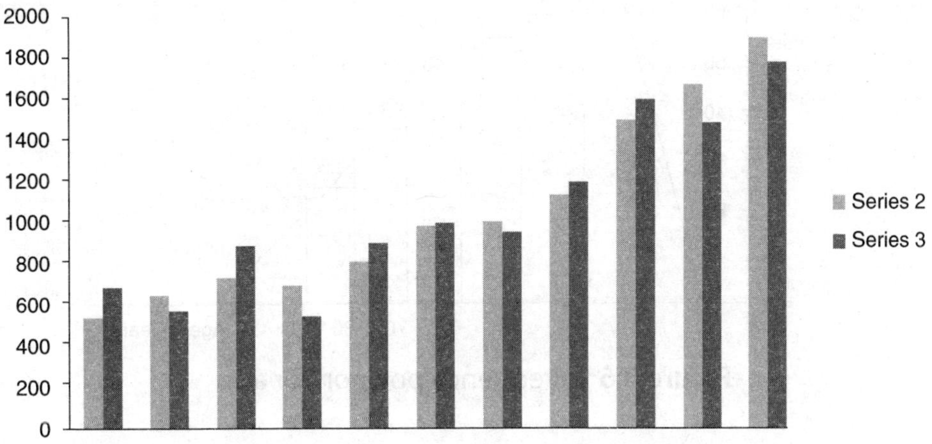

Figure 8.4 Compound bar graph

The component values are then expressed in terms of a percentage of the total to obtain the necessary length for each of these in the full length of the bars. The other rules regarding the shades, index and thickness are the same as mentioned earlier.

- A **frequency polygon** is formed by marking the midpoint at the top of the horizontal bars and then joining these dots using a series of straight lines. Frequency polygons are formed as a closed figure with the horizontal axis. A frequency polygon can also be converted into a histogram by drawing vertical lines from the bounds of the classes shown on the horizontal axis, and then connecting them with horizontal lines at the heights of the polygon at each midpoint. Fig. 8.6 shows the frequency polygon for the frequency distribution presented by the histogram in Fig. 8.2.

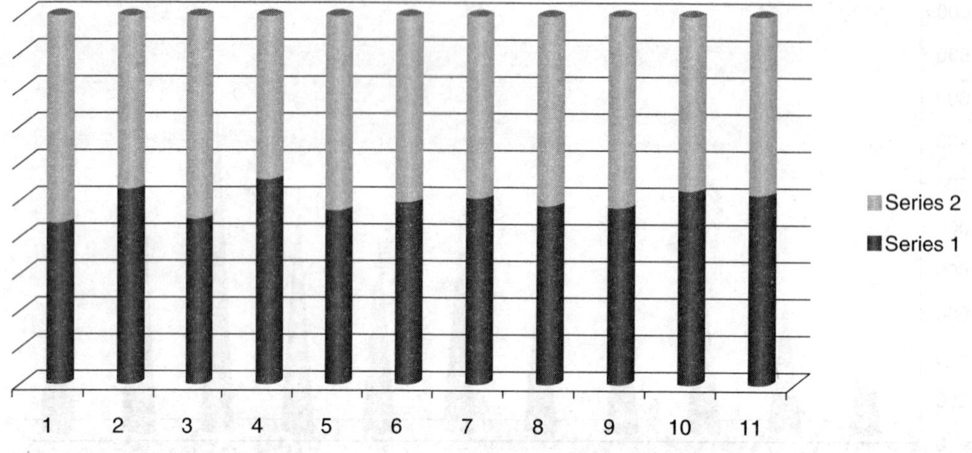

Figure 8.5 Subdivided bar graph

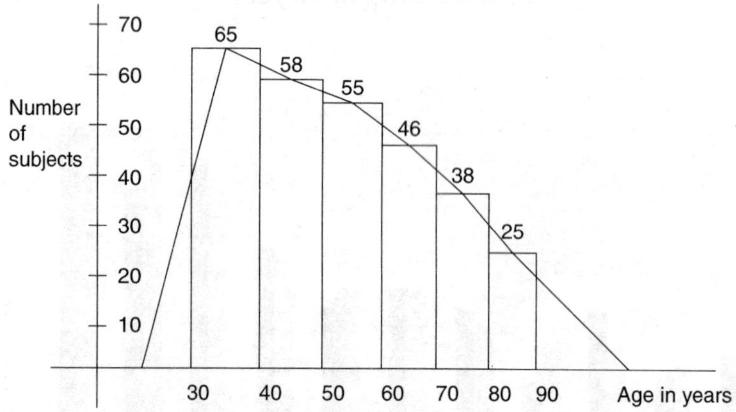

Figure 8.6 Frequency polygon for age

- **Cumulative frequency or Ogive** enables the researcher to see how many observations lie above or below certain values rather than merely recording the number of observations within intervals. Table 8.7 shows the cumulative frequency table for age of patients who attended OPD.
- **Pie diagrams** are frequently used to depict different types of observation in a data set on a percentage basis through the use of a circle. Usually, the largest percentage portion of data in a pie diagram is shown first, at the 12 o'clock position on the circle. Thereafter, the other observations in percent are shown in the clockwise direction in descending order of magnitude. The steps to draw a pie diagram are given below.
  1. Convert the observations in the data set (given in percentage) into corresponding degrees in the circle by multiplying each by 3.6.
  2. Draw a circle of desired size with a compass.

Table 8.7 Calculation of cumulative frequencies

Age in years	Upper class boundary	Number of patients (f)	Cumulative frequency	
			Less than	More than
10–15	15	6	6	40
15–20	20	11	17	34
20–25	25	9	26	23
25–30	30	7	33	14
30–35	35	5	38	7
35–40	40	2	40	2

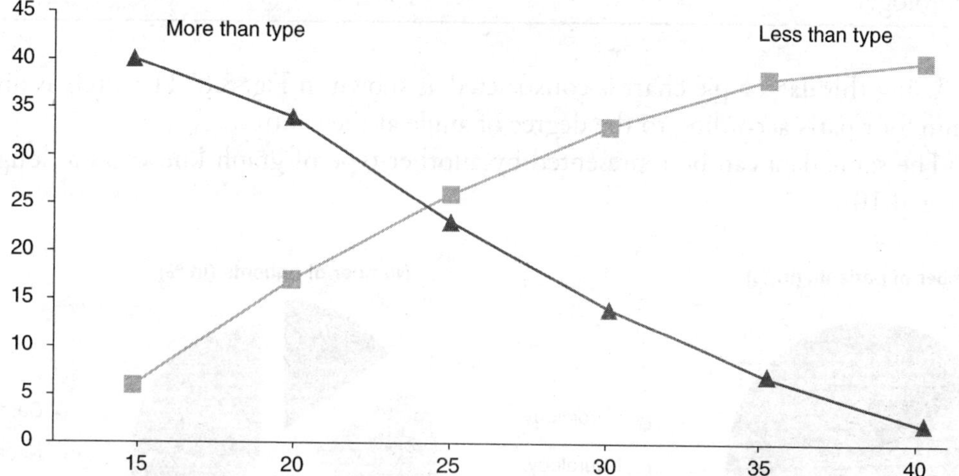

Figure 8.7 Ogive for age of patients who attended OPD in a year

3. Draw points on the circle according to the degree of each portion of the data and join each of these points to the centre of the circle.

For example, the number of patients (in percentage) who attended various speciality outpatient clinics in a particular year at a tertiary care hospital are given in Table 8.8.

Table 8.8 The number of patients (in percentage) who attended various speciality outpatient clinics in a particular year at a tertiary care hospital

Specialty outpatient clinic	Number of patient (in %)
Cardiology	40
Neurology	25
Oncology	20
Nephrology	15

To construct a pie diagram, each observation in the data set should be converted to the corresponding angle of the circle by multiplying it by 3.6 (Table 8.9).

Table 8.9 The number of patients (in percentage) who attended various speciality outpatient clinics in a particular year at a tertiary care hospital and their corresponding angle in a circle

Specialty outpatient clinic	Number of patient (in %)	Angle (degree)
Cardiology	40	144
Neurology	25	90
Oncology	20	72
Nephrology	15	54

Using this data, a pie chart is constructed as shown in Fig. 8.8. The circle is divided into four parts according to the degree of angle at the centre.

The same data can be represented by another type of graph known as a doughnut (Fig. 8.10).

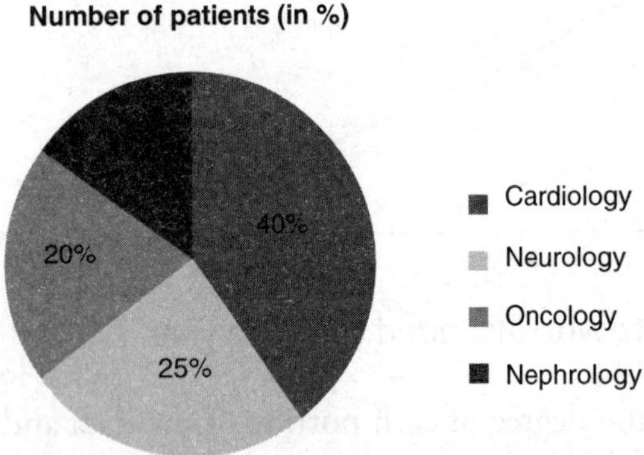

Figure 8.8 Percentage pie chart

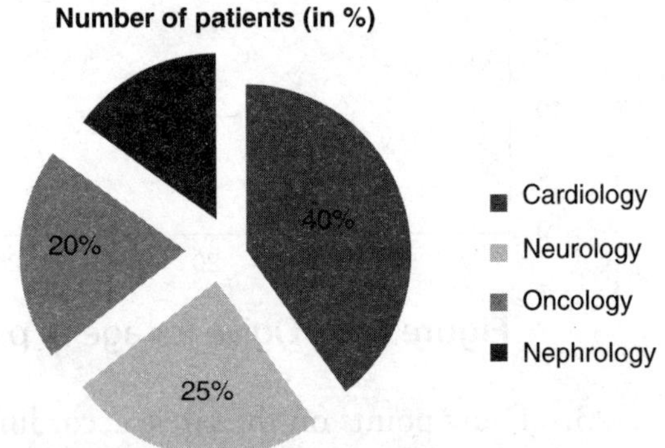

Figure 8.9 Exploded pie chart

Table 8.10 Number of cycles produced by a cycle manufacturer in a year

Year	2011	2012	2013	2014
Output	2000	2800	3200	4900

Number of patients (in %)

40%

20%

25%

Cardiology

Neurology

Oncology

Nephrology

Figure 8.10 Doughnut chart

- A **pictogram** is a pictorial bar chart used to present data to laypeople who cannot understand technical charts. Small symbols or simplified pictures are used to represent the size of the data. For example, Fig. 8.11 shows a pictographic presentation of the output of cycles produced by a cycle manufacturing company in a year (data given in Table 8.10).

  To represent the given data, the scale 1 cycle picture = 1000 cycles is selected for the pictogram. The cycle output figures are divided by 1000 to get 2, 2.8, 3.2 and 4.9, respectively.

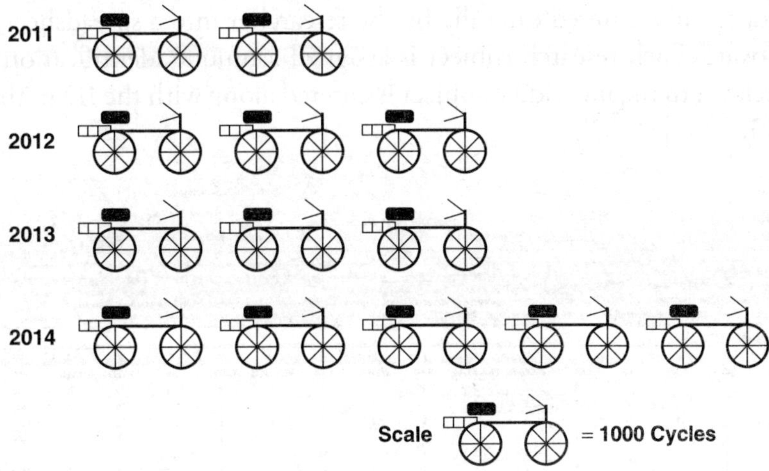

Figure 8.11 Output of cycles

ANALYSIS AND INTERPRETATION OF DATA

Analysis of data is an important step in the research process. It aims to provide meaning to the large data set collected to answer the research questions. Data analysis uses a number of statistical tests (parametric and non-parametric) depending on the type of variables and level of measurements used to collect information. Data related to categorical variables are first coded in numerical form to make them amenable to statistical analysis. However, variables on continuous and ratio levels of measurement can be entered directly in a spreadsheet according to their numerical value. Descriptive and inferential statistical tests are executed to analyse coded and organised data. Descriptive statistics includes measures of central tendency (mean, mode, median), measures of dispersion (range, standard deviation, variance, quartile range) and percentage to describe the pattern emerging from the data set. Inferential statistics is based on the law of probability and is used to test hypotheses. Parametric and non-parametric statistical tests are executed to calculate the p value and the significance of relationships between two or more variables under investigation. Given below are the steps in data analysis.

1. **Developing a coding system for data**: Coding is a method of categorising and indexing the data. As statistical operations can be executed only on numerical forms

of data, categorical information should be converted to numerical coded form so that it can be entered into spreadsheets for execution of analytical commands. For example, categorical data on the variable 'gender' can be coded as follows: Male-1; Female-2. Similarly, educational qualifications can be coded as: Illiterate-1; Primary-2; Middle-3; Secondary-4; Senior secondary-5; Graduate-6; Post-graduation and above-7. Continuous variable, ratio level data can be entered directly as exact values in the numerical form; for example, height, weight, temperature, pulse rate, respiratory rate.

2. **Entering data in a spreadsheet**: After developing a coding system for the entire range of the data set, it is entered carefully by the researcher into a spreadsheet, manually or using software. Each research subject is assigned a unique identification number and the data related to the individual subject is entered along with the ID in the spreadsheet (Fig. 8.12).

CODE NO	AGE	SEX	MS	RGN	ES	OCCU	INCOME	PLA STAY	DIAG.	NYHA	DOI	RHYTHM	CONDUC	EF	LVED	LVES	HT	WT	BMI
1	33	1	1	1	3	2	2	2	1	3	7	1	4	20	69	57	176	80	25.8
2	42	1	1	1	4	7	1	2	3	2	36	1	4	17.5	55	50	161.5	57	21.98
3	48	1	1	1	3	2	1	2	1	3	72	1	6	17.5	53	42	154.5	48	20.1
4	45	1	1	1	6	1	2	2	1	3	36	1	4	32.5	10	12	164	56	20.8
5	63	2	1	1	1	5	1	2	1	3	18	1	4	25	51	42	148	55	25.1
6	37	1	1	1	4	2	4	1	1	3	6	1	5	27.5	78	62	163.8	70	26.09
7	47	1	1	1	5	6	2	2	3	3	48	1	5	37.5	54	42	173	80	26.7
8	31	1	1	3	5	1	2	2	1	2	96	1	6	17	72	64	174	64	21.14
9	38	1	1	1	6	1	4	2	1	2	0.6	1	6	27.5	71	62	162	85	32.28
10	53	1	1	1	3	7	2	1	1	3	36	1	4	22.5	72	60	165	69	25.34
11	56	1	1	1	5	2	4	2	5	2	6	1	5	30	72	56	183	90	26.87
12	62	2	1	1	5	5	2	2	3	2	36	1	4	35	68	56	153.5	70	29.7
13	53	1	1	1	1	1	3	2	5	3	24	1	6	20	56	46	164	65	24.17
14	25	1	1	1	4	2	1	1	1	2	12	1	6	35	70	53	175	51.5	16.81
15	40	1	1	3	2	2	1	1	1	3	156	1	4	25	62	46	172	75	25.35
16	36	1	1	1	3	2	1	1	1	2	36	1	4	22.5	62	53	172.7	65	21.72
17	58	1	4	1	3	6	2	2	1	2	60	1	5	27	54	42	168	67	23.74
18	50	1	1	1	2	1	3	2	1	2	132	2	6	27	59	44	154	47	19.82
19	45	1	1	1	5	1	3	2	1	2	132	1	6	27.5	60	49	174	100	33.03
20	54	1	1	1	6	1	4	2	1	2	72	1	5	30	59	50	158	55	22.03
21	39	1	1	1	6	1	4	2	1	3	84	1	6	17	68	58	174	74	24.44
22	60	2	1	1	1	5	1	2	3	2	60	1	6	20	40	28	156	60	24.65
23	70	1	1	1	5	6	2	2	1	2	60	2	4	23	59	43	168	59	20.9
24	38	1	1	1	4	1	2	2	1	2	72	1	6	15	64	52	169.5	61	21.23

Figure 8.12 Data entry in MS Excel, a spreadsheet programme

3. **Data cleaning**: Data entry is prone to errors. It is good practice to enter the data each day as it is collected from the participants. It reduces the chances of errors in data entry. A colleague familiar with the coding system of the data can cross-check it for errors, missing values, outliers and wild code (code that is not possible).
4. **Handling missing values**: Sometimes, participants do not provide the required information related to some variables of interest in the questionnaire. For example, a participant did not provide information about his age and weight. The researcher

should systematically check for the extent and pattern of missing values in the data set. A number of strategies are available to handle the problem of missing values.

- **Delete the missing subjects**: All the data of the particular subject is deleted in its entirety if there is any missing information. It is the correct solution for missing values when one or two subjects are associated with most of the missing information in the data set.
- **Delete the variable**: The missing value variable is deleted for all the subjects. It is an appropriate strategy when a particular variable has the highest percentage of missing values.
- **Substitute with mean or median value**: The missing information can be substituted with the mean for the given variable. The researcher must judge whether the mean of the sample or the subgroup will be the best substitute for the missing value.
- **Delete cases pair-wise**: It is the most widely used strategy to handle the problem of missing values. Here, the researcher deletes cases selectively on a variable-by-variable basis. For example, the researcher has collected data of 100 subjects on age, height and weight; but there are missing values for 10 cases for age, 20 cases for height and 15 cases for weight. In this situation, the mean age is calculated from the available data of 90 subjects, mean height from the data of 80 subjects and so on. However, the drawback of this method is that the number of cases may fluctuate across the characteristics (90 for age, 80 for height and 85 for weight). Therefore, it is difficult to interpret the study result because the sample size is not constant.

5. **Transforming data**: This is referred to as data alternation or conversion. With the use of statistical software packages, it takes only a click to transform data to the desired format or measurement. For example, birth weight (in kg) of 100 neonates has been entered but to find out how many neonates are underweight, the given data must be transformed to a dichotomous variable (underweight and normal weight infant). SPSS software provides the Recode Into Different Variable command for this transformation. Compute is another command used for a similar purpose.
6. **Selecting appropriate descriptive and inferential statictics**: In this step, the reseacher has to look back to the research objectives and hypothesis to select the appropriate descriptive and inferential statistical operations to analyse the data. It will condense the data and generate the p value, the interpretation of which will provide answers to the research question. Descriptive and inferential statistics is described in detail later in the book.

To conclude, collection, organisation, transformation, cleaning of data and handling missing values are important tasks that make the data ready for statistical operations. The reseacher must prepare a detailed plan of data analysis while finalising the methodology of study. Analysis of empirical data collected in a research study produces meaningful information which answers the research questions under investigation.

CHAPTER SUMMARY

- Classification of data is the process of arranging data in groups/classes on the basis of certain characteristics/properties.
- A data array is used to organise the research data. Data is presented in raw form and is not arranged in any particular order or sequence.
- Frequency distribution is used to divide the data set into conveniently established numerically ordered groups or categories.
- Observations in the data set can be classified exclusively or inclusively. When the upper limit of a class interval is the lower limit of the succeeding class interval, it is the exclusive method; whereas, when both the lower and upper limits of a class interval are included in the interval itself, it is known as the inclusive method of classifying data.
- In the more than and less than cumulative frequency distribution, the frequencies of each class interval are added successively from bottom to top and top to bottom, respectively.
- Relative frequency of a class is the frequency of that class divided by the total number of observations.
- Tabulation is a way of summarising and presenting the given data in a systematic form in rows and columns.
- Figures and graphs can be used to present the data in pictorial form which provides a clearer meaning at a glance to a large group of data.
- A multiple bar (also known as grouped or compound) chart is useful for direct comparison between two or more sets of data. Each set is represented in different shades or colours on the same scale.
- A frequency polygon is formed by marking the midpoint at the top of horizontal bars and then joining these dots by a series of straight lines.
- Pie diagrams are frequently used to depict different types of observations in a data set on a percentage basis through the use of a circle.
- A pictogram is a pictorial bar chart that is useful in presenting data to laypeople who cannot understand technical charts. Small symbols or simplified pictures are used to represent the size of the data.
- Coding is a method of categorising and indexing the data to convert all the collected information into numerical form.
- Each research subject is assigned a unique identification number and the data related to the individual subject is entered along with the ID in the spreadsheet.
- Data entered in a spreadsheet should be checked for errors in data entry, missing values, outliers and wild code.
- Strategies used to handle missing values in a data set include deleting the missing subjects, deleting the variable, deleting cases pairwise and substituting with mean or median.

- Data transformation is referred to as data alternation or conversion from one level of measurement to another as per the requirements.
- Research objectives and hypotheses provide key information to determine the suitable descriptive and inferential operations for data analysis.

EVALUATE YOURSELF

Long Answer Questions

Q1: Analysis of data is one of the important steps in research. Write about a) Non-parametric test and its utilisation, and b) Organisation and level of data. Support your answer with examples.

Q2: List the steps in analysis of data.

Q3: Identify the guidelines for designing a table.

Q4: Explain the need for preparation of tables.

Q5: Explain the analysis and interpretation of data.

Q6: Calculate less than and more than cumulative frequency from the given data. Draw an Ogive.

Birth weight of neonates

Weight (in g)	Number of infants
500–1000	4
1000–1500	10
1500–2000	20
2000–2500	50
2500–3000	40
3000–3500	25
3500–4000	17

Short Answer Questions

Q1: Write short notes on

(a) Classification of data
(b) Types of bar graph
(c) Pie graph
(d) Handling missing values in data
(e) Cumulative frequency
(f) Ogive

Q2: Prepare a simple bar graph to depict the following data:

Profession	Number of subjects
Teacher	200
Doctor	250
Advocate	150
Nurse	350
Radiographer	50
Engineer	90
Architect	55
Beautician	100
Pharmacist	50

Multiple Choice Questions

Q1: Inclusive method of classifying data is:
(a) When both the lower and upper limits of a class interval are included in the interval itself
(b) When only the upper limits of a class interval are included in the interval itself
(c) When only the lower limits of a class interval are included in the interval itself
(d) All of the above

Q2: In greater than cumulative frequency distribution, frequencies of each class interval are:
(a) Added successively from bottom to top
(b) Added successively from top to bottom
(c) Subtracted successively from top to bottom
(d) Subtracted successively from top to bottom

Q3: In less than cumulative frequency distribution, frequencies of each class interval are:
(a) Added successively from bottom to top
(b) Added successively from top to bottom
(c) Subtracted successively from top to bottom
(d) Subtracted successively from top to bottom

Q4: Ogive is a:
(a) Relative frequency distribution (b) Cumulative frequency distribution
(c) Percentage frequency distribution (d) A type of pie graph

Q5: All of the following are strategies to handle the problem of missing values in a data set, *except*

(a) Delete the missing subjects
(b) Delete the missing variables
(c) Substitute the value with mean of a previous study
(d) Delete cases pair-wise

Answers

1. a **2.** a **3.** b **4.** b **5.** c

FURTHER READING

Allison PD. 2000. *Missing Data.* Sage, Thousands Oaks, CA.

Altman DG. 1992. *Practical Statistics for Medical Research.* Chapman & Hall, London.

Armitage P. 1989. *Statistical Methods in Medical Research.* Blackwell Scientific Publications, London.

Das R, Das PN. 2009. *Instant Medical Biostatistics.* Anne Books Pvt. Ltd, New Delhi.

Ferketich S, Verran J. 1994. An overview of data tranformation. *Research in Nursing & Health* 17: 393–396.

Harris ML. 1991. *Introduction to Data Processing, 3rd ed.* John Wiley & Sons, New York.

Kirkwood BR. 1988. *Essentials of Medical Statistics.* Blackwell Scientific Publications, London.

Mahajan BK, Khankal AB. 2010. *Methods in Biostatistics for Medical Students and Research Workers, 7th ed.* Jaypee Brothers Medical Publishers, New Delhi.

Negi KS. 2010. *Biostatistics, 2nd ed.* AITBS Publishers, New Delhi.

Polit DF. 1996. *Data Analysis and Statistics for Nursing Research.* Appleton & Lange, Samford, CT.

Rao S, Richard J. 2006. *Introduction to Biostatistics and Research Methods, 4th ed.* Prentice Hall of India, New Delhi.

Ress DG. 1989. *Essentials of Statistics.* Chapman & Hall, London.

Communication and Utilisation of Research

Chapter overview

- Introduction to communication of findings
- Disseminating research results at conferences
- Publishing a journal article
- Utilisation of research findings
- Barriers to research utilisation
- Facilitators of research utilisation
- Innovation diffusion model

INTRODUCTION TO COMMUNICATION OF FINDINGS

A research project is not considered complete until the findings have been communicated to others. The researcher should plan to communicate/disseminate the research findings after the project has been completed.

> *Failure to publish study findings is a form of scientific misconduct* –Winslow (1996)
>
> *Research not published is research not done* – Grady (2000)

Communication of research findings is the beginning of the most important phase of research, that is, the utilisation of research findings. If research findings are not utilised in nursing practice/education/administration, the conduct of research becomes a wasted effort. Therefore, nurse researchers need to understand the importance of implementing research findings.

HOW TO COMMUNICATE RESEARCH FINDINGS?

The findings of a research project can be communicated in two ways: orally or in writing. A nurse researcher may start the dissemination process by presenting study results to peers. Then, she may present the study results in an oral presentation or in a poster session at a local/national/international conference. Thereafter, she can publish the study results in a nursing journal. Sometimes, if the project has been funded by Trained Nurses Association of India (TNAI), Indian Council of Medical Research (ICMR), Sigma Theta Tau International Honour Society or by any other institution, the researchers are required to submit a written report of the study to the funding agency. If the researcher is pursuing the MSc Nursing/BSc Nursing/Post-basic BSc Nursing degree, she must present the research results in the form of theses and dissertations (Fig. 9.1).

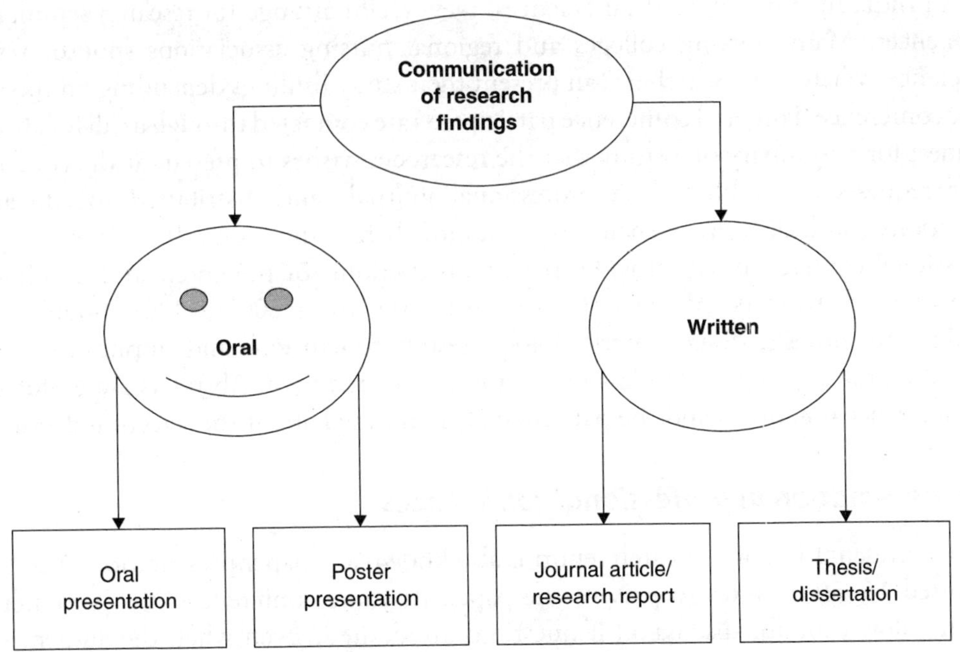

Figure 9.1 Communication of research findings

Nurse researchers must give priority to indexed journals as a publication medium. A research report is a written or oral summary of a study. It should be prepared in the order of the steps of the research process, beginning with the problem statement and ending with conclusions, implications and recommendations for future studies. While preparing the research report, due consideration should be given to **tense**—most of the research report will be written using the past tense because the study has already occurred. However, hypotheses and conclusions are written in the present tense, and implications and recommendations are focused towards the future. Hegyvary (2005) has stated that effective writing is not an innate skill; however, like any skill, it should be polished continually. It is the result of planning and organisation before the writing begins.

Disseminating Research Results at Conferences

Presentation of research findings at local, regional and national conferences enable quicker dissemination of study results to professional nurses. Research results can be communicated at professional conferences as oral presentations or poster presentations. Traditionally, oral presentation is preferred by nurse researchers; however, in the last two decades, poster presentations have become a popular mode of research dissemination at professional conferences.

Nursing organisations such as the TNAI, Indian Society of Psychiatric Nurses, Society of Community Health Nursing India, Society of Midwifery India, College of Nursing and All India Institute of Medical Sciences, New Delhi arrange for research seminars and conferences. Many nursing colleges and regional nursing associations sponsor research conferences where the researchers can present their study findings depending on the theme of the conference. Potential conference participants are contacted through a call for abstracts, a request for a summary of a study that the researcher wishes to present at the conference. These requests are published in professional journals and distributed to educational institutions and healthcare agencies 6–12 months before the event. The secretariat of the professional conference will provide specific instructions for presenters and deadlines for submission of abstracts. Abstracts (word limit varies from 200 to 300) should contain the aims, hypothesis, design, methodology, result, conclusions and implications. If the research is still in progress, the last two items are not required. Abstracts are evaluated by the conference organisers and the participants are notified about the selection decisions.

Oral presentation at professional conferences

The oral presentation of a research report is also known as a paper presentation. A presenter is allotted 15–30 minutes to present the paper. At some conferences, the presenter may have to allow time for discussion if questions are desired. Even when the audience does not get a chance to ask questions, presenters are usually willing to respond to questions during break or after the conference. In an article published in *Applied Nursing Research*, Miracle and King (1994) presented guidelines for both paper presentations and poster presentations (interested readers can refer this article). If the principal investigator is unable to attend the conference, a co-investigator or another person familiar with the study must present the paper.

The format of the oral presentation is similar to that of a journal article or other written research report of the study, as the steps of the research process are usually presented in chronological order. However, the material should be condensed to fit the time constraints of the conference. The style of presentation may vary from presenter to presenter; some prefer to attract the attention of the audience by reporting the findings first, then proceed to other parts of the study, and then return to discuss the findings in greater detail. The review of the literature should not be discussed in detail, and only pertinent studies should be mentioned. A written report of the study is usually published in the *conference proceedings*.

Presenting research results at a conference has some advantages over publishing them in a journal article. First, the investigator has the chance to present findings that are current. Because of the time lag in publishing, research published in journals may be outdated when it is printed. Second, the researcher will have the opportunity to interact with the interested audiences and will be able to locate other researchers who are studying similar phenomena.

Presenting a research poster

Research poster sessions are an excellent way for novice researchers to get an idea of how to present their findings at conferences and is also less intimidating than oral presentation. Poster sessions are generally held during professional conferences where oral presentations are also allowed. Usually, one or two hours of the conference are scheduled for poster presentation. This visual method of presentation may benefit a large number of people in a short time period. At a poster session, the presenters usually remain with their posters and interact with interested viewers. If posters are placed in a corridor of a clinical setting, patients and nursing staff can view the materials at their leisure.

Guideline for effective poster preparation

- A common poster size is 4 feet × 8 feet. However, the size of the poster may vary depending on the availability of space in the conference room/hall. Many conferences are held in hotels, and the size of the assigned rooms may dictate the number and size of the posters.
- Careful consideration should be given to the construction of posters. Technical help may be sought from a graphic artist (expert in CoralDraw), if required.
- Attractive eye-catching colour combinations should be used. For example, white on blue, black on tan, and white on black.
- Posters should contain the research problem statement, hypothesis/research question(s), sample description, material and methods, result and main conclusions.
- Diagrams, graphs and tables should be used to present certain aspects of the study, such as findings.
- Do not place too much material on a poster. A cluttered poster distracts the viewers. Material should be arranged and rearranged till the poster is eye-catching.
- The title should be in large letters, at least 1 inch high. Viewers should be able to see these letters from about 3 feet away.
- Typed material should be prepared with large letters. Many computer software programs have this capability.
- Letters may also be prepared freehand, with the use of a stencil or vinyl adhesive letters.

Publishing a Journal Article

Publishing an article in a journal has the potential to reach the largest percentage of nurses. It is considered a means of obtaining recognition for the author or authors. They aim for publication in professional research journals to ensure the most appropriate readership and potential for contribution to professional practice. The process of publishing a journal article takes time (six months usually); therefore, the researcher should plan accordingly. Peer-reviewed journals are considered the best platform for publication because the contents are scrutinised by peers for quality. Given below are the steps of the publication process in a peer-reviewed journal:

1. Submission of the manuscript to the journal—online, through CD-ROM or as a hard copy—according to the requirements of the journal.
2. The manuscript will be forwarded by the editor of the journal to two experts in the field (the author(s)' identity is not revealed) for review. Each reviewer will critique the manuscript and submit a report to the editor, referring to the article's relevance, the rigour of the research and its potential contribution to the profession. The reviewers will independently make recommendations as to whether it should be published or if it requires further work.
3. An editorial board then accepts or rejects the paper based on the reviewers' reports.
4. Authors may be required to incorporate suggestions given by reviewers and then resubmit to the same or a different journal for further consideration for publishing.
5. Once the article is accepted for publication, the authors are provided with *galley proofs* that are sheets of paper showing how the article will appear in typeset form. The authors are asked to proofread for errors and minor corrections.
6. When an author receives an acceptance letter from a journal, an approximate date or month of publication is usually included.

In an editorial published in *Research in Nursing and Health*, Patricia Becker (2004) reported some important data about publishing a journal article:

- The average time from first submission to notification of acceptance for publication is about 6.5 months.
- The acceptance rate for manuscripts varies among journals.
- Seven of the journals included in McConnell's (2000) survey of non-US nursing journals reported acceptance rates of less than 25%.
- The nurse editors of 90 journals in Freda and Kearney's (2005) survey reported the average acceptance rate for their journals to be 77%.

Therefore, authors should know the acceptance rates of the journals of interest before they submit their manuscripts.

Preparing the journal article

The length of journal articles varies a great deal, but most journals prefer manuscripts of 10–15 typed pages. The sections of the article and the format vary according to the journal. However, most articles contain these sections: introduction and background, materials and methods, findings and discussion. It is important for the researcher to carefully examine the target journal for style and format.

Selecting a journal: Selecting an appropriate journal for an article is an important decision. With each passing year, more open-access online nursing journals are coming into existence. After independence, *Nursing Journal of India* was the only journal devoted to the publication of nursing research studies in India. Since then, *Journal of Nursing Research and Midwifery, International Journal of Nursing Studies, Nightingale Times, International Journal of Nursing Education, International Journal of Nursing Care, Asian Journal of Cardiovascular Nursing, Indian Society of Psychiatric Nursing Journal, Baba Farid University of Health Sciences Nursing Journal* and *Kerala Nursing Forum* have been initiated. However, globally there are countless nursing journals fulfilling the publication needs of the Indian nurse researcher. The author is required to determine the journal most appropriate for the content of the article and then prepare the manuscript according to the guidelines of that particular journal. A manuscript that does not meet the needs of the journal's audience will not be accepted for publication in that particular journal. The author also needs to determine whether to select a refereed or non-refereed journal for publication. A refereed journal is one in which subject experts (selected by the journal's editorial staff) evaluate manuscripts. However, in a non-refereed journal, editorial staff members or consultants review the manuscripts. Final decisions about the publication of an article in both refereed and non-refereed journals are made by the journal editor.

The review of manuscripts by content or methodological experts who are professional colleagues is called peer review. The peer review process is considered the gold standard of scientific publishing because objective opinion about a manuscript is obtained from experts in the field. In a blind review, the reviewers are not told the author's identity before the manuscript is evaluated. This process provides equal chance to an unknown writer and a well-known author.

Reason for manuscript rejection
Poorly written manuscript
Content not comprehensive or inaccuracies in the content
Manuscript not appropriate for that particular journal
Journal has recently published a similar article
Methodology problems
Statistical problems, data interpretation problems

It is worthwhile mentioning to novice researchers that rejection of an article does not necessarily mean that it is not a good article. Rejection may be the result of strong competition for the limited space in nursing and allied health journals.

Preparing Theses and Dissertations

Theses and dissertations are an important means of communication of research studies conducted to fulfil educational requirements for an advanced degree in nursing. Because these documents serve a dual purpose of communicating research findings and providing evidence of the students' ability to carry out scholarly work, theses and dissertations are usually lengthy documents divided into several chapters. Graduate and postgraduate students should follow the guidelines provided by the concerned university for thesis preparation.

Writing the thesis and dissertation

Thesis or dissertation is a long piece of writing discussed in a logical way, completed by an undergraduate or postgraduate student based on her own original research for partial fulfillment of a university degree. Thesis is used interchangeably with dissertation; however, *thesis* implies that original research is involved, whereas *dissertation* implies that the researcher has looked into something and is setting down what she has found along with her thoughts on the same. Thus a *thesis* is what should be written to obtain a higher degree, but a *dissertation* is more likely to be a small part of a first degree.

Characteristics of good thesis

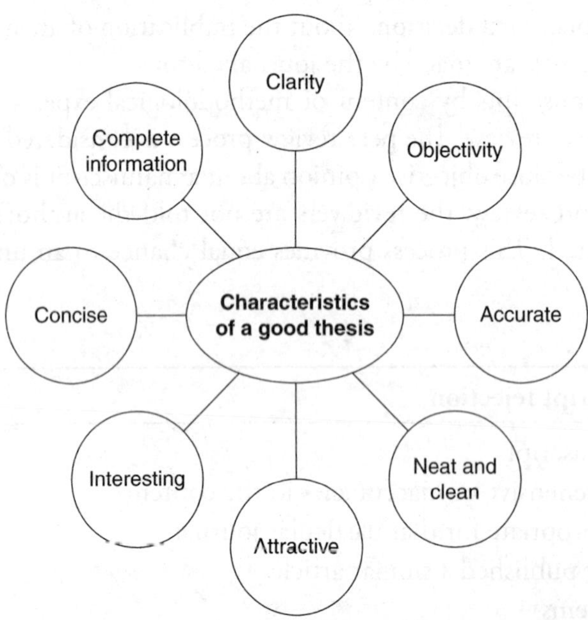

Figure 9.2 Characteristics of a good thesis

Table 9.1 Differences between thesis and manuscript (journal article) writing style

Thesis style	Manuscript style
■ Long literature review	■ Summary of past literature
■ Detailed description of statistical measures	■ Statistical measures explained
■ Short Implications section	■ Detailed Implications section
■ Focus on college requirements	■ Targeted at readers
■ Excessive use of references	■ Uses selected references
■ Academic writing style	■ Scholarly writing style
■ Excessive number of charts used	■ Selected charts to summarise data
■ 50 or more pages long	■ 10 to 20 pages long

Outline of thesis

Preliminary section: It includes the following information:

- Title page
- Endorsement by the HOD, principal/head of the institution
- Certificate by the guide, co-guide
- Declaration by the candidate
- Copyright certificate
- Acknowledgment
- Abstract
- Table of contents
- List of annexure
- List of tables
- List of figures
- List of abbreviations and symbols used

Acknowledgment: Persons who have made a substantial contribution to the study but whose contribution does not qualify them for authorship are included here. It may include the guide, co-guide, principle/HOD, faculty, statistician, friends, organisation, funding agency, family and patients or study participants. Ideally, it should be of one page and include the signature of the scholar with date and place.

List of abbreviations and symbols

- Use only standard abbreviations
- Do not use abbreviations in the title
- Specify abbreviation in full when it first occurs in the text
- Arrange in alphabetical order

For example, anon: anonymous; et. al: and others; illus: illustrated

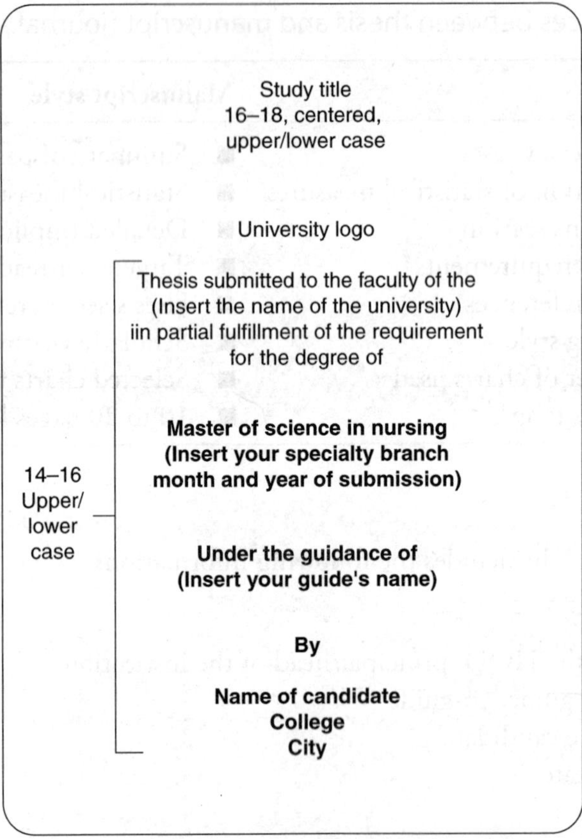

Figure 9.3 Format of title page of a thesis

Endorsement by the HOD, principal of the institution

This is to certify that the thesis entitled "<-- **study Title**------------------------------------>" is a bonafide research work done by **Name of the Candidate** under the guidance of **Name & designation of the Guide**

Seal & Signature of the HOD	**Seal & Signature of the Principal**
Name	**Name**
Date :	**Date :**
Place :	**Place :**

Figure 9.4 Endorsement by the HOD/Principal

Certificate by the guide

This is to certify that the thesis entitled "<------------------------------ **Study Title**---> " is a bonafide research work done by ----**Name of the Candidate**----- in partial fulfillment of the requirement for the degree of **Master of Science in Nursing** ------ **put your specialty**-----

Seal & Signature of the Guide	**Signature of the CO-Guide**
Name	**Name**
Designation & Department	**Designation & Department**

Date :
Place :

Figure 9.5 Certificate by the guide

Declaration by the candidate

I hereby declare that this thesis entitled " <------------------------------- **Study Title**--->" is a bonafide and genuine research work carried out by me under the guidance of ------**Name & designation of the Guide**--------.

Date :	**Signature of the Candidate**
Place :	**Name**

Figure 9.6 Declaration by the candidate

Copyright certificate

Declaration by the candidate

I hereby declare that the Rajiv Gandhi University of health sciences, karnataka shall have the rights to preserve, use and disseminate this thesis in print or preserve, use and disseminate this thesis in print or electronic format for academic / research purpose.

Date :	**Signature of the Candidate**
Place :	**Name**

© Rajiv Gandhi University of health sciences, karnataka

Figure 9.7 Copyright certificate

Abstract

It is the first point of contact with readers about findings, and so deserves careful attention. It should present a brief description of the research problem, methods and finding of the study so that readers can decide whether to read the entire thesis. There are two styles of writing abstracts: unstructured paragraph and structured abstract with subheadings.

Writing style of structured abstract (maximum 150–250 words)

- Background and Objectives
- Methods
- Results
- Interpretation and Conclusion
- Keywords (maximum 10, each keyword should be separated by a semicolon) will help others to locate the study online over the internet in databases

Table of contents: It should provide content details of the thesis along with the page numbers.

List of annexures: It provides information about the annexure used in the thesis along with the page number. Some of the commonly used annexures in postgraduate thesis are:

- Letter granting ethical clearance
- Patient information sheet
- Consent form
- Screening sheet
- Tool used in the study
- Certificate of competence
- List of experts
- List of statistical tests

List of tables: It should include table number and title of the table along with page number.

List of figures: Figure number and title, along with the page number.

Main body of the thesis: It includes

- Chapter I: Introduction
- Chapter II: Review of Literature
- Chapter III: Methodology
- Chapter IV: Analysis and Interpretation/Results
- Chapter V: Discussion and Summary

Chapter I: Introduction

- Introduction

- Background
- Need for the study and how this work will help
- Statement of the problem, research questions
- Aim of the study
- Objectives (1, 2, 3. . . .)
- Variables under study (IV, DV and EV), hypotheses,
- Delimitations, assumptions, opperational definitions
- Conceptual framework

At the end of each chapter, present a summary of the chapter and state

This chapter has dealt with ....

The next chapter will deal with ....

Chapter II: Review of Literature

- Divide all available reviews into different sections as per the study
- Arrange recent to old; in historical research, old to recent
- Follow the Vancouver style

Chapter III: Methodology

- Research design
- Setting
- Population
- Sampling technique and sample (IC and EC, sample size)
- Data collection tools and techniques (from tool no 1 to tool no n, with content validity and reliability, development of the tools)
- Translation of tools
- Researcher training for tool use
- Tools try-out
- Interventions, if any
- Ethical clearance
- Informed consent
- Data collection procedure (method of data collection)
- Pilot study
- Duration of data collection
- Problems in data collection (if any)
- Data analysis plan

Chapter IV: Analysis and Interpretation

- Results
- Specify coding of data, master data sheet and statistical package used in data analysis (SPSS 22)

- Present data in sections, objective-wise
- Present statistical significant *p* value in bold
- Emphasise only important observations from tables/illustrations in the text without undue repetition of data and provide interpretation of the findings
- Do not repeat the same data in tables and illustrations.
- Start with a description of sample characteristics, then present findings as per the objectives of the study, if any extra finding, place at the end.
- Write the *p* value exactly.

Chapter V: Discussion

- Provide a summary of the main findings at the beginning of the chapter. Do not repeat all the data.
- Provide a discussion of the study findings (reviews in support of your findings, defend your findings with available literature or logic).
- Conclusions (avoid conclusions for which adequate data has not been obtained)
- Implications (nursing education, administration, practice and research)
- Recommendations (present and future)
- Limitations

Supplementary Section

References

- Use Vancouver style to format the references
- References should be numbered consecutively in the order in which they are first mentioned in the text
- They should not be listed alphabetically by author or title or put in date order.

Appendices

Place after the reference section. The common appendices in an undergraduate and postgraduate thesis may include:

- Letter granting ethical clearance
- Informed consent and PIS
- Tools, original and translated
- Any developed protocols/guidelines
- Competency certificate
- List of experts
- CD containing the soft copy of the thesis

Specific instructions for writing a thesis

- Type on one side of the paper only
- Para indent 5–7 spaces

- Keep the text left aligned, do not justify lines
- Do not divide the words at the end of the line
- Leave 1–1.5" space on all sides of the paper (Lt 1.5", Rt 1", top and bottom 1")
- Number the tables/figures consecutively and not for each chapter separately
- Insert the figure in the text page itself instead of in a fresh page every time
- Do not break a table on two pages
- Obtain copyright permission to use photographs in the thesis
- Give a brief but clear title to each table/figure
- English editing ensures that the thesis is free from grammatical and spelling mistakes
- Avoid abstract terms and technical jargon as far as possible
- Use past or present perfect tense for review and discussion of past events
- Use past tense to discuss results
- Use present tense for conclusions
- Passive voice and impersonal pronouns should be used throughout as these suggest greater impartiality. Do not use I/We/Me/Us (personal pronouns)

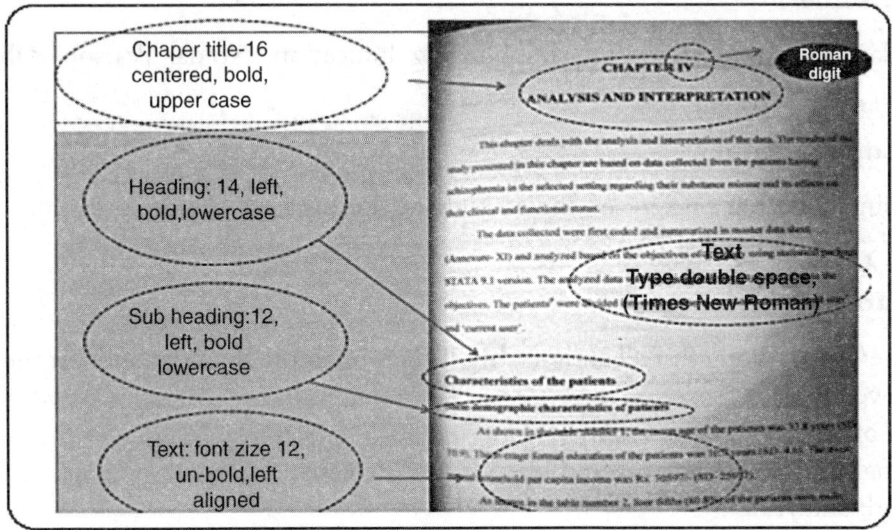

Figure 9.8 Font type, size for various section of thesis

Vancouver referencing style It is a numbered style of references that follows rules established by the International Committee of Medical Journal Editors. It is also known as Uniform Requirements for Manuscripts Submitted to Biomedical Journals. A list of references contains details only of those research papers cited in the text whereas a bibliography lists sources not cited in the text but which are relevant to the subject and were used for background reading.

Features

- In-text citing

- A number is allocated to a source in the order in which it is cited in the text
- If the source is referred to again, the same number is used
- Superscript as well as bracket format is acceptable for citing

Essential elements for referencing

For books

- Authors (list all authors, but if there are more than six, only list the first six followed by et al.)
  - Title
  - Edition
  - Place of publication
  - Publisher
  - Date (year)

Examples

Personal author

- Patidar AB. Communication and Nursing Education. Noida: Pearson Publication India; 2012.

Organisation as author

- Nursing Research Society of India. Nursing Research & Statistics. Noida: Pearson Publication India; 2013.

For a journal article

- Name/s of Author/s (list all authors, but if there are more than six, only list the first six followed by et al.).
- Title of article
- Journal title (abbreviated according to Index Medicus)
- Month and year
- Volume number
- Issue number
- Page numbers

Example

Patidar AB, Andrews GR, Seth S. Prevalence of obstructive sleep apnea, associated risk factors, and quality of life among Indian congestive heart failure patients: A cross sectional survey. *J Cardiovasc Nurs* 2011 Nov 26; 26(6):452–9.

No author given

Palliative and supportive care in advanced heart failure [editorial]. *Journal of Symptoms and Signs* 2012; 151–6.

Journal article in electronic format

Madden C. Service learning in nurse education: Teaching basic life support to school students. Response, University of Derby's online journal [Serial online] 2010[cited 2011 Sep 22];7:[2 screens]. Available from: URL: http://www2.derby.ac.uk/response/issue-7-new-horizons-pgr-conference-2010/71-cp/164-sl

Conference proceedings

Kumar S, Prabhakaran A, editors. Recent advances in clinical nursing. Proceedings of the 2nd National conference of nurse teacher association of India; 2015 Jan 15–19; Shimla, India; 1996.

Citing a newspaper article

Author. Title of article. Name of newspaper. Date of edition; Section if applicable (section abbreviated to Sect.); Page/s (1 space) Column number in round brackets (column abbreviated to col.).

RESEARCH UTILISATION

In the past, nursing care/practice has been based on tradition or authority. This is no longer acceptable in the era of evidence-based nursing practice. Nurses, being scientific professionals, must be able to justify the decisions they make and the care they provide to the patient. The situation in India is worrisome in this regard as the first-line care provider (GNM qualified nurses) lacks preparation in the research process, resulting in difficulties in using research in their practice. The main concern in the era of EBP is that the majority of practicing nurses have not experienced a formal research course. Thus, nursing research and EBP should be included in the RN-to-BSN curriculum and both the short-term and long-term effectiveness of the integration should be evaluated.

As the purpose of conducting nursing research is to endorse evidence-based nursing practice, study findings must be implemented in nursing practice. Research utilisation simply refers to the use of research findings in nursing practice. In the past few years, emphasis in the nursing literature has swung from research utilisation to evidence-based practice. While these terms are often used interchangeably, differentiation can be made between these two concepts. Evidenced-based practice is broader in scope than research utilisation as it encompasses not only evidence based on scientific findings but also evidence based on expert clinical opinion, patient and family preferences. Burns and Grove define research utilisation as, "The process of synthesizing, disseminating, and using research-generated knowledge to make an impact on or a change in the existing practices in society".

Barriers to research utilisation As pointed out by many nurse leaders and discussed at various scientific platforms, the utilisation of research findings in nursing practice is poor. There are many barriers to utilisation of research findings:

- **Nurses' negative attitude towards research**: Champion and Leach (1989) found that nurses' attitudes toward research were positively correlated to research utilisation (positive attitude towards research leads to positive attitude towards research utilisation). Similarly, Funk et al. (1991) reported in a study that slightly more than one-third of the respondents did not see the value of research in practice. Lewis et al. (1998) also reported similar findings in a study conducted on nephrology nurses.
- **Inadequate dissemination of research findings**: In India, most nursing research studies are never published or presented at professional conferences or workshops. Secondly, published or orally presented studies are often not explained at a level at which the practicing nurse can understand the findings. The journal articles are written in technical language that is not easily understood by practicing nurses.
- **Nurses' lack of knowledge of research**: Hutchinson and Johnston (2004) conducted a study on Australian nurses and reported that 66.2% listed lack of awareness of research as a barrier to research utilisation. Similarly, Paramonczyk (2005) reported lack of awareness of research findings as the second highest barrier to research utilisation among Canadian nurses.
- **Lack of organisational support for research**: Lack of institutional/organisational support has been recognised as a barrier to research utilisation in all of the published literature. Funk et al. (1991) conducted a study on approximately 2000 nurses in the United States and reported that the two greatest barriers to research utilisation were the nurses' report that they did not have "enough authority to change patient care procedures" and "insufficient time on the job to implement new ideas". Similarly, McCleary et al. (2003) surveyed 176 pediatric nurses in two teaching hospitals in Ontario, Canada. The study result highlighted lack of time to read research as the most frequent barrier to research utilisation. Paramonczyk (2005) also listed insufficient time on the job to implement new ideas as the greatest barrier to research utilisation.
- **Findings not ready to use in practice**: In an editorial in *Nursing Research*, Downs (1981) emphasised, "Research is not something that can be brewed overnight and ingested the next morning". She warned that research findings should not be consumed prematurely. Nursing practice cannot be changed on the basis of results of a single study. Polit (1996) also agreed that replication studies are needed because nurse researchers frequently use non-probability samples. It is also required for the continued development of the scientific basis of any discipline. Funk et al. (1989) stated that, "A crucial step in increasing the utilization of research results by practicing nurses is broad dissemination of research findings that are relevant and ready to use, in a form that is understandable to clinicians and with suggestions and support for implementation".

Facilitators of research utilisation

Organisation

- In-service facilities should have up-to-date research articles available at the nurse's station

- Willingness of the administrators to listen to nursing staff
- Encouragement shown by administrators for research utilisation/implementation of research findings

Research

- Making research easy to implement in a work setting

Communication/Presentation

- Communicating the research findings to applicable actions that can be implemented

Bridging the research and practice gap

Many nursing research utilisation projects have been described in literature. One widely known project is Conduct and Utilisation of Research in Nursing (CURN). Two models of research utilisation have also been described: innovation diffusion model proposed by Roger, and Stetler model of research utilisation.

CURN project CURN was a five-year project sponsored by Michigan Nurses Association. The main goal of the project was to increase the use of research findings in the daily practice of nurses. As a result of this project, nursing protocols were developed for nine clinical nursing practice problems. Horsley, Crane, Crabtree and Wood (1983) suggested the following steps for research utilisation:

1. Identify specific clinical nursing practice problems.
2. Assess the existing knowledge base on the issue.
3. Design a nursing practice innovation based on a scientific research base.
4. Implement clinical trials and evaluation of the innovation.
5. Decide to adopt, revise or reject the innovation.
6. Develop strategies to extend the innovation to other settings.
7. Determine means of continuing the innovation over time.

Innovation diffusion model This was developed by Roger. This model suggests five stages of innovation diffusion:

1. **Knowledge:** In this stage the nurse becomes aware of a research-based nursing intervention through conferences, journal articles and from discussions with colleagues.
2. **Persuasion:** In this stage, the nurse forms a positive or negative attitude towards the intervention based on the intervention's advantage, compatibility and complexity. After an attitude is formed, the decision stage is reached.
3. **Decision:** In this stage, the nurse decides whether or not to adopt the new intervention.
4. **Implementation:** In this stage, the nurse actually puts into practice the intervention or uses the knowledge indirectly, such as by discussing the findings with colleagues or citing it in one of their own publications.

5. **Confirmation:** In this stage, the intervention is evaluated for its effectiveness and a decision is made whether or not to continue using the intervention.

Stetler model of research utilisation This was first described in 1976. Stetler and Marram listed three phases of critical thinking:

1. Validation
2. Comparative evaluation
3. Decision-making

In 2001, Stetler revised the model and included two more steps:

1. Preparation
2. Validation
3. Comparative evaluation
4. Decision-making
5. Translation/Application and evaluation

The validation phase is also known as research utilisation critique. During this phase, an overall examination of the strengths and weaknesses of a study is undertaken, leading to a decision to accept or reject a particular study. The consumer must question every step of the research process. If a biased sample was used or invalid statistical procedures were used, the findings would be questionable. Stetler and Marram (1976) wrote that the consumer should look for, "What was found, about whom or what, under what conditions, by whom, when, where, and how". The nurse would also want to know how similar the research setting was to her own setting and how similar the study sample was to patients/clients with whom the nurse works. Comparative evaluation is undertaken to decide the feasibility of implementing the findings based on the constraints of the particular practice setting. Is there any legal risk to the patients, nurse or the organisation? Are resources available to adopt the innovation?

Once the nurse has assessed the feasibility, she must decide how to apply the findings. The nurse may choose a cognitive or direct application of the findings. Cognitive application implies that the nurse is not yet ready to implement the findings in practice but will use the information to enhance her knowledge base and may consider moving to direct application in the future. Direct application of research findings means that the nurse has decided to test the findings in practice.

CHAPTER SUMMARY

- A research project is not considered complete until the findings have been communicated to others.
- The findings of research can be communicated orally or in writing.

- While preparing the research report, due consideration should be given to tense, as most of the research report should be written in the past tense because the study has already occurred.
- Presentation of research findings at local, regional and national conferences enables quicker dissemination of study results to professional nurses.
- The oral presentation of a research report is also known as a paper presentation. A presenter is allotted 15–30 minutes to present the paper. At some conferences, the presenter may have to allow time for discussion if questions are desired.
- The format of the oral presentation is similar to that of a journal article or other written research report of the study, as the steps of the research process are usually presented in chronological order.
- Research poster sessions are an excellent way for novice researchers to get an idea of the presentation process and is less intimidating than oral presentation.
- Publishing an article in a journal has the potential to reach the largest percentage of nurses. It is considered a means of obtaining recognition for the author or authors.
- Once the article is accepted for publication, the authors are provided with galley proofs that are sheets of paper showing how the article will appear in typeset form. The authors are asked to proofread for errors and minor corrections in the galley proofs.
- The average time from first submission to notification of acceptance for publication is about 6.5 months.
- The length of journal articles varies a great deal, but most journals prefer manuscripts of 10–15 typed pages.
- Nurses, being scientific professionals, must be able to justify the decisions they make and the care they provide to the patient.
- Burns and Grove have defined research utilisation as, "The process of synthesizing, disseminating, and using research-generated knowledge to make an impact on or a change in the existing practices in society".
- Nurses' negative attitude toward research; inadequate dissemination of nursing research findings; lack of knowledge of nursing research; lack of institutional support for research, and study findings not ready for use in nursing practice are important barriers to research utilisation.
- Two models of research utilisation are innovation diffusion model proposed by Roger and Stetler model of research utilisation.

EVALUATE YOURSELF

Long Answer Questions

Q1: What do you mean by research utilisation? How will you improve research utilisation in your organisation?

Q2: How will you communicate your research findings? Explain in detail.

Q3: Explain the barriers in research utilisation in nursing.

Q4: How will you publish your research findings in a scientific journal?

Q5: Describe the conduct and utilisation of research in a nursing project.

Short Answer Questions

Write short notes on:

1. Peer-reviewed journal
2. Oral and poster presentation at professional conferences
3. Facilitator of research utilisation
4. Preparing an article for journals
5. Bridging the research and practice gap

Multiple Choice Questions

Q1: Which communication media can reach the largest percentage of nurses?
(a) Dissertation
(b) Journal article
(c) Paper presentation (oral)
(d) Poster

Q2: Which communication medium to disseminate research findings is probably the most appropriate for a novice researcher?
(a) Journal article
(b) Oral presentation
(c) Research paper
(d) Poster presentation

Q3: Which of the following is a reason for the rejection of a manuscript submitted to a journal?
(a) Manuscript is poorly written.
(b) Content of manuscript is inaccurate.
(c) Content of manuscript is not appropriate for the journal's readers.
(d) All of the above.

Q4: Which of the following is true for journal articles?
(a) Query letter should be sent before a manuscript is submitted.
(b) Format for research articles is usually the same for all journals.
(c) Journals do not accept manuscripts from novice researchers.
(d) Revisions are generally not needed in manuscripts submitted to journals.

Q5: The main aim of the CURN project sponsored by Michigan Nurses Association was
(a) To enhance methodological rigor in nursing research
(b) To find ways to improve the scientific status of nursing profession
(c) To put up the nurses' demand to the government
(d) To increase the use of research findings in the daily practice of nurses

Q6: Innovation diffusion model was proposed by

(a) Stetler (b) Roger
(c) Handeson (d) Orem

Q7: How many authors' names can be included in a journal article according to the Vancouver's style of referencing before inserting the word et al?

(a) Two (b) Four
(c) Six (d) Eight

Q8: Ideally, the abstract should be placed:

(a) In the middle of the thesis (b) At the end of the thesis
(c) At the beginning of the thesis (d) Anywhere in the thesis

Answers

1. b **2.** d **3.** d **4.** b **5.** d

6. b **7.** c **8.** c

FURTHER READING

Alcock D, Carroll G, Goodman M. 1990. Staff nurses perceptions of factors influencing their role in research. *The Canadian Journal of Nursing Research* 22(4): 7–18.

American Nurses Foundation Board of Trustees. 2005. American Nurses Foundation: Celebrating 50 years of service 1955–2005. *Nursing Research* 54:147.

Becker PT. 2004. What happens to my manuscript when I send it to *Research in Nursing & Health?. Research in Nursing & Health* 27: 379–389.

Berg JA. 2005. Creating a professional poster presentation: Focus on nurse practitioners. *Journal of the American Academy of Nurse Practitioners* 17: 245–248.

Bock LR. 1990. From research to utilization: Bridging the gap. *Nursing Management* 21: 50–51.

Burns N, Grove SK. 2005. *The practice of nursing research: Conduct, critique, and utilization, 5th ed.* Elsevier Saunders, St. Louis, MO.

Champion VL, Leach A. 1989. Variables related to research utilization in nursing: An empirical investigation. *Journal of Advanced Nursing* 14: 705–710.

Champion VL, Leach A. 1989. Variables related to research utilization in nursing: an empirical investigation. *Journal of Advanced Nursing* 14: 705–710.

Cronenwett LR. 1995. Effective methods for disseminating research findings to nurses in practice. *Nursing Clinics of North America* 30(3): 429–438.

Dougherty MC. 2005. Open peer review. *Nursing Research* 53:213.

Edwards-Beckett J. 1990. Nursing research utilization techniques. *Journal of Nursing Administration* 20(11): 25–30.

Fink R, Thompson CJ, Bonnes D. 2005. Overcoming barriers and promoting the use of research in practice. *Journal of Nursing Administration* 35: 121–129.

Fitzpatrick JJ. 2006. Challenges: The continued gap between research and professional practice. *Applied Nursing Research* 19:1.

Funk SG, Champagne MT, Tornquist EM, Wiese RA. 1995. Administrators' views on barriers to research utilization. *Applied Nursing Research* 8: 44–49.

Funk SG, Champagne MT, Wiese RA, Tornquist EM. 1991. Barriers: The barriers to research utilization scale. *Applied Nursing Research* 4(1): 39–45.

Gennaro S. 1996. Research utilization: An overview. *Journal of Gynecological and Neonatal Nursing* 23: 313–319.

Hutchinson AM, Johnston L. 2004. Bridging the divide: A survey of nurses' opinions regarding barriers to, and facilitators of, research utilization in the practice setting. *Journal of Clinical Nursing,* 13: 304–315.

Kajermo KN, Nordström G, Krusebrant Å, Björvell H. 1998. Barriers to and facilitators of research utilization, as perceived by a group of registered nurses in Sweden. *Journal of Advanced Nursing* 27: 798–807.

Kennedy MS. 2004. Not your grandma's nursing research. *American Journal of Nursing* 104:11.

McCleary L, Brown GT. 2003. Barriers to paediatric nurses' research utilization. *Journal of Advanced Nursing* 42: 364–372.

McConnell EA. 2000. Nursing publications outside the United States. *Journal of Nursing Scholarship* 32: 87–92.

Miracle VA, King KC. 1994. Presenting research: Effective paper presentations and impressive poster presentations. *Applied Nursing Research* 7: 147–151.

Retsas A. 2000. Barriers to using research evidence in nursing practice. *Journal of Advanced Nursing* 31: 599–606.

Rogers EM. 1995. *Diffusion of innovations, 4th ed.* The Free Press, New York.

Ryan NM. 1989. Developing and presenting a research poster. *Applied Nursing Research* 2: 52–55.

Stetler CB, Marram G. 1976. Evaluating research findings for applicability in practice. *Nursing Outlook* 24: 559–563.

Stetler CB. 1994. Refinement of the Stetler-Marram model for application of research findings to practice. *Nursing Outlook* 42: 15–25.

Stetler CB. 2001. Updating the Stetler model of research utilization to facilitate evidence based practice. *Nursing Outlook* 49: 272–279.

Taggart HM, Arslanian C. 2000. Creating an effective poster presentation. *Orthopaedic Nursing* 19: 47–52.

Winslow EH. 1996. Failure to publish research: A form of scientific misconduct? *Heart & Lung* 25: 169–171.

10 Critiquing Research Articles/Reports

Chapter overview

- Introduction to critiquing research articles
- Definition of terms
- Steps in quantitative research critiquing
- Steps in qualitative research critiquing

INTRODUCTION TO CRITIQUING RESEARCH ARTICLES

Research refers to a systematic inquiry that uses disciplined methods to answer questions or solve problems. Before applying the findings of a research study in clinical practice, the research methodology used to generate the findings must be critiqued. A critical appraisal of the strengths and limitations of a research study is necessary to ensure the dependability of the study results. Research critique refers to a systematic process of objectively reviewing a piece of research to ascertain both its strengths and its weaknesses, and its applicability in nursing practice.

The novice researcher must understand that research critiquing is not about finding errors in a study. Rather, it is a mechanism to provide feedback for improvement (Boswell and Cannon 2010). Most research studies have limitations and weaknesses therefore, the authenticity of the research findings should be assessed by careful critical analysis to determine evidence for improvement in nursing practice and to provide a background for conducting further study.

DEFINITION OF TERMS

A research critique is a carefully conducted thorough assessment of a study to evaluate its strengths, weaknesses, significance, scientific merit and application to clinical nursing practice, nursing theory or education.

It determines the authenticity of the information, assesses the credibility of the study results and weighs the evidence in terms of objectivity, utilisation, application and replication. The critique focuses on the key areas of methodology and determines whether the methodology undertaken to test an intervention or explore a problem is appropriate or ideal or if there are limitations that restrict the generalisability of the study findings. The process of critiquing is an impersonal/objective analysis of a piece of research work aimed at highlighting the strengths and weaknesses of the study. As nursing practice becomes increasingly evidenced-based, it is important that nursing care be based on sound research. All nurses should be competent enough to critically appraise research in order to identify what is the best practice.

Steps in Quantitative Research Critiquing

A quantitative research critique evaluates the quality of all steps of the quantitative research process undertaken by the researcher in the given research report. It also examines the organisation and presentation of the research report. The reviewer should be objective and realistic in identifying the study's strengths and weaknesses by providing specific examples of the same in the study. Feasibility of replication and usefulness of findings for clinical practice should be given due emphasis. The critique should begin with an understanding of the fundamental terms and concepts in the report, identifying the elements or steps of the research process such as problem, purpose, framework and design used by the researcher. Thereafter, every step is evaluated against the ideal criteria for the type of research undertaken. These guidelines are also helpful to a novice researcher while writing a research article for a journal.

Title

The ideal title should be between 10 and 15 words long. Titles that are too long or too short can be confusing or misleading (Parahoo 2006). The reviewer, while critiquing the title section of a report, should ask the following questions:

- Is the title of the research report too long or too short to provide accurate information about the study?
- Does the title clearly specify the purpose of the study?

Author(s)

The authors' qualifications and job title is a useful indicator to the researcher's knowledge of the area under investigation. The evaluator should ask the following questions:

- What are the author's professional qualifications?
- Has she published previously on a similar topic?

Abstract

Abstract is the summary that represents the entire article and is usually 150–250 words in length, depending on the journal's requirements. It should provide the necessary information to enable a reader to decide whether the article is of interest to her or not and whether or not to continue reading the entire article. It should provide a short and snappy overview of the article and include information regarding the purpose of the study, method, sample size, result, conclusion, discussion and recommendations. While reviewing the abstract, the reviewer should ask the following questions:

- Does the abstract explain the objectives of the paper?
- What methods were used to achieve the study objectives?
- What were the main findings?
- What conclusions were drawn based on the findings?

Introduction

The introduction should orientate the reader about the research questions/problem and develop the background of the study, including the purpose and need for research. The reviewer should focus on the following questions:

- Has the research question/problem been stated clearly?
- Does the problem statement express a relationship between two or more variables?
- Does the problem statement specify the nature of the population being studied?
- Is the problem significant enough to justify the enquiry?

Aims and objectives/research hypothesis

The aims and objectives of the study should be stated in clear and concise terms. Experimental and quasi-experimental studies should clearly state a hypothesis, including the dependent and independent variables and the population under investigation. The following questions should be considered:

- What is the purpose of the enquiry/study?
- Does the purpose of the study identify a relationship between two or more variables?
- What are the independent and dependent variables in the statement of hypothesis?
- What is the direction of the relationship in each hypothesis, if indicated?
- Are the hypotheses testable?

Theoretical framework

This should be presented following identification of the research problem. It should present the concepts being studied and the relationship between these concepts. The research study should then elaborate on this theory through empirical observation. Many research reports may not have a theoretical framework; however, nursing studies usually include a conceptual/theoretical framework depending on the requirement of the journal. The following questions should be considered:

- Are the concepts under study identified clearly?
- Does the theoretical framework inter-relate the concepts meaningfully?

Operational definitions

In a research study, the researcher needs to ensure that the reader understands the terms and concepts used in the research. The important variables and process of measuring them should be presented clearly.

Literature review

The literature review should provide an overview of the available literature related to the research problem being researched. It should cover an appropriate depth and breadth of reading around the topic being studied. Most of the studies included should be of recent origin and ideally less than five years old. However, there may be exceptions to this, for example, in areas where there is a paucity of research. Primary sources should be used more often than secondary sources. The literature review should begin with an introduction that identifies the keywords used to conduct the literature search and information about the databases (PubMed, CINHAL, Cochrane, etc.) used.

The reviewer, while critiquing the literature review, should ask the following questions:

- Is the literature review organised systematically (chronologically)?
- Is the literature review focused on the research problem?
- Does the review of literature also represent opposing views on the topic?
- Does it highlight gaps in knowledge which this study will fill?

Materials and methods

Methodology refers to the nuts and bolts of a research project. The materials and method section of the research report usually has subsections that describe the research approach, design, participants, sample size, sampling technique, randomisation procedure (in randomised control trials), full details of the intervention, validity and reliability, procedure for data collection and ethical clearance.

- *Research approach*—whether the chosen approach (quantitative or qualitative or mixed method) is justified for the given research problem.
- *Research design*—whether the researcher has adopted a research design best suited to answer the research question in the given research setting and other situational constraints. The design must seem to surge from the literature review, theoretical framework and hypothesis. Fig. 10.1 shows an example of a research design.

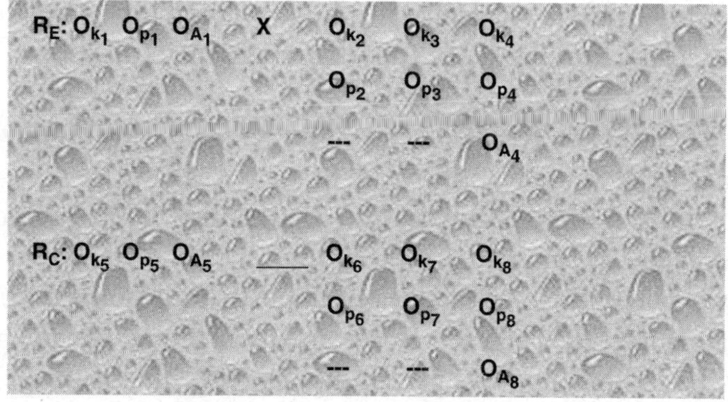

Figure 10.1 Research design

RE: Randomly assigned experimental group
OK$_1$: Pretest knowledge for experimental group
OP$_1$: Pretest practice for experimental group
OA$_1$: Pretest attitude for experimental group
X: BLS Training Programme
OK$_2$: Post-test knowledge for experimental group on Day 7
OP$_2$: Post-test practice for experimental group on Day 7
OK$_3$: Post-test knowledge for experimental group on Day 30
OP$_3$: Post-test practice for experimental group on Day 30
OK$_4$: Post-test knowledge for experimental group on Day 60
OP$_4$: Post-test practice for experimental group on Day 60
OA$_4$: Post-test attitude for experimental group on Day 60
OK$_5$: Pretest knowledge for control group
OP$_5$: Pretest practice for control group
OA$_5$: Pretest attitude for control group
OK$_6$: Post test knowledge for control group on Day 7
OP$_6$: Post test practice for control group on Day 7
OK$_7$: Post test knowledge for control group on Day 30
OP$_7$: Post test practice for control group on Day 30
OK$_8$: Post test knowledge for control group on Day 60
OP$_8$: Post test practice for control group on Day 60
OA$_8$: Post test attitude for control group on Day 60
RC: Randomly assigned control group

- *Participants or sample*—the number of participants/sample size, their inclusion and exclusion criteria and the selection process (sampling technique). If any participants dropped out from the study (usually in a longitudinal study), it should be mentioned clearly and the bias or possible distortion in results should be discussed. Details such as any reward/remuneration made to participants should be specified. The size of the sample is an important factor to determine the generalisability of the findings. Therefore, the sample size calculation should be mentioned clearly in the report. Ask the following questions:

- How was the sample recruited?
- Is the sampling technique appropriate to the design?
- Does the sample reflect the population as identified in the problem statement?
- Is the sample size appropriate for the study?

- *Randomisation*—the experimental research report should provide information about how the participants were assigned to the experimental and control groups.
- *Intervention*—basic information pertaining to the intervention, dose, frequency, withdrawal and re-institution of intervention at prescribed intervals and duration of the intervention should be given to provide a clear understanding of the intervention to the readers. If any apparatus was used, it should be described briefly and its utility in the research be explained.
- *Data collection procedure*—in a quantitative study, various strategies are used to collect data such as structured interviews, self-report questionnaires, attitude scales or observational checklist. Researchers can use a previously designed standardised tool or develop one for the study. However, this should be mentioned clearly in the research report. The data collection procedure should be explained step by step (see the example below).

Example: Steps in Data Collection

- Written permission for data collection was obtained from Principal, DMCH College of Nursing and the selected schools. The data was collected from students studying in selected schools of Punjab (April 2012–March 2013).
- Selected school was randomised by tossing a coin, either in control group or in experiment group.
- Students of Class 9, who fulfilled the inclusion criteria and were willing to participate in the study, were included in the study.
- Written informed consent was obtained from the students after explaining the nature, aims and purpose of the study.
- The students were administered the English version of the assessment tools in the following order:
    - In experiment group: Before intervention, the students were given a structured knowledge questionnaire and attitude scale. The investigator filled the observation checklist by observing student performance on the dummy. Post-intervention, Day 7, the students were again given Part II of the structured knowledge questionnaire and the investigator filled the observation checklist by observing the student performance on the dummy. Post-intervention, Day 30, the students were again given Part II of the structured knowledge

questionnaire and the investigator filled the observation checklist by observing the student performance on the dummy. Post-intervention, Day 90, the students were given the Part II of the structured knowledge questionnaire and attitude scale. The investigator filled the observation checklist by observing the student performance on the dummy. The same protocol was followed for the control group except that they were not given interventions.

- Students filled the structured knowledge questionnaire and attitude scale in the classroom itself in the presence of the investigator. During this, they were called one by one for height and weight measurement. Height was measured using a non-elastic inch tape mounted on the wall. Weight was measured using a spring balance weighing machine. The same machine was used throughout the study. Skill was assessed in a separate room using the training dummy. The student was asked to perform two cycles of cardiopulmonary resuscitation. The investigator observed the student's performance and filled the observation checklist. The collected data was entered in a master data sheet for analysis.

- *Validity and reliability*—validity is the ability of the instrument to measure what it is supposed to measure and reliability is the ability of the tool to consistently and accurately measure the concept under investigation. If a standardised tool has been used and not modified in any way, the validity and reliability will have been determined already and the researcher should just mention it. However, if the instrument has been modified or is being used for a new population, then previous validity and reliability will not be applicable. In this situation, the researcher should indicate the process of validity and reliability establishment of the modified tool.
- Ethics clearance—the process of obtaining ethics clearance and how ethical standards were maintained; whether the Institutional Ethics Committee/Institutional Review Board approved the study protocols.

The following questions should be considered while reviewing the material and methodology section:

- Is the chosen research approach design appropriate for the study?
- Is the research method proper for the research question?
- Is the tool used for data collection reliable and valid?
- What type of data collection methods are used in the study?
- Are the data collection procedures similar for all subjects?
- How have the rights of subjects been protected?
- Has informed consent been obtained from the subjects?
- Were the ethical considerations appropriate for the research and the participants?

Results

This section should contain the main results and findings, in enough detail (with statistical test value, *p* value and confidence interval). Tables and figures should be used for clear representation of data. The researcher should clearly identify what statistical tests were undertaken and why these tests were used.

Quantitative studies usually identify the lowest level of significance as 0.05. The percentage of the sample that completed the study is an important element in considering the generalisability of the results. The reviewer should ask:

- Has all the data has been taken into account? If not, why not?
- Are the results relevant to the research question?
- Do the results answer the research questions?
- What descriptive or inferential statistics are reported?
- Was the type of statistics used appropriate to the level of measurement for each variable?
- Are the inferential statistics used appropriately for hypotheses testing?
- Does the author report the level of significance set for the study? If so, what is it?
- Do the tables or figures have precise titles and headings?

Discussion

The results of the current study and those of other relevant previous studies should be discussed, and any suggestions for improvements or further research be made. There should be no repetition of points already made in other sections. The reviewer should check whether the results explain the connection between the theoretical framework and the research questions. A discussion of the findings should be related to the literature review, thus placing the study in context (Russell 2002). In this section, consideration should be given to external validity of the study. In addition, the researcher should make meaningful suggestions for future research in the area.

The following questions should be considered while reviewing the discussion section:

- Have the results been discussed in relation to the research question, and theoretical or conceptual frameworks?
- Have the results been compared with the results of previous studies?
- Have conclusions and/or recommendations been made appropriately from the data analysis?

Limitations

- Have the limitations been identified by the researcher?
- Have the implications of the limitations been discussed?

Conclusion

This section should summarise the main points and conclude the study results. However, it should not include any new information. The reviewer should check whether any new perspectives on the topic is demonstrated.

For conclusions, implications and recommendations, ask the following questions:

- Was/Were the hypotheses supported or not supported?
- Are the results interpreted in the context of the purpose, hypothesis/literature reviewed?
- Are the generalisations within the scope of the findings or beyond the findings?
- What recommendations for future research are stated or implied?
- How and under what circumstances are the findings applicable to nursing practice?
- Should these results be applied to nursing practice?
- Would it be possible to replicate this study in another clinical practice setting?

Reference list or bibliography

Sources referred to in the article should be compiled in the reference list; sources actually accessed in preparation for the article should be included in the bibliography. The research study should conclude with an accurate list of all the books, journal articles, reports and other media referred to in the article (Polit and Beck 2006).

Many tools can help novice and advanced reviewers critique research studies. Ryan-Wenger (1992) proposed a method for research critique in which they included two types of questions for critiquing a research article: credibility questions and integrity questions. Credibility questions ask how believable the work is. They focus on the researcher's qualifications and ability to undertake and accurately present the study findings. Integrity questions are concerned with the robustness of the research method.

Steps in Qualitative Research Critiquing

Qualitative research is different from quantitative research; therefore, for critiquing qualitative research, the researcher should have adequate understanding of qualitative research methods like grounded theory, phenomenology and ethnography.

The qualitative research critique focuses on the following criteria:

- **Descriptive vividness:** Quality study requires a rich description that is vivid (lively) to readers of the report. The purpose of the study, significance and interpretations must be clearly articulated so that the reader has the sense of personally experiencing the event so that they can clearly understand the significance of the study findings.
- **Methodological congruency:** The critique should judge whether the approach used in the study is consistent with the philosophical base of the study. Is adequate documentation of the participants and rationale for their selection clearly described? Is the context and location depicted fully?

- **Analysis and interpretation preciseness**: The analytical process involves a series of interpretations and data transformations so that data can be converted to several levels of abstraction. Data analysis and interpretation conveys meaning to the phenomenon under study. It requires the researcher to involve others in the interpretative process (data interpretation triangulation) so that a meaningful picture of the phenomenon under study can be presented.
- **Theoretical connectedness**: Theoretical connectedness critique focuses on study assumptions, methodological procedure, interpretative and analytic approach. These must be consistent with the philosophical or theoretical basis of the study.
- **Heuristic relevance**: This is reflected in the reader's ability to recognise the phenomenon under study, its applicability to nursing practice and its persuasion on future research. Heuristic relevance critique asks the following questions:
  - Will the readers be able to recognise the phenomenon and its connection to their personal and professional experiences and to nursing practice (intuitive recognition)?
  - What are the similarities between the current knowledge base and the study findings? Are the findings applicable to nursing practice, research and education?

CHAPTER SUMMARY

- Research critique refers to a systematic process of objectively reviewing a piece of research to as certain both its strengths and its weaknesses, and its applicability to nursing practice.
- A research critique is a careful complete assessment of a study to evaluate its strengths, weaknesses, significance, scientific merit and application to practice, theory or education.
- A quantitative research critique evaluates the quality of all the steps of the quantitative research process taken by the researcher in the given research report; it also examines the organisation and presentation of the research report.
- The ideal title should be between 10 and 15 words long.
- Abstract is a representative summary of the entire article and is usually 50–250 words in length, depending on the journal's requirements.
- Aims and objectives of the study should be stated in clear and concise terms.
- Theoretical framework should present the various concepts being studied and the relationship between those concepts.
- Review of literature should cover an appropriate depth and breadth of reading around the topic being studied. Most of the studies included should be of recent origin and ideally less than five years old.
- The materials and method section of the research report usually has subsections that describe the research approach, design, participants, sample size, sampling technique, randomisation procedure, details of intervention and ethical clearance.

- The result section should contain the main results and findings, in enough detail (with statistical test value, *p* value, confidence interval).
- The discussion section should include the results of the current study and those of other studies, and any suggestions for improvements or further research are made here.
- The conclusion section should summarise the main points and conclude the study results.
- The research study should conclude with an accurate list of all the books, journal articles, reports and other media referred to in the work.
- Qualitative research critique focuses on descriptive vividness, methodological congruency, analysis and interpretation preciseness, theoretical connectedness and heuristic relevance.

EVALUATE YOURSELF

Long Answer Questions

Q1: What is research critiquing? How it is used to support evidenced-based nursing practice?

Q2: What are the important steps of qualitative research critiquing?

Q3: Elaborate the important steps of quantitative research critiquing?

Short Answer Questions

Write short notes on:

1. Need for research critiquing
2. Descriptive vividness in qualitative research
3. Critiquing methodology section in quantitative research
4. Criteria for critiquing abstracts
5. Criteria for critiquing review of literature
6. How you will critique the discussion section in a research report

Multiple Choice Questions

Q1: A research critique should be:

(a) Subjective
(b) Objective
(c) Confidential
(d) Both a and c

Q2: An ideal study title should be written in:

(a) 20–30 words
(b) 10–15 words
(c) 20–25words
(d) 20–30 words

Q3: The word limit for an ideal abstract is:

(a) 150–250 words (b) 250–500 words
(c) 350–400 words (d) 400–500 word

Answers

1. b **2.** b **3.** a

FURTHER READING

Bassett C, Bissett J. 2003. Reading and critiquing research. *Br J Perioper Nri K* 13(4): 162–164.

Beauchamp T, Childress J. 2001. *Principles of Biomedical Ethics, 5th ed.* Oxford University Press, Oxford.

Burns N, Grove S. 1997. *The Practice of Nursing Research: Conduct, Critique and Utilization, 3rd ed.* WB Saunders Company, Philadelphia.

Burns N, Grove S. 1999. *Understanding Nursing Research, 2nd ed.* WB Saunders Company. Philadelphia.

Burns N, Grove SK. 2007. *Understanding Nursing Research, 4th ed.* Elsevier, New Delhi.

Mateo MA, Kirchhoff KT. 1999. *Using and Conducting Nursing Research in the Clinical Setting, 2nd ed.* WB Saunders Company, Philadelphia.

Parahoo K. 2006. *Nursing Research, 2nd ed.* Palgrave, New York.

Polit D, Beck C, 2006. *Essentials of Nursing Care: Methods, Appraisal and Utilization, 6th ed.* Lippincott Williams and Wilkins, Philadelphia.

Polit DF, Hungler BP. 1995. *Nursing Research: Principles and Methods, 6th ed.* JB Lippincott, Philadelphia.

Polit H, Beck CT. 2008. *Nursing Research, 8th ed.* Williams and Wilkins, New Delhi.

Russell C. 2005. Evaluating quantitative research reports. *Nephrol Nurs J* 32(1): 61–4.

Ryan F, Coughlan M, Cronin P. 2007. Step-by-step guide to critiquing research. Part 2: Qualitative research, *British Journal of Nursing* 16 (12): 738–743.

Ryan-Wenger N. 1992. Guidelines for critique of a research report. *Heart Lung* 21(4): 394–401.

Stockhausen L, Conrick M. 2002. Making sense of research: A guide for critiquing a paper, *Contemporary Nurse* 14 (1): 38–45.

Talbot LA. 1995. *Principles and Practice of Nursing Research.* Mosby, St. Louis.

Tanner J. 2003. Reading and critiquing research. *Br J Perioper Nurs* 13(4): 162–164.

Wood GL, Haber J. 2002. *Nursing Research Methods, Critical Appraisal and Utilization, 5th ed.* Mosby, St Louis.

11 Research Proposals

Chapter overview

- Introduction to research proposals
- Types of proposals
- Writing a research proposal
- Steps in developing a research proposal
- Characteristics of a quality research proposal
- Budget plan, action plan
- Final proofreading and editing
- Common reasons for proposal rejection

INTRODUCTION TO RESEARCH PROPOSALS

According to their curriculum, students of MSc Nursing are required to write a synopsis/ research proposal for their proposed thesis to be submitted to the University. Research proposals are usually developed after the institutional research committee selects an appropriate research problem. Alternatively, the seasoned researcher can develop the same in response to a call placed by a funding agency. The research proposal formally describes the research process for the proposed problem statement. A well-written research proposal ensures that scholars have done sufficient preliminary work in the proposed area of research. It is an **intellectual scholastic contract** between the scholar and the research committee of the organisation/university/funding agency. The research committee judges the scientific merit and feasibility of the research proposal before approving the same. It is noteworthy that a well-planned and worked out research proposal is the backbone of a successful thesis, whereas a vague, poorly conceptualised proposal may be a disaster for the scholar.

While writing the proposal, the researcher should aim to convince the research committee that the proposal has scientific merit and that she has identified the methodology best suited to carry out the proposed study within the given time frame and resources. Further, the results of the proposed study will be useful to professionals in solving current practice issues. The researchers are advised to visit the website of the university/funding agency and carefully read the instructions to be followed while writing the proposal. The format of a formal research proposal may vary (length/word limit, structure and format) from university to university; however, the basic content remains the same. Research proposals can be of many types, so the content will vary accordingly.

TYPES OF PROPOSALS

Solicited/Request for proposals

Solicited/Requested proposals are those prepared and submitted in response to a call for a proposal by a funding agency in the specified area of interest. The proposal submitted in response to this call is known as a solicited proposal. Researchers are advised to visit the website of the particular agency before writing the formal proposal. For example, Indian Council of Medical Research solicits research proposals in specified areas of interest, such as HIV/AIDS, tuberculosis, epidemiology of malaria, kala azar, and so on.

Unsolicited proposals

This type of research proposal is prepared by the researcher in her area of interest. Thereafter, it may be submitted to a funding agency that the researcher believes has an interest in the proposed research area.

Pre-proposals

Pre-proposals are usually solicited before a full-length research proposal. The purpose of the pre-proposal is to minimise an applicant's effort in preparing a full-length proposal. Also, the funding agency can perform a quick review of the brief pre-proposal. If the agency is interested after such a review, the researcher can then submit the full-length proposal.

Continuation proposals

As the name suggests, this type of research proposal is submitted for a proposal that the funding agency has already accepted and for which it has provided initial funding. It is submitted to request for the release of further funds, and the acceptance of the same usually depends on satisfactory work progress as well as availability of funds with the sponsoring agency.

WRITING A RESEARCH PROPOSAL

The format of a research proposal may vary according to the requirements and format of the university or funding agency. However, the general outline and content of a research proposal is as follows:

- Title page
- Abstract
- Introduction and background of the study
- Need for the study
- Problem statement
- Aims and objectives
- Literature review
- Material and methods
  - Study approach, study design
  - Research subject, population, sample size, power of the study, sample size calculation, sampling technique, inclusion/exclusion criteria
  - Study variables
  - Interventional protocols
  - Data collection tools and techniques
  - Ethical considerations
  - Consent form
  - Pilot study/try out
  - Statistical methods/tests/level of significance
- Budget plan
- Work plan
- Dissemination plan

Title page

This is the first page of the research proposal and should include the following information.

Personal information about the researchers

- Name
- Academic title (Dr, Prof)
- Position held by the researcher, for example, Assistant Professor/Associate Professor/ Professor
- Nationality (for proposals to be submitted to international funding agencies)
- Office/Home address
- Telephone/Fax and e-mail

Title of the proposed research study This should be stated clearly and concisely. The title is usually brief and hence immense care must be taken for the selection of appropriate words and their association with one another.

For example: An experimental study to evaluate the effectiveness of a training programme on the knowledge, attitudes and practice of Basic Life Support techniques among students of Class 9 from selected schools in Punjab.

Abstract

This provides a clear and concise snapshot of the proposed study. It can be formatted or not, depending on the requirements of the agency. However, the researcher must pay great attention while writing the abstract as it should provide condensed information related to the study within a limited word count. All the important information must be incorporated in the abstract and it should be stimulating enough to stir the interest of the reader to go through the entire proposal.

Introduction and background of the study

This section should introduce the research topic by providing the scientific background of the proposed research problem. It should inform the reviewer about the current trends and literature upon which the proposed study is based, and it should expose the unanswered questions and explore the existing gap in the literature. The introduction should start with a broad overview of the topic and gradually focus on the proposed research area.

Need for the study

Research is a labour-intensive task that requires investment of time, energy and money. Therefore, the researcher must justify why the proposed study must be undertaken and explain the benefits of carrying out this project. She must also elaborate on the new information it might yield, how it can improve the practice of nursing and benefit mankind at large. In this section, the researcher should present arguments to justify why it is important to undertake the proposed research project by providing relevant references from the literature. The researcher must also explain how the proposed study will fill gaps in existing knowledge or resolve current controversies.

For example, the need for the above cited research title may be written as follows:

In India there is paucity of work in this direction. The current study is aimed at evaluating the effectiveness of the training programme on the knowledge, attitudes and practice of Basic Life Support techniques among Class 9 students from selected schools in Punjab. In India, increasing the number of lay BLS providers is the need of the hour because of the alarming rise in the prevalence of coronary artery disease (CAD), which in turn is responsible for most out-of-hospital sudden cardiac deaths. As the prevalence of CAD is rising among the young who are economically productive, it may have a negative impact on the economy of the nation. The finding of the current study will also provide baseline data to plan for other interventional strategies to improve BLS techniques among school children.

Problem statement

The research question or problem should be stated clearly and concisely. It should be an attention-grabbing statement.

For example: A descriptive study to assess the level of assertiveness among staff nurses working in tertiary care hospitals of Bhopal, MP.

Aims and objectives

Aims are the broad general statements indicating the goals of the project. The aims should be stated clearly. Objectives are more specific and should be given separately. They should incorporate the key study variables, relationship/association/correlation between two or more study variables and the type of the population of interest. For example, for the problem statement given above, the aims and objectives can be as follows:

Aims The current study aims to assess the level of assertiveness among staff nurses working in a tertiary care hospital in Bhopal, Madhya Pradesh.

Objectives

- To assess the level of assertiveness among staff nurses working in a tertiary care hospital in Bhopal
- To determine the association between the level of assertiveness and professional qualification among staff nurses
- To determine the association between the level of assertiveness and professional experience among staff nurses
- To determine the association between the level of assertiveness and selected socio-demographic variables among staff nurses

The research objectives should be followed by a hypothesis in an experimental study. It should tentatively predict or explain the relationship between two or more variables. The researcher can state the research problem or statistical hypothesis, indicating the level of significance.

Sometimes, research questions can replace the research objectives. Research questions are interrogative statements that reflect the objectives of the research project, directly or indirectly. Both research objectives and research questions may be stated sometimes, depending on the requirements or format of the research proposal. For example, research questions for the research problem stated above may be as follows:

1. What is the level of assertiveness among staff nurses working in a tertiary care hospital in the city of Bhopal?
2. Are graduate nurses more assertive than diploma nurses?
3. Are experienced nurses more assertive than novice nurses?
4. Are nurses working in critical care settings more assertive than nurses working in other clinical areas?

Literature review

This section should provide a brief account of the most recent studies related to the research area. It should critically appraise the work done in the past to prepare a background/context and need for the proposed research study. The review should be logical, comprehensive, complete and up to date; however, recitation of every study ever conducted is not required.

Material and methods

This is the heart of the research proposal and requires a lot of consideration before the methodological aspects of the proposed project are finalised. It should clarify the following questions:

1. What research approach will be adopted for the proposed project?
2. Which research design is to be used?
3. What sampling technique is to be used for the recruitment of the study subjects?
4. What is the sample size and how is it to be calculated?
5. What are the inclusion and exclusion criteria for sampling?
6. What intervention will be tested? What are the details of each intervention?
7. What are the variables under study? (outcome variable, independent variable, research variable)
8. What are the ethical issues? Will the proposal be submitted to the IEC?
9. What are data collection tools and which techniques will be employed to collect data?
10. What is the data analysis plan? Which statistical tests will be used to analyse data?

Research approach

Based on the nature of the phenomenon under investigation, the researcher should decide whether quantitative, qualitative or a mixed method approach will be suitable for the proposed project.

Research design

This is the overall blueprint of the research study—to obtain answers to the research question. The researcher must give due consideration to the research question, feasibility, time frame, strengths and weaknesses of alternative designs, resources available and ethical considerations. Standard terminology must be used to label the study design. For example, randomised control trial, pre-test post-test experimental study, quasi-experimental study, case-control study. Please see *Chapter 4, Research Approaches and Designs* for more information about study designs. Research design can be explained with the use of a flow chart that presents a clearer picture of the study design.

Research subject, population, sample size, power of the study

- *Research subjects:* Subjects are the group of individuals/patients/objects on whom the research is conducted. In the proposal, the researcher should provide specifications about the subjects and define the target as well as accessible population. Personal attributes, disease conditions, age, gender and any other condition of interest must be stated while defining research subjects.

- *Sample size:* Sampling is the process of selecting a portion of the population to represent the entire population of interest (target population). Determination of the sample size can be a difficult job for the novice researcher. However, she must give due consideration to the availability of the subject, time and resources before determining the actual sample size. Power analysis is required to calculate the actual sample size to obtain significant results. Accurate sample size and rationale for the same should be mentioned in the proposal. The data necessary to calculate the sample size and the method of estimation of sample size should also be included.
- *Power of the study:* It is the complement of beta that determines the possibility of reducing type II errors in hypothesis testing. It is also used while calculating the sample size. More study power requires a large sample size. However, the researcher must find the right balance between alpha and beta, as increasing beta may cost alpha, which increases the chances of type I error in hypothesis testing. Usually, the power of 0.80 is selected; the researcher must mention this in the proposal.

Sampling technique

These are of two types: probability sampling and non-probability sampling. Probability sampling is considered superior and more scientific then non-probability sampling. The researcher must give due consideration before selecting the appropriate sampling strategy as per the needs of the study and other factors that influence the sampling process. The selected sampling technique should be mentioned clearly in the research proposal. However, the rule of thumb is that probability sampling techniques should be used if possible as they are considered more scientific than non-probability sampling. In true experimental studies, along with the sampling technique, the process of randomisation should also be discussed. The purpose of randomisation is to maximise the probability that groups receiving differing interventions will be comparable. Some methods of randomisation are:

- Drawing from a hat/lottery/flipping a coin
- Table of random numbers
- Computer generated (www.randomization.com)

Inclusion and exclusion criteria

Inclusion criteria are those that, if fulfilled by a research subject, make him eligible to be included in the study. Similarly, exclusion criteria are those that render a person not eligible for recruitment into the study as a subject. The research proposal should list the inclusion and exclusion criteria after due consideration is given to ethical and other aspects of the study.

Study variables

A variable is defined as the characteristic or quality that varies from person to person. The research proposal should identify the variables under study and define them operationally if needed. In a randomised control trial or true experiment, the following types of variables should be identified and described clearly by the researcher:

- Dependent/Outcome variable
- Independent variable/intervention/experiment
- Extraneous/Confounding variable

In studies other than experimental ones, the variables are classified as demographic variables, research variables and so on.

Independent variable/outcome variable/interventional protocols The researcher should provide every detail of the intervention in the experimental study. The literature review can provide useful insight to determine the dose, frequency and time of administration, risk, benefit and other aspects of interventions. The intervention must be described clearly in the proposal with a full description of various aspects of the experiment. Brainstorming is required to carefully design the various aspects of the intervention. The investigator should also list the main outcome variables and the method of measurement of the same.

Data collection tools and techniques

Data collection tools and techniques are important aspects of a research proposal. The researcher needs to determine the type of information to be collected and how it will be collected. If standardised tools are available to collect information about a variable of interest, then they should be used after obtaining due permission from the author of the tools. However, if standardised tools are not available, the researcher needs to develop the appropriate tools and state how the reliability and validity of these tools will be established. Selection of appropriate data collection tools and techniques determines the authenticity and quality of the data collected.

For further information about data collection tools and techniques, please see *Chapter 7, Data Collection Tools and Techniques.*

Ethical considerations

The research proposal should address the following ethical principles:

- Principle of respect for persons
- Principle of non-maleficence
- Principle of beneficence
- Principle of justice

It is important that the researcher mention in the research proposal whether she will submit the proposal to the Institutional Ethical Committee/Institutional Review Board.

Consent form The consent form is an important aspect of ethical consideration and needs to be developed while submitting the proposal to the IEC/IRB. It should include a clause that the subject has been provided full disclosure of the study and is willing to participate in the study voluntarily. The consent form should have provision for the signature of the participant and two witnesses. It should be developed in languages that can be understood (read/write) by the research participants.

CONSENT FORM

Code no

The subject ______________________ has been fully informed about the nature and purpose of the study. The subject has been asked if any questions have arisen regarding the study and these questions have been answered to the best of the investigators' ability. A signed copy of this form will be made available to the subject.

Investigators' signature: Date: ____________

____

I agree to participate in the study, **"A Study to evaluate the effectiveness of the training programme on the knowledge, attitudes and practice of Basic Life Support techniques among Class 9 students in selected schools of Punjab".**

I have had the study explained to me.

- I have been given the opportunity to ask questions and have been answered to my satisfaction.
- I furthermore recognise the fact that I am free to withdraw this assent and to discontinue participation in this project at any time without prejudice to my academic study.
- I voluntarily give consent to participate in this study.

Name of the Respondent:	**Name of witness:**	**Name of the witness:**
____________	____________	____________
Signature/Thumb impression:	Sign/Thumb Impression	Sign/Thumb impression
____________	____________	____________
Date: ____________	Date: ____________	Date: ____________
Address:	Address: ____________	Address: ____________
____________	____________	____________

Pilot study/try out

A pilot study is a full dress rehearsal of the actual research project to identify the difficulties the researcher might encounter in the research setting. The proposal should specify whether the pilot study will be carried out or not. If yes, then on how many subjects. Newly constructed tools should undergo a try-out process to identify difficulties faced by participants in understanding/comprehending the tool.

Statistical methods/tests/level of significance

The procedures for recording, storing and reducing data should be explained. How data quality will be ensured and what statistical tests (descriptive and inferential) will be employed for data analysis must be stated. The analysis section should correspond to the specific objectives of the study. A description of planned analysis for the primary study objectives and for any secondary objectives must be included. The level of significance that will be used in the proposed study should also be stated. Usually, alpha is kept at 0.05; however, the researcher may choose the level of 0.01 or 0.001 depending on the nature of the intervention.

Budget plan

Budget planning is required for different segments of expenses likely to be incurred in project planning, execution and dissemination. The costs of the project should not be unnecessarily inflated. The use of costly equipment and other facilities should be justified. Once all the project activity costs are listed, the costs must be split according to the format of the funding agencies:

- Expenses for personnel (salary and benefits)
- Expenses for consultants (salary)
- Equipment to be utilised in the study and expenses for the same
- Laboratory tests and their cost
- Travel expenses
- Patient care costs
- Other expenses, if any

The year-wise break-up must be kept in mind while preparing the budget. The budget requirement will be low in the initial phase, increases rapidly during the execution phase and then fall rapidly at the end.

Action plan

The action plan of the project should depict the delegation of work to be carried out in the specified period of time. The researcher needs to anticipate the time requirement for each step of the research process and prepare an action plan, as depicted below.

ACTION PLAN

Activity	**2010**		**2011**				**2012**				**2013**			
Months	6–9	10–12	1–3	4–6	7–9	10–12	1–3	4–6	7–9	10–12	1–3	4–6	7–9	10–12
Rev. of Lit.	√	√	√	√	√	√	√	√	√	√	√	√		
Finalisation of protocols	√	√	√	√										
Pretesting of protocols					√									
Pilot study						√								
Data collection								√	√					
Data analysis										√				
Chapter writing									√	√	√	√		
Submission of thesis													√	

Final proofreading and editing

Careful editing of the proposal is mandatory to refine it and to reduce any chance of error. The title, abstract and contents of the proposal must correspond to each other. The writing style must be reasonable, clear and declarative. The text must be structured using section headings and charts/diagrams should be provide to enhance the clarity of the content. Grammatical/Spelling mistakes must be checked for and corrected; if required, help must be sought from an experienced academic to proofread the proposal to ensure institutional and international academic standards for the research proposal. The novice researcher should provide an answer to the million dollar question: Why should the funding agency fund this research? Why should the institutional research committee accept it? How will the research benefit the wider society or contribute to the research community?

COMMON REASONS FOR PROPOSAL REJECTION

Novice researchers should avoid some of the common mistakes leading to rejection of the study proposal. Some of the factors leading to rejection, identified by National Institutes of Health (NIH), are as follows:

Factors leading to proposal rejection
Nature of the problem
Generation of new or useful knowledge by the project is uncertain
Unclear and unsound statement of the hypothesis
Inappropriate approach to the research problem
Research plan lacks complete concrete details
Research method adopted to carry out inquiry is inappropriate
The investigator not adequately trained in the proposed area of research
The investigators will be required to devote too much time to teaching or other non-research duties

Similarly, based on a sample of 353 research grant applications, The Bureau of Occupational and Vocational Education listed the following reasons for rejection of research proposals:

Important reasons for proposal rejection
Forgot to number the pages
Forgot to include a table of contents
No abstract given
Failed to provide resumes of proposed consultants
Failed to list the objectives of the project
No resume of the principal investigator

Therefore, investigators are required to focus on these common flaws to avoid the disappointment of proposal rejection.

CHAPTER SUMMARY

- A research proposal is a formal description of the research process for the proposed problem statement. It ensures that the candidates have done sufficient preliminary reading/research in their area of interest and are able to provide more than a broad description of the topic that they are planning to research.
- Solicited proposal, unsolicited proposal, pre-proposal and continuation or non-competing proposal are different types of research proposals.
- The title page of the research proposal should include the personal data of the researcher and the title of the planned dissertation.
- Need for the study should present an argument to explain why this study should be carried out.

- Literature review should present a critical summary/appraisal of previous research studies to place a research problem in context or to identify gaps in knowledge and weaknesses in prior studies so as to build a case for the proposed study.
- The research proposal must identify the dependent or outcome variables, independent or predictor variables (the presumed cause) and extraneous variables (confounding variables).
- While selecting a research design, due consideration must be given to the research question, strengths and weaknesses of alternative designs, feasibility, time frame, resources and ethical considerations.
- Random allocation/randomisation is an important feature of randomised clinical trials that refers to the assignment of subjects to treatment conditions in a manner determined by chance alone.
- The proposed sample size must be justified and the data necessary to calculate sample size must be provided. The researcher must also state how the estimates were obtained.
- Every detail of the intervention in the experimental study must be included.
- An appropriate data collection tool should be selected for the given research study based on the objective of the study; definitions of concept and measuring model; reliability (i.e., internal consistency, test–retest reproducibility, inter-observer reliability) of the tool; validity (i.e., content validity, concurrent validity and construct validity) of the tool; sensitivity; and interpretability (the degree to which one can assign qualitative meaning to an instrument's quantitative scores).
- The procedures for recording, storing and reducing data must be explained. How data quality will be ensured and what statistical tests (descriptive and inferential) will be employed for data analysis should be stated.
- A budget plan must be prepared for different segments of expenses likely to be incurred in project planning, execution and dissemination. Costs of the project should not be unnecessarily inflated.
- Careful editing of the proposal is mandatory to refine it and to reduce any chance of error. The title, abstract and contents of the proposal must correspond to each other.
- The National Institutes of Health (NIH) identified various reasons leading to rejection of a research proposal—the most important reason being the incompetence of the researchers.

EVALUATE YOURSELF

Long Answer Questions

Q1: Define research proposal. What are the steps in research proposal development? Explain in detail.

Q2: What are the components of the methodology section in a research proposal?

Q3: What factors will you keep in mind while preparing the budget of your research proposal?

Q4: Prepare a sample research proposal for the problem: A descriptive study to assess the patient's satisfaction with nursing care in a tertiary care hospital in Bhopal, MP.

Q5: Which common errors would you like to focus on to prevent rejection of the research proposal by the funding agency?

Short Answer Questions

Q1: List the common reasons leading to rejection of research proposals.

Q2: What is the purpose of writing a need for the study in a research proposal?

Q3: Explain the types of research proposals.

Multiple Choice Questions

Q1: A solicited research proposal is one which is prepared:
(a) In response to a call for proposals from a funding agency
(b) In response to errors in the previous proposal
(c) To solicit cooperation among nurses and other healthcare professionals
(d) In an emergency

Q2: Which of the following is a common reason for rejection of a proposal?
(a) Inappropriate approach to the research problem and research methodology
(b) Research plans lack complete concrete details
(c) The investigator is not adequately trained in the proposed area of interest
(d) All of the above

Answers

1. a **2.** d

FURTHER READING

Cuca JM, McLouglin WJ. 1987. Why clinical research grant applications fare poorly in review and how to recover. *Cancer Investigation* 5: 55–58.

Denzin NK, Lincoln YS. 1994. *Handbook of Qualitative Research.* Sage Publications, Thousand Oaks, CA.

Gitlin LN, Lyons KJ. 1996. *Successful grant writing. Strategies for health and human service professionals.* Springer Publishing Co., New York.

Lock LF, Spirduso WW, Silverman SJ. 1993. *Proposals that work.* Sage Publications, Newbury Park, CA.

Polit DF, Hungler BP. 1995. Nursing *Research: Principles and Methods, 5th ed.* JB Lippincott Company, Philadelphia.

Ries JB, Leukefeld CG. 1995. *Applying for research funding. Getting started and getting funded.* Sage Publications, Thousand Oaks, CA.

Streiner DL. 1996. While you're up, get me a grant: A guide to grant writing. *Can J Psychiatry* 41: 137–143.

Woodward DK, Clifton GC. 1994. Development of a successful research grant application. *Am J Hosp Pharm* 51: 813–822.

12 Introduction to Statistics

Chapter overview

- Introduction
- Basic statistical terminology
- Types, significance and scope of statistics
- Applications of statistics in health—ratios, rates, vital health statistics (birth and death rates, measures related to fertility, morbidity and mortality)
- Types and levels of data and their measurement

INTRODUCTION

The data collected in a study does not by itself answer research questions or hypotheses. Systematic analysis of data is required to identify trends and patterns of relationships among variables.

Statistic or *datum* (plural: *statistics* or *data*) refers to a piece of information or a measured fact stated in figures, such as the pulse rate of a person. It is concerned with methods of collection, classification, organisation, presentation and summarisation of data, drawing inferences from the data and testing hypotheses. Statistics in any form deals with all aspects of data. It processes jumbled data to bring out the information a researcher is looking for to answer the research questions.

Biostatistics is a branch of statistics that involves the application of statistical tools to classify, organise, summarise and interpret data generated in the biological sciences, such as medicine, surgery, public health, biology and other health sciences. It helps ascertain whether the difference in the dependent variable is due to different treatments or due to chance, measurement errors or characteristics of study subjects. Therefore, biostatistics is particularly concerned with the validity of inferences from the sample about the population from which it was drawn. As the primary purpose of research in any discipline is advancement of knowledge, without the application of statistics to analyse the research data, this advancement is not possible.

BASIC STATISTICAL TERMINOLOGY

Data Plural of datum, and refers to facts, symbols, quantities and information collected from the subjects in a research project, such as height, weight, pulse rate, blood pressure, respiratory rate and oxygen saturation.

Variable A characteristic, attribute, property, measurement or value that varies from one subject or object to another, such as height and weight.

Sample A subset of the population that represents it in a research study. It is a group of subjects recruited for the study purpose as it is not always feasible to study the entire population.

Parameter A value described in relation to the population, such as mean, standard deviation, variance and proportion. The researcher applies statistical tests to the sample data, which results in values known as sample statistics. With the application of inferential statistics, the researcher infers population parameters from sample statistics. This may be a point estimation (single value) or interval estimation (interval values). Sample statistics is represented in Roman letters whereas population parameters are denoted by Greek letters (Table 12.1).

Table 12.1 Population parameters and samples statistics

Values	Population parameters	Sample statistics
Mean	μ	$\bar{x}$
Standard deviation	σ	s
Variance	σ^2	s^2
Proportion	P	p

Point estimation Estimation of population parameters from sample statistics in the form of a single value.

Interval estimation The use of sample data to calculate the interval of values within which the true population parameters are believed to lie. It is represented by an upper confidence limit and a lower confidence limit within which the population mean is estimated to be present.

Level of significance (α) The probability of committing a type I error in hypothesis testing (rejecting the null hypothesis when in fact it is true). Level of significance also informs how willing the researcher is to take the risk of committing a type I error. It is usually established by the researcher beforehand (0.05, 0.01 and 0.001). For example, 0.05 level of significance can be interpreted as 'If we recruit 100 samples from the same population and test the same hypothesis from the data of 100 samples separately, there is a possibility of committing a type I error only five times'.

Statistically significant result When the calculated test statistics falls beyond the critical limit, or when the calculated *p* value of a test statistics is less than the established level of significance. For example, to know whether the difference between pretest knowledge mean score and post-test knowledge mean score after the BLS workshop is significant or due to chance, the researcher must apply inferential test to compute the *p* value. Suppose the computed *p* value is 0.03, which is less than the pre-established level of significance (0.05), we can state that the results are statistically significant and the increase in post-test knowledge score is caused by the BLS workshop.

One-tailed test When one end of the sampling distribution is used in hypothesis testing to determine improbable values. One-tailed test may be appropriate for directional hypothesis.

Two-tailed test When both ends of the sampling distribution are used in hypothesis testing to determine improbable values.

Beta (β) Refers to the probability of committing a type II error in hypothesis testing.

Power of study The ability of a study design to detect relationships that exist among variables. It is the complement of beta $(1 - \beta)$.

Confidence interval A range of values within which the unknown population parameter is estimated to lie. The level of confidence of the confidence interval would indicate the probability that the confidence range captures this true population parameter, given a distribution of samples. It is represented by a percentage in the research reports, such as 95%, 99% confidence interval. A confidence interval of 95% at the level of 0.05 means that the researcher is 95% confident that the true value of the population parameter is in the confidence interval and 95% of the observed confidence intervals will hold the true value of the parameter.

Critical region The set of values in the sampling/theoretical distribution that leads to rejection of the null hypothesis if the test statistics fall at or beyond the critical regions.

Statistical power of a test The probability that a test correctly rejects the null hypothesis when the null hypothesis is false.

Outliers Values in a data set that are outside the normal range of values.

Degree of freedom (df) The number of sample values that are free to vary. Different formulas are used to calculate the degree of freedom in different statistical tests; however, often it is N – 1.

Factor analysis A statistical procedure used to reduce a larger data set of variables to a smaller set with common characteristics.

Bivariate statistics Statistical procedures applied to analyse the empirical relationship between two variables; for example, factor analysis, multiple regression and ANOVA.

Sampling distribution A theoretical distribution showing the values of statistics computed from an infinite number of samples as data points in the distribution.

Standard error The standard deviation of the sampling distribution of the mean.

TYPES OF STATISTICAL METHODS

Two important statistical methodologies are used in data analysis: descriptive statistics and inferential statistics.

Descriptive statistics describes and summarises the data collected from a sample using measures of central tendency (mean, mode and median), measures of variation (range, variation and standard deviation), percentage and frequency distribution. Measures of central tendency represent the central value in a distribution, whereas measures of variation provide information about the extent to which the data is dispersed around the central value and each other.

Inferential statistics is based on the theory of probability and draws inferences from data subject to random variation. Researchers usually collect data from the sample; however, to generalise the findings to the entire population and to draw meaningful conclusions about the entire population, inferential statistics is needed. These inferences may take the form of hypothesis testing, correlation and association between variables.

It helps the researcher determine if the difference detected between two or more groups such as an experimental and control group is real or if it is due to chance, because of an unrepresentative sample. Inferential statistics generates the *p* value to determine whether or not the null hypothesis should be rejected. The *p* value provides the probability of getting results by chance, if in fact the null hypothesis were true. If the *p* value is smaller than the chosen level of significance (usually < 0.05), the null hypothesis is rejected and it is accepted that the groups are truly different with regard to the outcome. Similarly, if the *p* value is larger than the level of significance (> 0.05), the researcher accepts the null hypothesis and concludes that the intervention had no effect on the outcome.

There are two classes of inferential statistics: parametric and non-parametric statistics. Inferential statistics that evaluate nominal and ordinal data are categorised as non-parametric tests, while those that evaluate interval and ratio data are categorised as parametric tests.

Parametric tests

Parametric tests are applicable to data following a particular probability distribution. They are powerful tests used to estimate the population parameters from the sample statistics. Compared to non-parametric tests, parametric tests have more underlying assumptions. If a parametric test meets these assumptions, it produces more accurate and precise results. The statistical power of parametric tests is higher than that of non-parametric tests. However, if the underlying assumptions are violated, parametric tests can be very misleading. They are applicable when the data level is continuous or a ratio. Examples of parametric tests are t-test, z-test, Pearson product moment, ANOVA and ANCOVA.

Non-parametric tests

Non-parametric tests are also called distribution-free statistics as these tests do not require data to follow the normal distribution. They can describe some attribute of a population, its relationship with some other attribute, test hypotheses about that attribute, and require no assumptions about the form of the population data distribution. Non-parametric tests are applicable when the sample size is small, the assumptions of parametric tests cannot be fulfilled or data is on nominal or ordinal level. Examples of non-parametric tests include Chi-square test, Mann–Whitney, Wilcoxon rank sum test and Kruskal–Wallis test.

APPLICATION AND SCOPE OF STATISTICS IN HEALTH

Statistical methods have wide scope in all fields that involve data collection and decision-making based on analysis and interpretation of data. Statistical methods are applied in a wide range of scientific and social research, including nursing, biology, sociology, social science, government and business. Some specialised fields of inquiry use statistics so extensively that they have specialised terminology such as biostatistics, business statistics, demography, engineering statistics, epidemiology (statistical analysis of disease), psychological statistics, social statistics and medical statistics.

Application of statistics in the health sciences is of great importance as it summarises trends, ratio and rates of occurrence of events that have a significant impact on the health of the population.

Applications in nursing

- To compare the efficacy of a particular nursing intervention or line of nursing care
- To compare the efficacy of an innovative teaching method over a traditional one

- To find associations between two variables, for example, unprotected sex and AIDS
- To identify signs and symptoms of a disease, for example, cough in myocardial infarction is found by chance and chest pain is present in almost every case

Applications in pharmacology

- To check the efficacy of a new drug to treat a disease; the drug is administered to animals or humans to check whether the change in the dependent variable is by chance or due to the drug
- To check how potent a new drug is compared to the standard drug
- To explore the adverse effects of a drug; for example, dry cough is frequently associated with the use of calcium channel blockers, but weakness is a chance finding

Applications in anatomy and physiology

- To define the normal range of physiological parameters such as mean pulse rate is 72 but the normal range is 60–100. Any value of pulse rate that falls between 60 and 100 is considered normal; pulse rate below the lower limit is called bradycardia and that beyond the upper limit is termed tachycardia.
- To find out the limit of normality in variables such as height and weight

Applications in pathology

- To define normality of variables such as normal serum sodium level and normal blood glucose level
- To define pathologic lesions in a disease; papule in chickenpox is a characteristic lesion but the presence of a macule is a chance finding.

Application in microbiology

- To define the normality and range of variables such as the size and shape of bacteria, virus and parasites

Applications in public health

- In epidemiological studies, the role of causative factors can be statistically tested; for example, smoking is correlated statistically with cancer—the prevalence of cancer is higher in those who smoke as compared to those who do not.
- To describe the incidence and prevalence of disease, disease-specific mortality and morbidity rate, death rate and other statistics of vital events in a population

VITAL HEALTH STATISTICS

Vital health statistics is the application of statistical methods to determine various rates, ratios and trends pertaining to birth, death, maternal death and infant mortality which are considered vital to determine the health status of a community.

Rate A proportion where the numerator represents the occurrence of an event in the given population and the denominator represents the population. It is multiplied by 1000, 10,000 and 100,000 as per the required magnification. It may be a crude rate or specific rate when all of the population or a specific group of the population, respectively, are taken into consideration. Similarly, the rate is termed quinquennial and decennial when it is calculated for a period of five years and ten years, respectively.

Specific rate This is computed for a specific group of a population such as for a particular gender, occupation and educational status.

Crude birth rate The ratio of the total number of live births to the total mid-year population in a specified year. It is expressed as total live births per 1000 of the population in a specified year.

$$\frac{\text{Total number of live birth in a year}}{\text{Mid-year population}} \times 1000$$

Measures relating to fertility

Fertility-related statistics in a given population can be measured by a number of indicators such as birth rate, general fertility rate, total fertility rate, marriage rate and pregnancy rate.

General fertility rate refers to the total number of live births during a year in an area per 1000 women in the reproductive age group (15–44 or 49 years).

$$\text{GFR} = \frac{\text{Number of live births during a year}}{\begin{array}{l}\text{Mid-year number of females in}\\ \text{reproductive age group in the same year}\end{array}} \times 1000$$

Total fertility rate refers to the average number of children a woman is likely to have throughout her reproductive years, bearing children at the same rate as the women now in each age group.

Marriage rate refers to the number of marriages in a year per 1000 population.

Pregnancy rate refers to the ratio of the number of pregnancies in a year to married women in the reproductive age group.

Measures relating to morbidity

Incidence rate The number of new cases of a disease in a specified period of time in the population. It may be weekly, monthly or yearly.

$$\text{Incidence Rate} = \frac{\text{Total number of new cases during a specified period}}{\text{Population at risk in the same period}} \times 1000$$

Prevalence rate It takes into consideration new as well as old cases of disease in a specified period of time.

$$\text{Prevalence Rate} = \frac{\text{Total number of new and old cases during a specified period}}{\text{Population at risk in the same period}} \times 1000$$

Prevalence may be of two types: point and period. Point prevalence is computed for a specific point of time whereas period prevalence is computed for a specified duration of time, for example, three months and six months.

Measures relating to mortality

Crude death rate The ratio of the total number of deaths to the total mid-year population in a specified time frame. It is expressed as total deaths per 1000 of the population in a specified year.

$$\frac{\text{Total number of deaths}}{\text{Mid-year population}} \times 1000$$

Specific death rate The ratio of the number of deaths in a specified age group/ gender/section of the population to the total mid-year population of that specified group in a year.

$$\frac{\text{Total number of deaths in specified group of the population}}{\text{Mid-year population of the group}} \times 1000$$

Maternal mortality rate The total number of deaths of women while pregnant or within 42 days of child birth from puerperal causes and not from accidental or incidental causes. It is expressed as the total number of deaths of mothers as defined above per 100,000 live births in a year.

$$\frac{\text{Total number of female deaths while pregnant or within 42 days of termination of pregnancy from puerperal causes during a given year}}{\text{Total no. of live births in the same year}} \times 100000$$

Infant mortality rate The ratio of the total number of deaths of children less than one year of age to the total number of live births in a year. It is expressed as the total number of deaths per 1000 live births in a specified year.

$$\frac{\text{Number of deaths of children} < 1 \text{ year of age in a given year}}{\text{Number of live births in the same year}} \times 1000$$

Demography It is the scientific study of the human population. It focuses on population change, and composition and distribution of the population. The main source of population data is the census, carried out every 10 years by the Census Commissioner of India.

Sex ratio It is computed as the number of females per 1000 males.

$$\frac{\text{Number of females}}{\text{Number of males}} \times 1000$$

TYPES AND LEVELS OF DATA AND THEIR MEASUREMENT

SS Stevens published an article in *Science* titled 'On the theory of scales of measurement' in which he proposed his typology of levels of measurement. Stevens claimed that all measurement in science uses four types of scales: nominal, ordinal, interval and ratio. Some statistical operations/tests are possible for a particular level of measurement.

Nominal scale This is the lowest level of measurement. Nominal data deals with names or categories; therefore, it is used to collect qualitative data. For example, religion (measured as Hindu, Sikh, Christian, Jain, Buddhist and so forth); time of day (morning, afternoon, evening, night); gender (male, female, unspecified); type of automobile (sedan, SUV, sports car, and so on). Data at this level cannot be ordered in a meaningful way, and therefore the calculation of mean and standard deviation has no merit.

Ordinal scale It is the next level of measurement in which data is arranged according to the relative standing/distance/ranking. Data at this level can be ordered, but meaningful magnitudnal; differences between the data cannot be calculated. For example, ranking an experience as a '5' on a scale of 1 to 7 tells the researcher that it is higher than an experience ranked as '2'. The ordinal scale indicates the relative standing or increase or decrease in the order of the categories. For example, mild, moderate and severe are examples of ordinal levels of measurement. It does not allow precise measurement but represents the relative standing of the categories.

Interval scale This deals with data that can be ordered, and differences between the pair of values can be meaningfully interpreted. Interval scale lacks an absolute zero and therefore a number of statistical operations and interpretations are not possible. The Fahrenheit and Celsius scales of temperature are examples of data at the interval level of measurement. The difference between 100° and 40° temperature is 60°, which equals the difference between 70° and 10°. However, 0° (in both scales) temperature does not represent the total absence of temperature. Similarly, it cannot be said that 90°C is three times as hot as 30°C. Zero in the interval scale is arbitrarily placed, which is a point on the scale with numbers both above and below it (for example, –10°F).

Ratio scale This is highest level of measurement that has all of the features of the interval level along with an absolute zero value that signifies the point at which the characteristic being measured vanishes (absolute zero). Due to the presence of the absolute zero, comparison of data is possible; therefore, the use of phrases such as 'three times' and 'four times' is meaningful at the ratio level.

For example, a distance is a ratio level measurement. Ten kilometres is twice as far as five kilometres. Zero kilometre means lack of distance or no length. So ratios can be formed between the data. Similarly, income (measured in rupees, with 0 equal to no income) and years of formal education are ratio level measurements.

Interval and ratio data are amenable to parametric statistics (mean, standard deviation, t-test, ANOVA, correlation) which is considered more powerful than non-parametric statistics. As a rule, more statistical technique options are available for the analysis of parametric data. Non-parametric data (nominal and ordinal) is lacking in some parameters and cannot be added, subtracted, multiplied or divided. Non-parametric data is analysed using non-parametric statistics (mode, median, interquartile range, Chi-square, Wilcoxon rank sum, Kurskal–Wallis, Friedman test and Fisher's exact test).

CHAPTER SUMMARY

- Statistics is concerned with methods of collection, classification, organisation, presentation and summarisation of data, drawing inferences from the data and testing hypotheses.
- Biostatistics is a branch of statistics that applies statistical tools to classify, organise, summarise and interpret data generated in the biological sciences, such as medicine, surgery, public health, nursing and other health sciences.
- Data refers to facts, symbols, quantities and information collected from the subjects in a research project.
- Parameters are the values described in relation to the population such as mean, standard deviation, variance and proportion.
- Level of significance refers to the probability of committing a type I error in hypothesis testing.

- When the calculated test statistics fall beyond the critical limit, or when the calculated *p* value of test statistics is less than the established level of significance, the results are said to be statistically significant.
- Power of the study refers to the ability of a study design to detect a relationship that exists among variables. It is the complement of beta (1 – β).
- Descriptive statistics describes and summarises data collected from a sample.
- Inferential statistics is based on the theory of probability and draws inferences from the data subject to random variation.
- There are two classes of inferential statistics: parametric and non-parametric. Inferential statistics that evaluate nominal and ordinal data are categorised as non-parametric tests, while those that evaluate interval and ratio data are categorised as parametric tests.
- Application of statistics in health sciences is of great importance as it summaries trends, ratios and rates of occurrence of events which have significant impact on the health of the population.
- Vital health statistics is the application of statistical methods to determine various rates, ratios and trends pertaining to birth, death, maternal death and infant mortality which are considered vital to determine the health status of a community.
- Nominal scale is the lowest level of measurement. Nominal data deals with names or categories and is therefore used to collect qualitative data.
- Ordinal data is arranged as per its relative standing/distance/ranking. Data at this level can be ordered, but meaningful magnitudinal differences in the data cannot be calculated.
- The interval level of measurement deals with data that can be ordered, and differences between the pair of values can be meaningfully interpreted.
- Zero in the interval scale is arbitrarily placed, which is a point on the scale with numbers both above and below it (for example, –10°F).
- Ratio is the highest level of measurement and has all of the features of the interval level and an absolute zero value that signifies the point at which the characteristic being measured vanishes (absolute zero).
- Interval and ratio data are amenable to parametric statistics (mean, standard deviation, t-test, ANOVA, correlation) which is considered more powerful than non-parametric statistics.

EVALUATE YOURSELF

Long Answer Questions

Q1: Define statistics. Explain the scope and application of statistics in health.

Q2: Explain the difference between parametric and non-parametric tests.

Q3: Define biostatistics. What is vital health statistics?

Q4: Differentiate descriptive and inferential statistics.

Q5: What are the levels of measurement? Explain with examples.

Short Answer Questions

Q1: Define the following terms:
(a) Confidence interval (b) Level of significance
(c) Critical regions (d) Interval estimation
(e) Point estimation (f) Sample
(g) Variable (h) Power of a study
(i) Statistically significant result (j) Parameter

Q2: Define crude birth rate, death rate, maternal mortality rate and fertility rate.

Multiple Choice Questions

Q1: Income (in rupees where 0 means no income) belongs to which level of measurement?
(a) Nominal level (b) Ordinal level
(c) Continuous level (d) Ratio level

Q2: Temperature belongs to which level of measurement?
(a) Nominal level (b) Ordinal level
(c) Continuous level (d) Ratio level

Q3: Computation of mean and standard deviation has no merit for which of the following variables?
(a) Gender (b) Height
(c) Weight (d) Blood pressure

Q4: Which of the following is a parametric statistical test?
(a) ANOVA (b) t-test
(c) z-test (d) all of the above

Q5: Which of the following is a non-parametric test?
(a) Chi-square (b) t-test
(c) ANOVA (d) All of the above

Q6: The standard deviation of the sampling distribution of the mean is known as:
(a) Theoretical distribution (b) Population parameter
(c) Standard error (d) Confidence interval

Q7: Which of the following is not a population parameter?
(a) σ (b) P
(c) μ (d) s

Answers

1. d **2.** c **3.** a **4.** d **5.** a **6.** c **7.** d

FURTHER READING

Anderson DR, Sweeney DJ, Williams TA. 1994. *Introduction to Statistics: Concepts and Applications.* West Group.

Chance BL, Rossman AJ. 2005. Preface. *Investigating Statistical Concepts, Applications, and Methods.* Duxbury Press.

Cox DR. 2006. *Principles of Statistical Inference,* Cambridge University Press.

Freedman DA. 2005. *Statistical Models: Theory and Practice.* Cambridge University Press.

Geisser S, Johnson WM. 2006. *Modes of Parametric Statistical Inference,* John Wiley & Sons.

Mahajan BK. 2006. *Methods in Biostatistics, 6th ed,* Jaypee, New Delhi.

Schervish MJ. 1995. *Theory of Statistics.* Springer, New York.

13 Measures of Central Tendency

Chapter overview

- Introduction to measures of central tendency
- Mean
- Median
- Mode
- Selecting the appropriate measure of central tendency
- Position of measures of central tendency

INTRODUCTION TO MEASURES OF CENTRAL TENDENCY

In any research study, the researcher collects large quantities of a wide range of data. For example, a researcher may collect height and weight data from 100 subjects. But each of these 100 individual values of height and weight cannot be used to interpret the study results. What is required is a single value that can represent the whole of the data set. Measure of central tendency, also known as measure of central location, is that single value that represents the central position of the given data set. Researchers describe the whole data set using this single value. In the example mentioned above, the researcher cannot use the individual readings of height and weight to describe the study results. Rather, she needs to obtain one single value to describe the height and weight of 100 study subjects. Measure of central tendency is a summary measure that attempts to describe a whole set of data with a single value that represents the middle or centre of its distribution.

Three measures of central tendency are frequently used by nurse researchers: **mean**, **median** and **mode**. All three are valid measures of central tendency, but which measure would be most appropriate in a particular situation depends on the type of the data set.

MEAN (ARITHMETIC)

The mean (or average) is the most popular and well-known measure of central tendency. It is the most frequently and widely used measure of central tendency in nursing research reports. It is calculated by summing the value of each observation in a distribution and dividing the sum by the total number of observations. It is noteworthy here that the population mean is indicated by the Greek symbol μ, whereas sample mean is indicated by the symbol $\overline{x}$. This is because, in statistics, sample and population have different meanings. Mean can be calculated for two types of data: discrete and continuous.

As mentioned earlier, mean is equal to the sum of all the values in the data set divided by the number of values. So, if there are n values in a data set and they have values x_1, x_2, ..., x_n then mean can be calculated using the formula given below.

$$\overline{x} = \frac{(x_1 + x_2 + \cdots + x_n)}{n} \qquad \mu = \frac{\Sigma x}{n} \qquad \overline{x} = \frac{\Sigma x}{n}$$

This formula for mean shows that each value in the data set is included in the calculation, which makes it a favourable measure of central tendency in most situations.

Characteristics of Mean

- Mean is the arithmetic average of a data set.
- A given data set has only one mean.
- Its value is influenced by extreme measurements.
- The sum of the deviations of each value from the mean is always zero.

Mean calculation for ungrouped data

Example 13.1

Calculate the mean of the given data set

54, 54, 54, 55, 56, 57, 57, 58, 58, 60, 60

1. First, add all the values given in the data set

   $54 + 54 + 54 + 55 + 56 + 57 + 57 + 58 + 58 + 60 + 60 = 623$

2. Divide the total generated in the first step by the number of observations or values. In this example, the number of values is 11. Therefore, $623/11 = 56.6$.
3. Mean of the given data set is 56.6.

Mean calculation for grouped data

Sometimes, researchers present the data in the form of a frequency. The mean of the grouped data is calculated by dividing the sum of all observations by the number of observations.

So if, x_1, x_2, x_3 … x_n are the given observations, with their respective frequencies f_1, f_2, f_3 … f_n, then sum of observations $= f_1x_1 + f_2x_2 + f_3x_3 + \cdots + f_nx_n$.

The number of observations $= f_1 + f_2 + f_3 + \cdots + f_n$

$$\text{Mean} = \frac{f_1 \times X_1 + f_2 \times X_2 \cdots + f_n \times X_n}{f_1 + f_2 + \cdots f_n}$$

Example 13.2

Calculate the mean of following data:

Observation (x)	10	20	30	40	50	60	65	70	79	80
Frequency (f)	4	5	4	4	3	2	2	6	10	3

To calculate mean, as explained above, the following steps must be carried out.

Step 1: Calculate the sum of the given frequencies (Σf) and sum of $f \times X$ (Σfx)

f	X	$f \times X$
10	4	040
20	5	100
30	4	120
40	4	160
50	3	150
60	2	120
65	2	130
70	6	420
79	10	790
80	10	800
	$\Sigma f = 50$	$\Sigma fx = 2830$

Step 2: Calculate mean by putting the values in the formula

$$\text{Mean } (\bar{X}) = \frac{\Sigma fx}{\Sigma f}$$

$$\text{Mean} = \frac{2830}{50}$$

$$= 56.6$$

Mean calculation for class interval data

When data is presented in tabular form, with a class interval, and each class has its frequency, then mean can be calculated from the formula given below.

$$\bar{X} = \frac{\Sigma fx}{\Sigma f}$$

where, x is the midpoint of the class interval.

Example 13.3

Calculate the arithmetic mean of the given data set:

Class interval	Frequency (f)
10–20	3
20–30	9
30–40	5

Step 1: Calculate the sum of frequency (Σf)

Here, $\Sigma f = 17$.

Step 2: Calculate the midpoint (X) for each class interval.

$$\text{Here, Midpoint } (X) = \frac{(10+20)}{2}, \frac{(20+30)}{2}, \frac{(30+40)}{2} = 15, 25, 35$$

Step 3: Multiply the midpoint with its corresponding frequency (fX).

Step 4: Find ΣfX.

$$\Sigma fX = (3 \times 15) + (9 \times 25) + (5 \times 35) = (45 + 225 + 175) = 445$$

Class interval	Frequency (f)	Midpoint (X)	Xf
10–20	3	$(10 + 20)/2 = 15$	$3 \times 15 = 045$
20–30	9	$(20 + 30)/2 = 25$	$9 \times 25 = 225$
30–40	5	$(30 + 40)/2 = 35$	$5 \times 35 = 175$

Step 5: Put the values in the formula

$$\text{Arithmetic mean} = \frac{\Sigma fX}{\Sigma f} = \frac{445}{17} = 26.17$$

Alternatively, the step deviation method can be used to calculate mean for the data presented in the form of a class interval. This method is explained using the following example.

Example 13.4

Calculate the mean of the following data with the help of the step deviation method.

CI	10–20	20–30	30–40	40–50	50–60	60–70	70–80	80–90	90–100	100–110
F	4	5	4	4	3	4	16	13	11	16

CI	Midpoint (x)	f	$d = x - a$	$U = d/h$	fd
10–20	15	4	–40	–4	–160
20–30	25	5	–30	–3	–150
30–40	35	4	–20	–2	–80
40–50	45	4	–10	–1	–40
50–60	55	3	0	0	0
60–70	65	4	10	1	40
70–80	75	16	20	2	320
80–90	85	13	30	3	390
90–100	95	11	40	4	440
100–110	105	16	50	5	800
		$\Sigma f = 80$			$\Sigma fd = 156$

Here, $a = 55$ (assumed mean) and $h = 10$ (class interval).

$$\bar{X} = a + \frac{\Sigma fu}{\Sigma f} \times h$$

$$= 55 + \left(\frac{156}{80}\right) \times 10$$

$$= 55 + 19.5$$

$$= 74.5$$

Advantage of mean

- It can be used for both continuous and discrete numeric data.

Limitations of mean

- It includes every single value in the dataset in its calculation; therefore, it is sensitive to the influence of extreme values and skewed distributions.
- It cannot be calculated for categorical data.

As listed above, one limitation of mean is that it is susceptible to the influence of extreme values/outliers. Therefore if in a data set, there are outliers, mean cannot be considered a good measure of central tendency because it fails to depict the central position of the data set. For example, consider the weight of 10 nursing students:

Student	1	2	3	4	5	6	7	8	9	10
Weight (in Kg)	50	55	53	48	52	54	**75**	55	**80**	51

The mean weight for these 10 students is 57.3. However, inspecting the raw data suggests that this mean value may not be the best way to accurately reflect the typical weight of a student, as most students weigh in the range of 50–55 kg. Mean is being skewed by the two high values. Therefore, in this situation, another measure of central tendency is used instead of mean.

In a normally distributed data set, mean, median and mode all are identical and represent the most typical value in the data set. However, in skewed distribution, mean loses its ability to provide the best central location for the data because the skewness in the data drags it away from the typical central value. However, median best retains this position and is not as strongly influenced by the skewed values. This is explained in more detail in the skewed distribution section later in this chapter.

MEDIAN

Median is the 'middle value' of a data set when all the observations are arranged in ascending/descending order. It divides the frequency distribution into two exact halves. Fifty percent of observations in a distribution have scores at or below the median. Hence, median is also termed as the 50th percentile. Median is the preferred measure of central tendency for a skewed distribution.

Median calculation

Step 1: Arrange the data in order (either ascending or descending).

Step 2: If the number of observations is odd, then the $(n + 1)/2$th observation (in the ordered set) will be the median. When the number of observations is even, the mean of the $n/2$th and the $(n/2 + 1)$th observation will be median.

Example 13.5

Calculate the median of the data set given below:

65	55	89	56	35	14	56	55	87	45	92

Step 1: We first need to arrange the data in ascending order:

14	35	45	55	55	*56*	56	65	87	89	92

Step 2: As the number of observation is odd, the median will be the $n + 1/2$th value in the ordered data. So, $11 + 1/2 = 6$th value in the data set is median, and in this case, it is 56.

Example 13.6

Calculate the median of the data set given below:

65	55	89	56	35	14	56	55	87	45

Step 1: Rearrange the data in ascending order:

14	35	45	55	55	*56*	56	65	87	89

Step 2: As the number of observations is even, the median will be the mean of the $n/2$th and the $n/2 + 1$th value in the ordered data. So, $10/2$th = 5th and 6th value's mean will be median, which is 55.5.

Advantages of median

- Median is preferred over mean when the distribution is asymmetrical or skewed as it is not distorted by outliers/skewed data.
- It is easier to compute and comprehend median than mean.
- It can be determined for ratio, interval and ordinal scale.

Limitations of median

- It cannot be calculated for nominal data.

- It does not take into account the exact value of each observation and hence does not use all the information available in the data set.
- Unlike mean, median is not amenable to further mathematical operations and hence its use in statistical tests is limited.

MODE

Mode is defined as the value that occurs most frequently in the data. Some data sets do not have a mode because each value occurs only once. On the other hand, some data sets can have more than one mode. It represents the highest bar in a bar chart or histogram. It is possible to have more than one mode, and to have **no** mode also.

Calculation of mode

Example 13.7

Find the mode of the given data set:

54, 54, 54, 55, 56, 57, 57, 58, 58, 60, 60

Step 1: Prepare a frequency distribution table of the given data set:

Age	Frequency
54	3
55	1
56	1
57	2
58	2
60	2

Step 2: Identify the most frequently occurring value. In this example, it is 54.Therefore, the mode of this distribution is 54.

Mode is used as a measure of central tendency for categorical data where the most frequently occurring category must be determined, as shown in Fig. 13.1.

Figure 13.1 depicts the most commonly preferred fast food in Bhopal, which is samosa. However, one of the problems with mode is that it is not unique, so this creates a problem when two or more values share the highest frequency, such as given in Fig. 13.2.

Figure 13.2 depicts fast food preferences among the people of Indore. Here, the highest frequency is shared equally by kachori, samosa and pakora; therefore, there are three modes in this distribution. But which mode best describes the central tendency of this

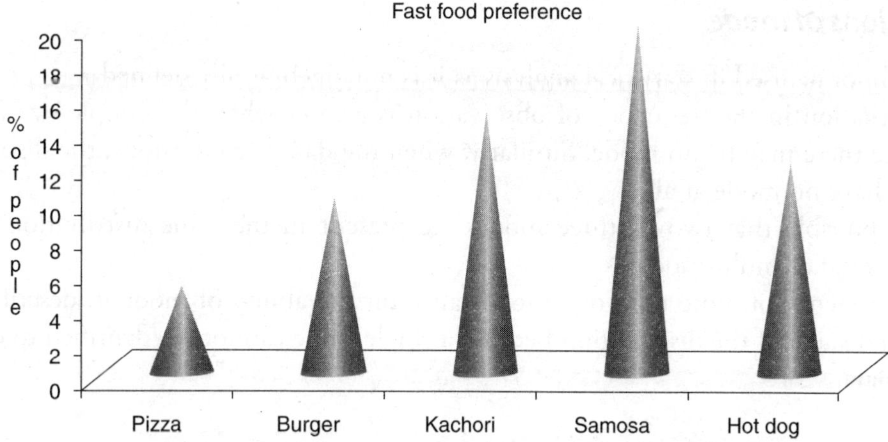

Figure 13.1 Fast food preference among people of Bhopal

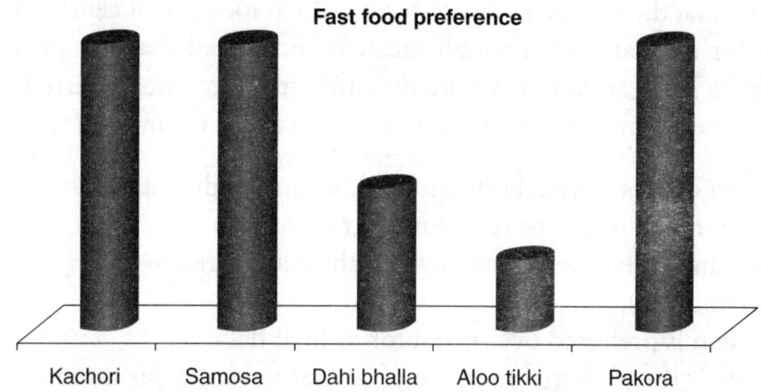

Figure 13.2 Fast food preference among people of Indore

data? Further, using mode as a measure of central tendency with continuous data may be problematic because it is unlikely to have any one value that is more frequent than the other.

For example, consider measuring the height of 20 students to the nearest 0.1 cm. Now the question is 'How likely is it that we will find two or more students with exactly the same height (150.2 cm)'. It is hardly possible in such a small sample (20 students) and with a large range of possible heights, it would be difficult to find two students with exactly the same height; that is, to the nearest 0.1 cm. This is why mode is very rarely used with continuous data.

Advantages of mode

- It is the only measure of central tendency that can be used for data measured in a nominal scale.
- Calculation of mode is very simple.

Limitations of mode

1. It cannot be used in statistical analysis as it is not algebraically defined.
2. Fluctuation in the frequency of observation is greater when the sample size is small, hence there may be no mode. Similarly, when the data is continuous, the distribution may have no mode at all.
3. It is possible that two or three modes are present in the same distribution of data (bi-modal or multi-modal).
4. The presence of more than one mode can limit the ability of mode in describing the central value of the distribution because a single value cannot be identified to describe the data.

SELECTING THE APPROPRIATE MEASURE OF CENTRAL TENDENCY

While analysing data, the researcher must decide which measure of central tendency would be appropriate for the data set. Though mean is considered the best measure of central tendency, there are some situations where the other measures are preferred. The following rules help determine the most appropriate measure of central tenancy for specific conditions:

- **Rule 1:** When data is normally distributed, mean, median and mode are all identical and hence any measure can be used for central position.
- **Rule 2:** Median is preferred to mean when there are extreme scores in the distribution (skewed distribution).
- **Rule 3:** Median is preferred over mean for ordinal data.
- **Rule 4:** Mode is the preferred measure of central tendency for nominal data.

POSITION OF MEASURES OF CENTRAL TENDENCY

The relative positions of the measures of central tendency (mean, median, and mode) depend on the shape of the distribution. As mentioned earlier, in a normal distribution, all the measures of central tendency are equal. However, in a skewed distribution, the relative position of mean, median and mode changes, as follows (Fig. 13.3):

- Mean is pulled towards the extreme observations (at the tail of the distribution)
- Median lies between mean and mode.
- Mode lies in the hump of the skewed distribution.

Skewed distributions

If the curve has one tail that is longer than the other, it is termed a skewed distribution. If the longer tail of the distribution is on the left, it is called **negatively skewed;** similarly, if the longer tail is on the right, it is called **positively skewed**.

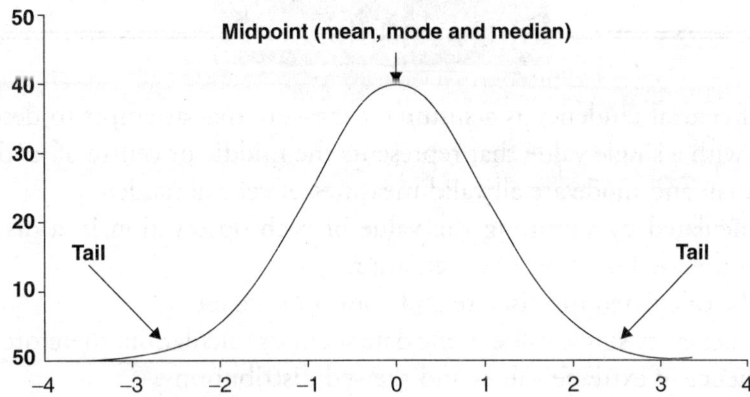

Figure 13.3 Normal distribution curve (mode, median and mean coincide in the middle of the distribution)

In a skewed distribution, mode remains the most commonly occurring value, median remains the middle value, but mean is 'pulled' in the direction of the tails. Therefore, in a skewed distribution, median is a preferred measure of central tendency, as depicted in Fig. 13.4.

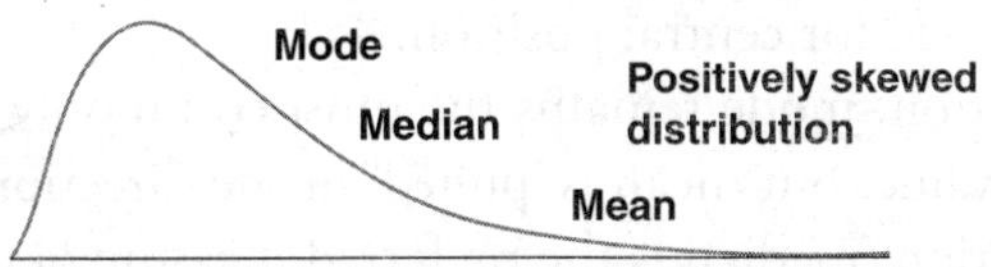

Figure 13.4 Positively skewed distribution

The value of mean is highest, median has middle value and mode has least value in a positively skewed distribution.

Negative skewness

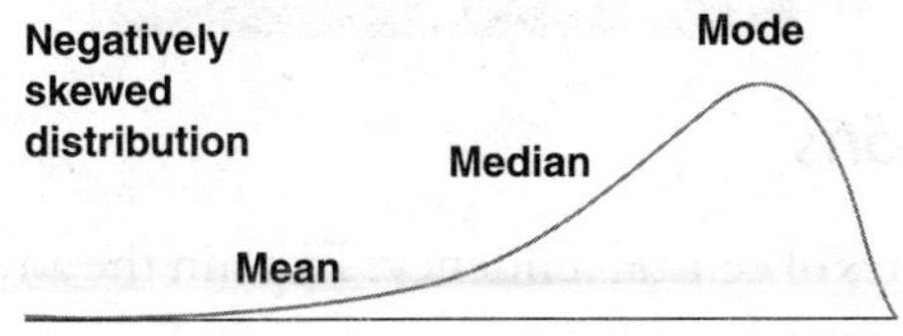

Figure 13.5 Negatively skewed distribution

Negatively or left-skewed distribution is characterised by a longer tail on the left side of the distribution than the right side. Mean is 'pulled' toward the left tail of the distribution. The value of mean is least, median has middle value and mode has highest value in this situation (Fig. 13.5).

CHAPTER SUMMARY

- Measure of central tendency is a summary measure that attempts to describe a whole set of data with a single value that represents the middle or centre of its distribution.
- Mean, median and mode are all valid measures of central tendency.
- Mean is calculated by summing the value of each observation in a distribution and dividing by the total number of observations.
- Mean can be calculated for discrete and continuous data.
- Mean includes every single value in the data set in its calculation; therefore, it is sensitive to the influence of extreme values and skewed distributions.
- Median is the 'middle value' of a data set when all the observations are arranged in ascending/descending order.
- Median is the preferred measure of central tendency for skewed distributions.
- Median can be determined for ratio, interval and ordinal scale.
- Unlike mean, median is not amenable to further mathematical operations and hence its use in statistical tests is limited.
- Mode is defined as the value that occurs most frequently in the data.
- Two or three modes may exist in the same distribution of data (bi-modal or multi-modal).
- When data is normally distributed, mean, median and mode are all identical, hence any measure can be used for central position.
- In a skewed distribution, mode remains the most commonly occurring value, median remains the middle value, but mean is 'pulled' in the direction of the tails.
- In a skewed distribution, median is the preferred measure of central tendency.
- The value of mean is highest, median has middle value and mode has least value in a positively skewed distribution.
- The value of mean is least, median has middle value and mode has highest value in a negatively skewed distribution.

EVALUATE YOURSELF

Long Answer Questions

Q1: What are the measures of central tendency? Explain the advantages and disadvantages of each measure of central tendency.

Q2: Calculate mean, mode median from the following data:

5, 10, 6, 8, 9, 5, 11, 3, 2, 7, 4, 11, 5, 6, 8, 9

Q3: What is the relative positioning of different measures of central tendency? Explain in detail.

Q4: Calculate the mean of the following data:

Observation (x)	10	20	30	40	50	60	65	70	79	80
Frequency (f)	6	8	5	9	2	1	5	6	8	3

Q5: Calculate the median of the data set given below:

45	15	29	46	65	34	86	95	87	15	72

Short Answer Questions

Q1: In a skewed data set, which measure of central tendency is preferred and why?

Q2: Write a short note on measures of central tendency for nominal data?

Q3: What are the advantages and disadvantages of mean?

Q4: What are the advantages and disadvantages of mode?

Q5: What are the advantages and disadvantages of median?

Multiple Choice Questions

Q1: Which of the following is a measure of central tendency for nominal data?
(a) Mean (b) Mode
(c) Median (d) All of the above

Q2: Which of the following is the preferred measure of central tendency for a skewed data set?
(a) Mean (b) Mode
(c) Median (d) All of the above

Q3: In normally distributed data,
(a) Mean, mode and median values are the same
(b) Mean value is more than median value
(c) Median value is more than mean value
(d) Mode value is more than median and mean value

Q4: In a positively skewed distribution, which of the following is the preferred measure of central tendency?
(a) Mean (b) Mode
(c) Median (d) Standard deviation

Q5: In a negatively skewed distribution, which of the following is the preferred measure of central tendency?

(a) Mean (b) Mode
(c) Median (d) Variance

Answers

1. b **2.** c **3.** a **4.** c **5.** c

FURTHER READING

Dawson B, Trapp RG. 2004. *Basic and Clinical Biostatistics, 4th ed.* Mc-Graw Hill, New York.

Glaser AN. 2000. *High Yield Biostatistics, 1st ed.* Lippincott Williams and Wilkins, New Delhi.

Gravetter FJ, Wallnau LB. 2000. *Statistics for the Behavioral Sciences, 5th ed.* Thomson Learning, Belmont Wadsworth.

Measures of Central Tendency. Laerd Statistics. (https://statistics.laerd.com/statistical-guides/measures-central-tendency-mean-mode-median.php)

Norman GR, Streiner DL. 2000. *Biostatistics, the Bare Essentials, 2nd ed.* BC Decker Inc. Hamilton.

Petrie A, Sabin C. 2009. *Medical Statistics at a Glance, 3rd ed.* Wiley-Blackwell, Oxford.

Sundaram KR, Dwivedi SN, Sreenivas V. 2010. *Medical Statistics Principles and Methods, 1st ed.* BI Publications Pvt Ltd, New Delhi.

Sundar Rao PS, Richard J. 2006. *Introduction to Biostatistics and Research Methods, 4th ed.* Prentice Hall of India Pvt Ltd, New Delhi.

Swinscow TD, Campbell MJ. 2003. *Statistics at Square One, 10th ed.* Viva Books Private Limited, New Delhi.

14 Measures of Variability

Chapter overview

- Introduction to measures of variability
- Range
- Interquartile range
- Variance
- Standard deviation
- Choosing the appropriate measure of variability

INTRODUCTION TO MEASURES OF VARIABILITY

In the previous chapter, the measures of central tendency were used to identify the midpoint of a distribution. However, within a data set, the actual values usually differ from one another and from the midpoint value itself. Therefore, what is required is a measure or single value that can express the variability within the given distribution. Measures of variability provide a mechanism to scholars to find out how much variation and diversity there is in a distribution. They represent the dispersion or variation among the values in a given data set. When the values in a distribution are considerably higher or lower than the mean value, it signifies the presence of high dispersion. The most commonly and frequently used measures of variability are range, interquartile range variation and standard deviation.

Range

Range is defined as the difference between the largest and smallest values in a data set. It is the most elementary measure of variation. Even though range is the easiest measure of variability to compute, it is not widely used because it is based on only two of the items in the data set and is thus highly influenced by extreme data values.

For example, the weight (in kg) of 14 male and 14 female nursing students is given in Table 14.1. Find out the weight range of male and female nursing students separately and identify which group has more dispersion.

Table 14.1 Comparison of weight of male and female nursing students

Male group	55	44	60	65	80	90	45	43	100	50	49	43	62	67
Female group	40	47	50	45	42	58	55	56	57	48	51	59	62	60

In the male group, the highest weight is 100 kg, while the lowest value is 43 kg. Therefore, the weight range of the male group is 100 – 43 = 57. Likewise, in the female group, the highest weight is 62 kg and lowest is 40 kg, which yields a range of 62 – 40 = 22. This indicates that there is wider variation in the weight of male nursing students than among female nursing students.

The problem associated with range is that, it is based exclusively on the two most extreme values within the data set; therefore, if any one of these values is an outlier, it will result in an atypical range that is not representative of the variability within the data set. In order to reduce the problems caused by outliers in a data set, the interquartile range is often calculated instead of range.

Advantages

- Easy to calculate
- Makes conceptual sense

Disadvantages

- Only uses the two extreme scores
- Not resistant to outliers

Interquartile Range

The interquartile range as a measure of variability corresponds with median, a measure of central tendency. The interquartile range indicates the extent to which the middle 50% of values within the data set are dispersed. The following steps explain the calculation of interquartile range.

Step 1: Arrange the data in descending order of magnitude.

Step 2: Identify the median of the distribution

Step 3: Identify the upper and lower quartiles. The upper quartile lies halfway between median and the highest value in the data set, while the lower quartile lies halfway between median and the lowest value in the data set.

Step 4: The interquartile range is found by subtracting the lower quartile from the upper quartile.

For example, Table 14.2 shows the age of CHF patients arranged in order of magnitude.

Table 14.2 CHF patients (age) arranged in order of magnitude

LQ — Median — UQ

CHF Patients	A	B	C	D	E	F	G	H	I	J	K	L	M	N	O	P	Q	R	S	T
Age	60	62	64	66	68	70	72	74	76	78	80	82	84	86	88	90	92	94	95	96

Step 1: The median lies at the midpoint between the two central values (10th and 11th) = halfway between 78 and 80 = 79
Step 2: The lower quartile lies at the midpoint between the 5th and 6th values = halfway between 68 and 70 = 69
Step 3: The upper quartile lies at the midpoint between the 15th and 16th values = halfway between 88 and 90 = 89
Step 4: The interquartile range for this data set is therefore 89 – 69 = 20, whereas the range is 96 – 60 = 36.

Another method of calculating interquartile range is by splitting the distribution into 'quarters or fourths'.

Q1 = value at 25 percentile
Q2 = value at 50 percentile (median)
Q3 = value at 75 percentile
Q4 = value at 100 percentile

In this method, the formula used to calculate the interquartile range is Q3 – Q1.
Steps to calculate interquartile range using the quarters or fourth method:

Step 1: Arrange the scores from lowest to highest.
Step 2: Find the location of the median value.
Step 3: Find the locations of the quartile (Q1 and Q3).
Step 4: Find the exact values of the quartiles.
Step 5: Calculate the difference between Q1 and Q3.

Quartile location in orderly data can be identified using the following formula:

$$\text{Quartile location} = \frac{\text{Median location} + 1}{2}$$

Note: In some cases, median location may be a fractional value (when *N* is even); in this situation, the fraction should be dropped before computing the quartile location.

Example 14.1

Compute the interquartile range of the given data set (*N* is odd).

1	2	3	5	7	8	10	11	12

Step 1: Median location: $(N + 1)/2 = (9 + 1)/2 = 5^{th}$ observation (see the arrow).

1	2	3	5	7	8	10	11	12

Step 2: Quartile location = $(5 + 1)/2 = 3$.

Count 3 up from the bottom value (for Q1) and 3 down from the top value for the quartiles (for Q3).

		Q1				Q3		
1	2	3	5	7	8	10	11	12

Interquartile range: Q3 – Q1 = 10 – 3 = 7

Example 14.2

Compute the interquartile range of the given dataset (*N* is even).

1	2	4	5	7	8	10	11

Step 1: Median location: $(N + 1)/2 = (8 + 1)/2 = 4.5$.

1	2	4	5	7	8	10	11

$$\text{Median} = \frac{5+7}{2} = 6$$

Step 2: Quartile location = (4 + 1)/2 = 2.5.
Count up 2.5 from the bottom value and 2.5 down from the top value for the quartiles.

	Q1 ↓					Q3 ↓	
1	2	4	5	7	8	10	11

Q1 = Average of 2 and 4 = 3

Q3 = Average of 8 and 10 = 9

Interquartile range = 9 − 3 = 6

Advantages

- Not influenced by outliers
- Good measure of variability for skewed distributions

Disadvantages

- Uses only two scores (Q3 and Q1) for calculation
- Entire distribution is not used in the computation of interquartile range

The main drawback of interquartile range is that, it is based on only two values from the data set. Therefore, standard deviation (discussed later in the chapter) is considered a more powerful measure of dispersion because it takes into account every value in the data set.

Variance

Variance is defined as the degree to which the scores in a distribution vary around the mean. It is also known as mean square, which is the average of the squared deviation around the mean. As depicted in Table 14.3, the sum of the deviation of individual values from the mean is always zero (Σd). Because Σd is always zero, the average of the deviations will also always be zero. To overcome this problem, each deviation is squared and the sum is computed. This sum is divided by the number of observation to compute the variance. Large values of σ^2 indicate more variability around the mean. The disadvantage of variance is that it uses squared values instead of original values in its calculation.

Table 14.3 Standard deviation

Deviation (d) = ($X - \mu$)

X	$d = X - \mu$	d
3	3 – 2	1
0	0 – 2	–2
4	4 – 2	+2
1	1 – 2	–1

Mean (μ) = 2 $\Sigma d = 0$

$$\text{Variance } \sigma^2 = \frac{\Sigma(X-\mu)^2}{N}$$

Example 14.3

Compute the variance of the following data:

3	4	5	4

Step 1: Calculate the mean of the given data set
Mean = 4.

Step 2: Find the deviation (D) of each value from the mean using the formula ($D = X - \mu$).

Step 3: Square each value of D (see table below)

Step 4: Sum each squared value of D ($\Sigma D^2 = 1 + 0 + 1 + 0 = 2$).

Step 5: Divide the sum by the number of observations (N): 2/4 = 0.5.
So, the variance (σ^2) of the given data set is 0.5.

X	$d = X - \mu$	D	d^2
3	3 – 4	–1	1
4	4 – 4	0	0
5	5 – 4	+1	1
4	4 – 4	0	0

Standard Deviation

Standard deviation is simply defined as the square root of the variance. It is the most widely used measure of variability as it takes into account every value in a data set. It provides a single value that indicates the average amount by which every observation within a data set varies from the mean. A small standard deviation indicates that values in the data set are tightly clustered together. When the values are spread apart, the standard deviation will be relatively large. In research reports, standard deviation is presented in conjunction with mean and is measured in the same units.

In statistics, population and sample are treated differently; therefore, the formula used for the computation of population and sample standard deviation is different. The standard deviation of an entire population is known as σ (sigma) and is calculated using the following formula:

$$\text{Population standard deviation } (\sigma) = \sqrt{\frac{\Sigma(X-\mu)^2}{N}}$$

where:

- X represents each value in the population
- μ is the mean value of the population
- N is the number of values in the population

The standard deviation of a sample is known as S and is calculated using the following formula:

$$\sigma = \sqrt{\frac{\Sigma(x-\bar{x})^2}{n-1}}$$

where

- X represents each value in the sample
- X bar is the mean value of the sample
- $n - 1$ is the sample size minus 1 (also known as degree of freedom)

The researcher's main goal is to estimate population parameters based on the sample statistics so that they can generalise their findings to the target population. As sample tends to have less variability than population, sample variance underestimates the true population variance. Therefore, to overcome this problem, the formula is adjusted by taking $(n - 1)$ instead of N to make the sample variation unbiased.

$$S^2 = \sqrt{\frac{\Sigma(X-\bar{X})^2}{n-1}}$$

Shortcut method

A shortcut method of calculating variance and standard deviation requires two quantities, given as follows:

Σx = Sum of the values

Σx^2 = Sum of the squares of the values

For example, use the four values: 3, 1, 2, 5.

Here,

$\Sigma x = 11$

$\Sigma x^2 = 39$

Now, $\Sigma(x - \bar{x})^2$ is determined using a shortcut formula:

$$\Sigma(x - \bar{x})^2 = \Sigma x^2 - \frac{(\Sigma x)^2}{n} = 8.75$$

The variance and standard deviation are now calculated using the same formula:

$$S^2 = \sqrt{\frac{\Sigma(X - \bar{X})^2}{n - 1}}$$

$$S^2 \text{ (variance)} = \frac{8.75}{3} = 2.91$$

S (standand deviation) = 1.70

Calculating standard deviation using Microsoft Excel

Excel is a utility of Microsoft Office that includes functions to calculate population and sample standard deviations. The appropriate commands are entered into the formula bar towards the top of the spreadsheet and the corresponding cells in the spreadsheet are updated to show the result. The command to find the population standard deviation in Excel is = STDEVP(VALUES) and in the screenshots (Figs 14.1 and 14.2) given below, the command = STDEVP(A2:A6) gives an answer of 7.39.

The same data can be used to demonstrate how to calculate the sample standard deviation in Excel. The sample standard deviation is calculated using = STDEV(VALUES),

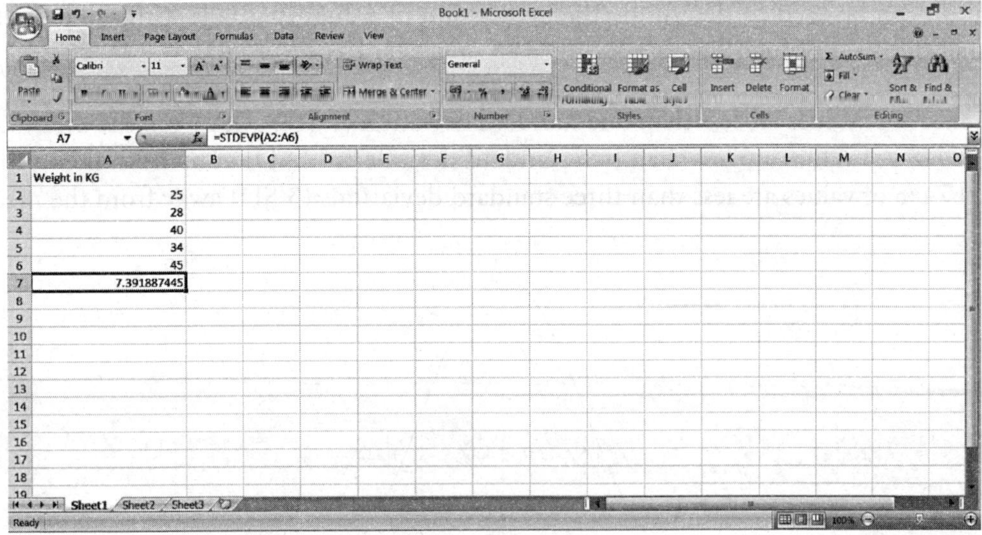

Figure 14.1 Using Microsoft Excel to compute population standard deviation

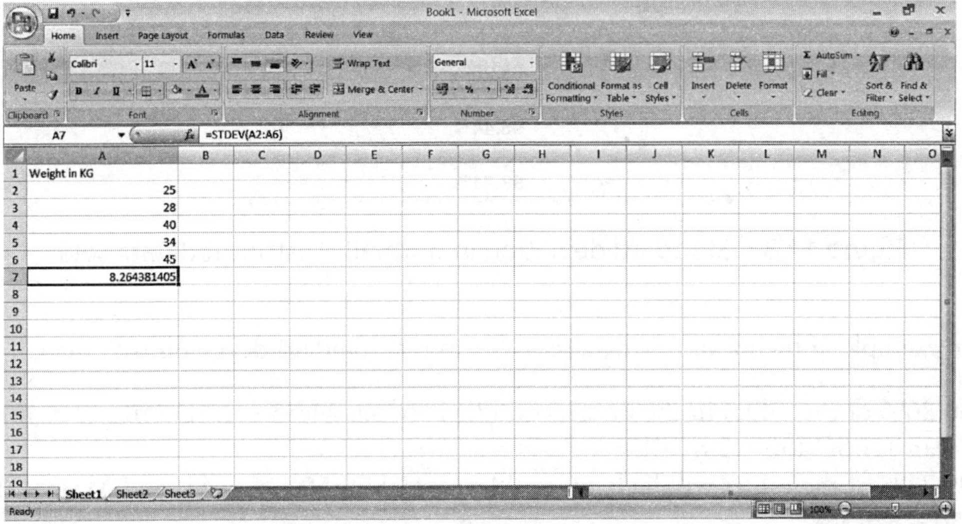

Figure 14.2 Using Microsoft Excel to compute sample standard deviation

and in this case, the command is = STDEV(A2:A6), which produces an answer of 8.26 (sample standard deviation is always greater than the estimated population standard deviation, if used for the same data set).

Standard deviation in normal distribution data set

In a normally distributed data set, most values are bunched around the mean, whereas very few values tend to be extremely high or low. In normally distributed data sets, standard deviation can be used to determine the proportion of values that falls within a particular range of the mean value (Fig. 14.3).

- 68.26% of values are less than one standard deviation (1 SD) away from the mean value
- 95.44% of values are less than two standard deviations (2 SD) away from the mean
- 99.74% of values are less than three standard deviations (3 SD) away from the mean.

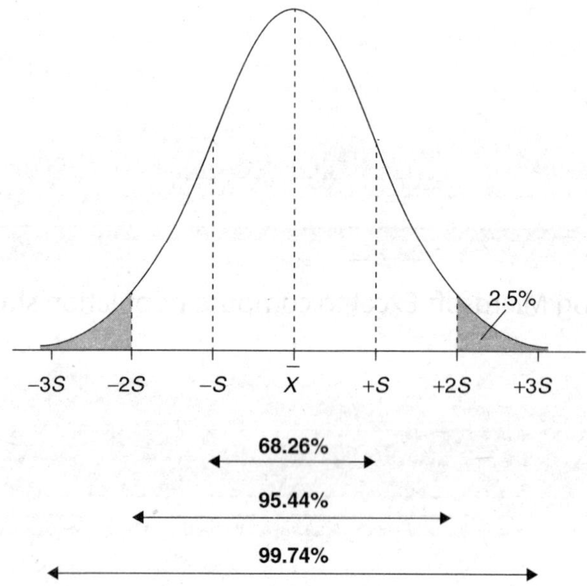

Figure 14.3 Standard deviation in normally distributed data sets

For example, if the mean of a data set is 50 and its standard deviation is 2, then

- 68.26% of the values in the data set will lie between Mean – 1 SD (50 – 2 = 48) and Mean + 1 SD (50 + 2 = 52).
- 99.74% of the values will lie between Mean – 3 SD (50 – 6 = 44) and Mean + 3 SD (50 + 6 = 56).

Choosing the appropriate measure of variability While analysing data for a study, the nurse researcher must select the appropriate measure of variability. Which measure of variability is suitable for a particular group of data is determined by the level of measurement of the data. In addition to this, the skeweness of the distribution also plays an important part in the selection of the measure of dispersion. Interquartile variation is used for nominal scales, whereas range and interquartile range are used for ordinal scales. Similarly, variance and standard deviation are computed for a normally distributed ratio and interval scale, whereas range and interquartile range may be used for seriously skewed data (Fig. 14.4).

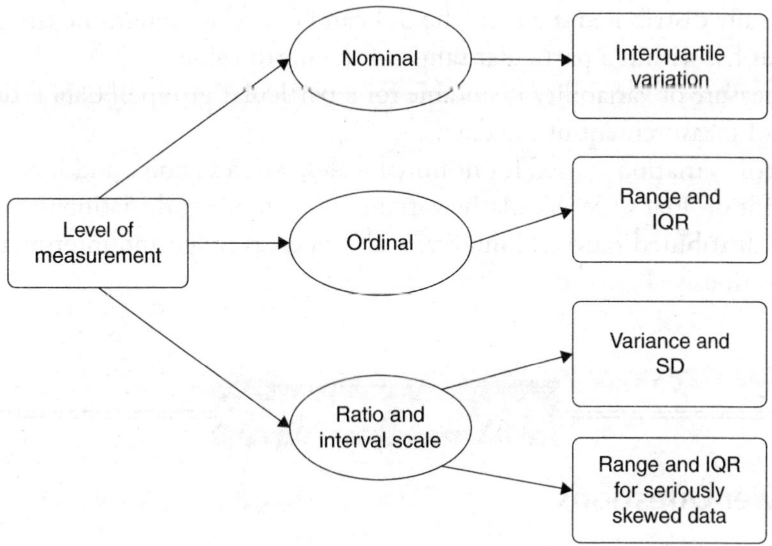

Figure 14.4 Selecting the appropriate measure of variability

CHAPTER SUMMARY

- Measures of variability represent the dispersion or variation among the values in a given data set.
- Range is defined as the difference between the largest and smallest values in a data set.
- The interquartile range indicates the extent to which the middle 50% of values within the data set are dispersed.
- The main drawback of interquartile range is that it is based on only two values from the data set.
- Variance is defined as the degree to which the scores in a distribution vary around the mean. It is also known as mean square, which is the average of the squared deviation around the mean.
- Standard deviation is simply defined as the square root of the variance. It is the most widely used measure of variability as it takes into account every value in a data set.
- A small standard deviation indicates that values in the data set are tightly clustered together. When the values are spread apart, the standard deviation will be relatively large.
- In statistics, population and sample are treated differently; therefore, the formulae used for the computation of population and sample standard deviation are different.
- The command to find the population standard deviation in Microsoft Excel is = STDEVP(VALUES) and the command for sample standard deviation is = STDEV(VALUES).

- In a normally distributed data set, the SD can be used to determine the proportion of values that fall within a particular range of the mean value.
- Which measure of variability is suitable for a particular group of data is determined by the level of measurement of the data.
- Interquartile variation is used for nominal scales, whereas range and interquartile range are used for ordinal scale. Similarly, variance and standard deviation are computed for normally distributed ratio and interval scale, whereas range and interquartile range are used for seriously skewed data.

EVALUATE YOURSELF

Long Answer Questions

Q1: Define the measures of variability. Explain the advantages and disadvantages of each.

Q2: Calculate interquartile range for the following data set:

MI Patients	A	B	C	D	E	F	G	H	I	J	K	L	M	N	O	P	Q	R	S	T
Age	54	60	64	66	63	71	75	76	76	75	90	32	74	76	78	60	72	44	45	66

Q3: Compute the variance of the following data set:

6	5	3	4

Q4: What important factors will you consider before selecting the appropriate measure of dispersion?

Q5: Compute standard deviation for the following data set:

12, 15, 20, 25, 30, 56, 40, 50

Short Answer Questions

Q1: Write a short note on interquartile range.

Q2: Advantages and disadvantages standard deviation

Q3: Variance

Q4: Range

Multiple Choice Questions

Q1: Which of the following is a measure of dispersion?
(a) Variance (b) Mean
(c) Mode (d) Median

Q2: For normally distributed ratio level data, the appropriate measure of dispersion is:
(a) Standard deviation (b) Range
(c) Interquartile range (d) Variance

Q3: 68.26% of the values in a normally distributed data set lies within:
(a) Mean ± 1SD (b) Mean ± 2SD
(c) Mean ± 3SD (d) Mean ± 4SD

Q4: What percentage of values lies between mean ± 3SD in normally distributed data?
(a) 68.26% (b) 99.74%
(c) 95.44% (d) 70.45%

Q5: Interquartile variation is used as a measure of dispersion for:
(a) Nominal data (b) Ordinal data
(c) Ratio data (d) Continuous data

Q6: For a seriously skewed data set, which of the following is an appropriates choice as a measure of dispersion?
(a) Interquartile range (b) Range
(c) Both a and b (d) Standard deviation

Answers

1. a **2.** a **3.** a **4.** b **5.** b **6.** c

FURTHER READING

Dawson B, Trapp RG. 2004. *Basic and Clinical Biostatistics, 4th ed.* Mc-Graw Hill, New York.
John WB, James VK. 2002. *Research in Education, 7th ed.* Prentice Hall India.
Mahajan BK. 2011. Methods in Biostatistics, *6th ed.* JayPee Brothers Publishers.
Sundaram KR, Dwivedi SN, Sreenivas V. 2010. *Medical Statistics Principles and Methods, 1st ed.* BI Publications Pvt Ltd, New Delhi.
SundarRao PS, Richard J. 2006. *Introduction to Biostatistics and Research Methods, 4th ed.* Prentice Hall India.

Measures of Relationship

Chapter overview

- Meaning and need for correlation
- Scatter diagram method
- Product moment correlation
- Rank order correlation
- Simple linear regression analysis and prediction

CORRELATION: MEANING AND NEED

When an academic paper states that the height and weight of a person are correlated with each other, it means that both these variables have a reciprocal relationship and changes in one variable will lead to changes in the other.

Correlation is defined as a measure that determines the type (positive or negative) and magnitude (strength) of the association between two quantitatively measured variables. It is denoted by *r* (correlation coefficient), and the value of *r* ranges from −1 to +1 (Fig. 15.1). However, *r* does not take into account prior knowledge of whether one variable is dependent on the other. The aim of correlation statistics is only to quantify the association. Many decisions in the nursing sciences depend on the idea of causal relationships; therefore, understanding the concept of relationships between two or more variables is important for identifying the limitations of the conclusions presented in the literature.

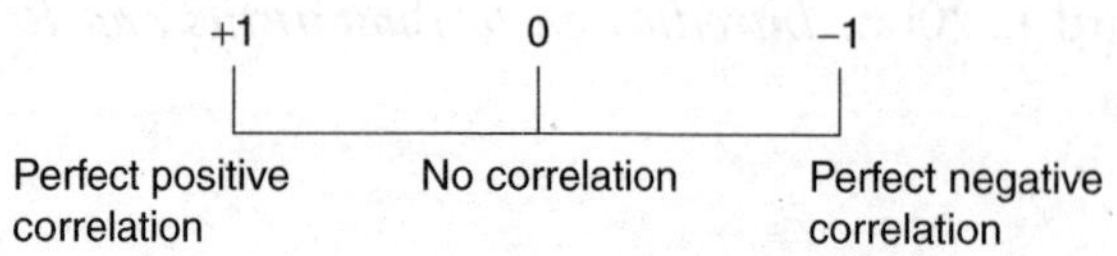

Figure 15.1 Correlation relationship

Table 15.1 Interpretation of correlation coefficient (*r*)

Correlation coefficient value (*r*)	Interpretation
±0.8 and above	Higher correlation coefficient
±0.4 to ±0.7	Moderate correlation coefficient
±0.3 and below	Weak correlation coefficient
0	No correlation

SCATTER DIAGRAM METHOD

Correlation data is represented on a special type of graph called a scatter plot (or scatter diagram). On a scatter plot, one variable (X) is placed on the horizontal axis (abscissa) and the other variable (Y) is placed on the vertical axis (ordinate). The plot reveals how the values on the vertical axis are scattered for a given value on the X axis and how the values on the X axis are scattered for a given value on the Y axis. As it shows the scatter of the two variables with respect to each other, this diagram is called a scatter diagram. The pattern of clustering of observations provides information about the type of correlation between the two variables.

Scatter diagrams help visualise the type of relation that exists between two variables, whether linear or non-linear or no relation. However, they do not help quantify the relationship. If the relation appears as linear or near linear, it can be quantified by a measure called the correlation coefficient (*r*).

TYPES OF CORRELATION

- Positive and negative
- Simple and multiple
- Linear and non-linear

Positive correlation

When two variables are positively related to each other, then a positive correlation is said to exist between them. Change in one variable will lead to change in the other variable in the same direction (whether positive or negative). In other words, the ups and down in both variables occur in a similar fashion, i.e., if one variable ascends, the other will also rise; if there is a decrease in one variable, the other variable will also decrease. When the correlation is perfect ($r = +1$), both variables will increase or decrease to the same extent. Perfect correlation is very rare in nature. On a scatter diagram, a positive correlation appears, as given in Fig. 15.2, which shows the correlation of knowledge score with skill score about Basic Life Support. A subject who scores higher on knowledge also scores higher on skills for Basic Life Support. The change in both the variables is at the same rate.

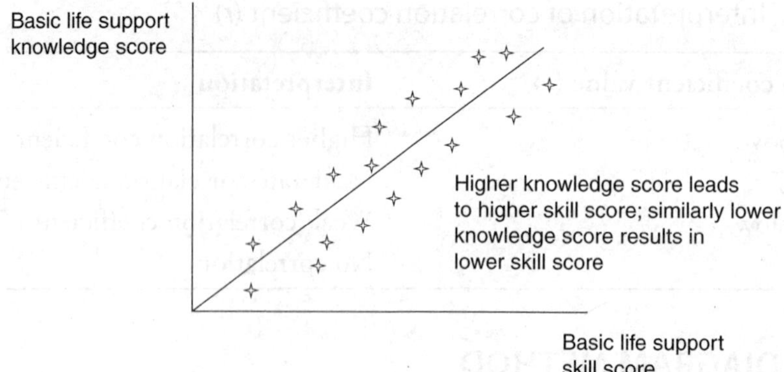

Figure 15.2 Positive correlation

Negative correlation

When two variables are negatively related to each other, a negative correlation is said to exist between them. Change in one variable will lead to change in the other variable in the opposite direction; i.e., if there is an increase in one variable, the other variable will show a decrease, and vice versa. When the correlation is perfect ($r = -1$), the increase and decrease in both variables will be of the same extent. For example, body weight and hours of physical activity are negatively correlated, as shown in Fig. 15.3.

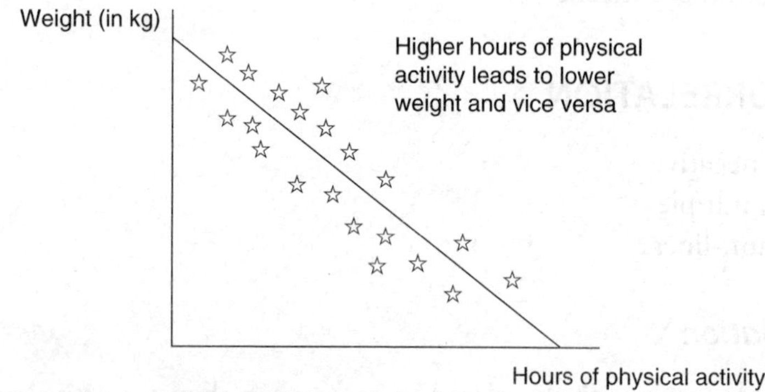

Figure 15.3 Negative correlation

Simple and multiple correlations

The terms simple and multiple correlations are used according to the number of variables in the study. Simple correlation is defined as the relationship between two variables only; for example, the correlation between blood pressure and age. In contrast, multiple correlations are relationships among three or more variables; for example, correlation among age, blood pressure and cholesterol level.

Linear and non-linear correlations

When observations on two related variables are scattered around the central straight line in a scatter diagram, it is known as a linear correlation. In this type of correlation, change in one variable leads to change in the other variable at a ratio that is constant (Fig. 15.4). For example, consider the data given below:

Variable X	Variable Y	Constant change ratio in X and Y
4	7	–
8	14	2
12	21	3

In this data set of two related variables, change in both the variables is in ratio, that is, constant at each step. In non-linear correlation, change in one variable tends to lead to a varying change in the correlated variable (Fig. 15.5). Consider the following example:

Variable X	Variable Y	Variable change ratio	
		X	Y
4	7	–	–
5	14	1	2
6	21	1	3

No correlation

If the correlation coefficient is zero or nearly zero, it means that both the variables do not have any relationship or that no correlation exists between them. Consider Fig. 15.6, which depicts no correlation.

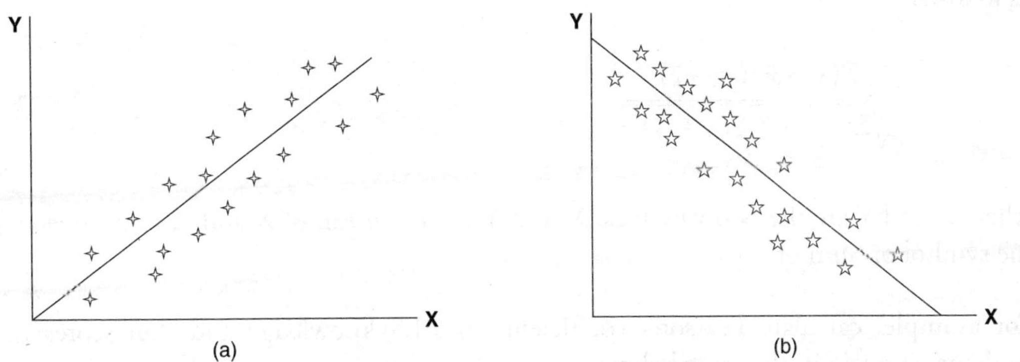

Figure 15.4 (a) Positive and linear correlation (b) Negative and linear correlation

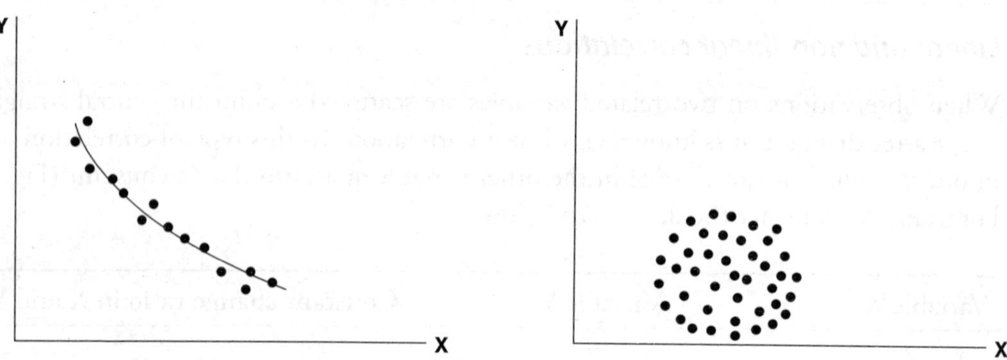

Figure 15.5 Negative non-linear correlation

Figure 15.6 No correlation

CORRELATION STATISTICS

Correlation statistics is applicable for ordinal, continuous and ratio level measurements. However, the method of calculating differs according to the level of measurement for which the data is collected. Correlation statistics is both descriptive and inferential. Therefore, it can be used to describe or test a hypothesis about the relation between two variables. The methods of correlation coefficient calculation and the applicability of each method are now discussed.

Karl Pearson's Product Moment Method

This method of calculating the correlation coefficient is used for variables that are measured on continuous or ratio level (for example, height, weight, pulse rate, systolic blood pressure, respiratory rate, temperature and so on) and are normally distributed in the population. It not only describes the magnitude and direction of correlation (descriptive statistic) but is also used to test hypotheses (inferential statistic) about whether the correlation is significant or not. It can be used for both within the group and between groups situations. It is denoted by the symbol *r*. The formula used to compute Pearson's correlation coefficient is as follows:

$$r = \frac{\Sigma(x - \bar{x})(y - \bar{y})}{\sqrt{\Sigma(x - \bar{x})^2 \, \Sigma(y - \bar{y})^2}}$$

where X and Y are the two variables; $\bar{X}$ and $\bar{Y}$ are the mean of X and Y, respectively; Σ is the symbol of 'sum of'.

For example, calculate Pearson's coefficient for BLS knowledge and skill scores of 10 students, as given in the table below:

Subject	BLS knowledge score (X)	BLS skill score (Y)
1	15	8
2	17	8
3	12	6
4	18	7
5	20	9
6	11	4
7	10	3
8	09	4
9	05	2
10	08	4

Step 1: Calculate the mean of X and Y and insert the values in the last row of columns 1 and 2 of the table, as given below:

Subject ID	X	Y	$X-\bar{X}$	$Y-\bar{Y}$	$(X-\bar{X})(Y-\bar{Y})$	$(X-\bar{X})^2$	$(Y-\bar{Y})^2$
	(1)	(2)	(3)	(4)	(5)	(6)	(7)
1	15	8	$15-13=02$	$8-6=2$	$2\times 2=4$	04	4
2	17	8	$17-13=04$	$8-6=2$	$4\times 2=8$	16	4
3	12	6	$12-13=-01$	$6-6=0$	$-1\times 0=0$	1	0
4	18	7	$18-13=05$	$7-6=1$	$5\times 1=5$	25	1
5	20	9	$20-13=07$	$9-6=3$	$7\times 3=21$	49	9
6	11	4	$11-13=-02$	$4-6=-2$	$-2\times -2=4$	4	4
7	10	3	$10-13=-03$	$3-6=-3$	$-3\times -3=9$	9	9
8	09	4	$09-13=-04$	$4-6=-2$	$-4\times -2=8$	16	4
9	10	7	$10-13=-03$	$7-6=1$	$-3\times 1=-3$	9	1
10	08	4	$08-13=-05$	$8-6=2$	$-5\times 2=-10$	25	4
	$\sum X=130$ Mean = 13	**$\sum Y=60$ Mean = 6**			**$\sum(X-\bar{X})(Y-\bar{Y})=47$**	**$\sum(X-\bar{X})^2=158$**	**$\sum(Y-\bar{Y})^2=40$**

Step 3: Compute the deviations $(X-\bar{X})(Y-\bar{Y})$ from the mean for each observation of X and Y (see columns 3 and 4). Multiply the deviation of X with the deviation of Y and finally sum it (see column 5).

Step 4: Square the deviation of each observation from mean for both variables. Compute the sum of both the columns separately (columns 6 and 7).

Step 4: Multiply $\Sigma(X - \overline{X})^2$ and $\Sigma(Y - \overline{Y})^2$.

Step 5: Use Pearson's formula to find the correlation coefficient.

$$r = \frac{47}{\sqrt{158 \times 40}}$$

$$= 0.519$$

Interpretation: The resultant correlation coefficient between the knowledge score and skill score is moderate; hence it can be concluded that higher knowledge score leads to higher skill score for BLS. However, we cannot ascertain with this descriptive statistics whether this correlation is significant or not (whether the results are by chance only or if it is a real situation in the population).

For hypothesis testing, as inferential statistics, Pearson's correlation is symbolised by the Greek letter rho (ρ). Therefore, the null hypothesis states that rho is 0, whereas the alternative hypothesis states that rho is not equal to 0.

$H_0: \rho = 0$ $H_A: \rho \neq 0$

It must also be ascertained whether the calculated value of $r = 0.519$ is significant at the significance level of 0.05 for a two-tailed test.

For hypothesis testing, the degree of freedom must be computed. It is equal to the number of subjects minus 2 (N – 2) for the correlation coefficient. In the above example, it will be $10 - 2 = 8$. Thereafter, the tabulated value of r must be referred to for the degree of freedom of 8, level of significance 0.05 and two-tailed hypothesis testing. The tabulated value is found to be 0.6319 which is more than the calculated value of r. Hence, the null hypothesis is accepted and the alternative hypothesis is rejected.

NOTE

- r is a pure number without any units.
- Absence of correlation or poor correlation only means that there is no linear relation between the variables. It may not mean that the two variables are unrelated.
- Computation of r is logical only when the scatter diagram indicates a linear relationship and there is biological plausibility of relation between the two variables.
- Presence of high correlation should also be not interpreted as the two variables are directly related. Both may be due to the presence or absence of other common factor(s).

Use of Microsoft Excel to compute

1. Enter the data for the X and Y variables.
2. Click Formula, then Statistics and finally select Pearson. The Function Argument window will be displayed.
3. Enter data in Array 1 and Array 2 (Array 1 is the number of first row: last row in which data on the X variable is entered, here it is A2:A11; similarly Array 2 is B2:B11).
4. Click OK. *r* will be displayed on the spreadsheet.

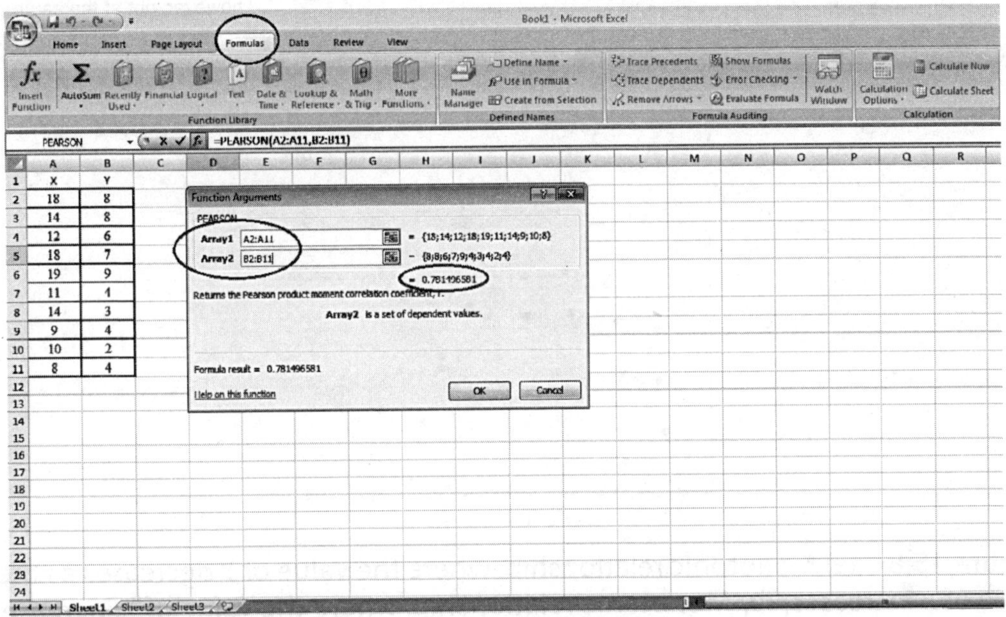

Figure 15.7 Using MS Excel to compute

Spearman Rho (ρ)

Spearman rho is used to compute the correlation for ranked or ordinal variables. Ranks are assigned to the observations in the X and Y data set. It is a non-parametric bivariate descriptive as well as inferential statistics which shows the strength and direction of the relationship between two ranked variables and confirms whether the relationship is different from zero (hypothesis testing). The sign (plus or minus) of the Spearman correlation indicates the direction of the relationship between X and Y. If Y tends to increase when X increases, the Spearman correlation is positive. Similarly, if Y tends to decrease when X increases, the Spearman correlation is negative. A Spearman correlation of zero indicates that there is no association of increase or decrease between the X and Y variables. The Spearman correlation coefficient becomes 1 when X and Y are perfectly monotonically related. Spearman correlation is used when assumptions of the Pearson correlation are violated (data is not normally distributed). Secondly, it is used when there is a monotonic relationship between the variables. A monotonic relationship exists if when the value of one variable increases, the value of the other variable either increases or decreases (Fig. 15.8).

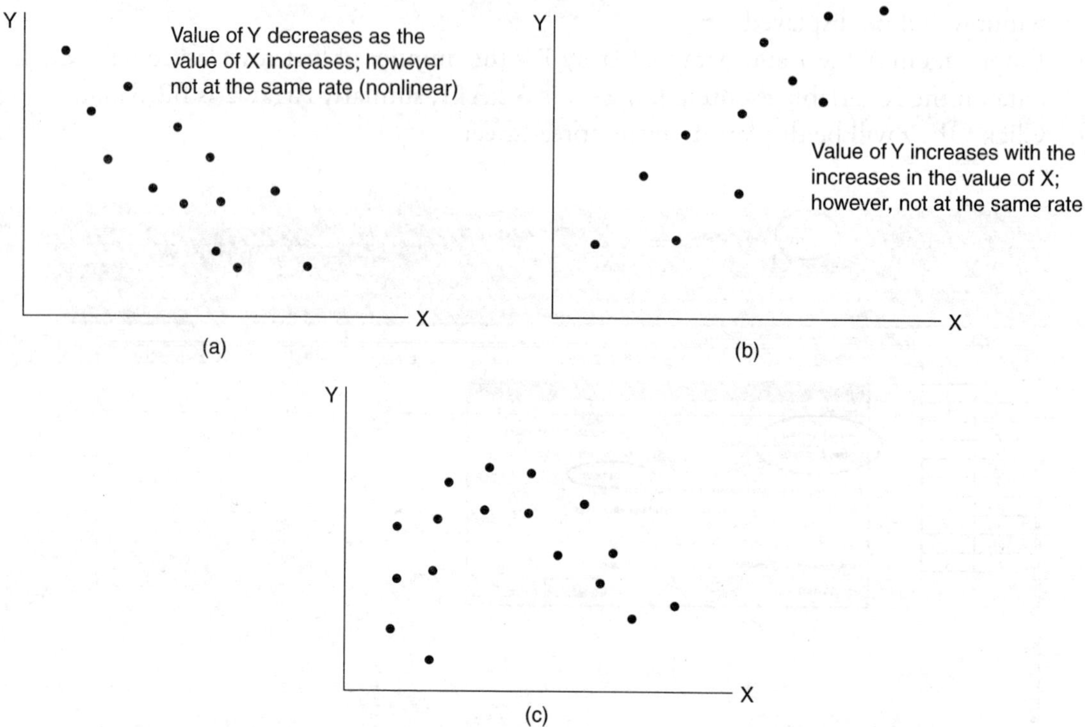

Figure 15.8 (a) Monotonic relationship, where the value of *Y* decreases as the value of *x* increases; (b) Monotonic relationship, where the value of *Y* increases as the value of *x* decreases (c) Non-monotonic relationship

The formula for calculating the Spearman rho correlation coefficient is as follows.

$$\textbf{Spearman's rho } (\rho) = \frac{1 - 6\sum d^2}{n(n^2 - 1)}$$

where n is the number of paired ranks and d is the difference between the paired ranks.

How to rank the data

Ranking of each observation of the X and Y variables is undertaken systematically. Rank 1 is assigned to the highest value; rank 2 to the second highest value and so on. There will be as many ranks as the number of observations. Whenever there are two identical values in the data set, it is known as a tie. In this situation, the **average** of the ranks that the identical values would have otherwise occupied is used, for example, ranks 7 and 8 will be divided into 7.5 and 7.5 for each of the tied observations. The next rank to be assigned in the data set will be 9.

For example, the theory and practical marks in six subjects are given below:

Theory marks	Practical marks	Rank (Theory marks)	Rank (Practical marks)
55	50	2	3
40	60	4.5	1
40	45	4.5	4
45	40	3	5
60	55	1	2
35	30	6	6

There are two identical values in the theory marks, i.e., 40 marks. Therefore, the rank for the ties is calcuated as follows:

$$4+5=\frac{9}{2}$$
$$=4.5$$

Given below are the marks in Pathology and Microbiology obtained by five nursing students. Calculate Spearman's correlation coefficient.

Pathology	20	15	11	16	10
Microbiology	15	14	10	13	12

The calculation is explained in the table given below:

Pathology marks	Microbiology marks	Rank (Pathology)	Rank (Microbiology)	d	d^2
20	15	1	1	0	0
15	14	3	2	1	1
11	10	4	5	−1	1
16	13	2	3	−1	1
10	12	5	4	1	1
					$\sum d^2 = 4$

Inserting values in the formula, as given below:

$$\textbf{Spearman's rho } (\rho) = \frac{1-6\sum d^2}{n(n^2-1)}$$

$$= \frac{1-6\times 4}{5(25-1)}$$

$$= \frac{1-24}{120}$$

$$= 1 - 0.2$$

$$= 0.8$$

The formula for tied ranks is:

$$\rho = \frac{\sum_i (x_i - \bar{x})(y_i - \bar{y})}{\sqrt{\sum_i (x_i - \bar{x})^2 \sum_i (y_i - \bar{y})^2}}$$

where i = paired score.

Kendall's Tau

This is another test used to compute the correlation coefficient between ordinal level variables. It is named after Maurice Kendall, who developed it in 1938. The value of Kendall's tau ranges from +1 to –1. It also describes the magnitude and direction of the relationship and confirms whether the relationship is different from zero. It is a non-parametric hypothesis test for statistical dependence based on the tau coefficient. It is symbolised by tau (τ). The similarity between Spearman's and Kendall's correlation is that both are non-parametric tests used for ranked observations. However, Kendall's correlation differs in the interpretation of the correlation value. Unlike Pearson's and Spearman's correlation, which represent a similar magnitude of the correlation coefficient, this represents a probability. It is the difference between the probability that the observed data is in the same order versus the probability that the observed data is not in the same order.

$$\tau = \frac{\text{Concordant pairs} - \text{Discordant pairs}}{\frac{1}{2}N(N-1)}$$

A concordant pair is one where the rank of the second variable is greater than the rank of the first variable. A discordant pair is when the rank is equal to or less than the rank of the first variable.

The following data represent a teacher's ranking of 10 cardiac nursing students as to their suitability for a career in and knowledge of cardiology:

Student code	Career	Cardiology knowledge
Student 1	1	1
Student 2	2	4
Student 3	5	2
Student 4	3	3
Student 5	4	5

Step 1: Sort these in order such that one of the variables is in the proper order. Here, Career will be sorted and then Cardiology knowledge will be examined for the value of S (Number of concordance – Number of discordance).

Student code		Career	Cardiology knowledge
Student 1	a	1	1
Student 2	b	2	4
Student 3	c	5	3
Student 4	d	3	5
Student 5	e	4	2

Step 2: Calculate the number of pairs of concordance and discordance.

Pair (a,b) = + 1 (C) (for career variable a < b; for cardiology knowledge a < b)
Pair (a,c) = + 1 (C)
Pair (a,d) = + 1 (C)
Pair (a,e) = + 1 (C)

Pair (b,c) = – 1 (D) (for career variable b < c; for cardiology knowledge b > c)
Pair (b,d) = + 1 (C)
Pair (b,e) = – 1 (D)
Pair (c,d) = + 1 (C)
Pair (c,e) = – 1 (D)
Pair (d,e) = – 1 (D)

Step 3: Insert the values in the formula

$$\frac{6-4}{\frac{1}{2}5(5-1)}$$

$$= \frac{2}{10} = 0.2$$

If there are tied (same value) observations, then τ_b is used:

$$t_b = \frac{S}{\sqrt{\left[n(n-1)/2 - \sum_{i=1}^{t} t_i(t_i - 1)/2\right]\left[n(n-1)/2 - \sum_{i=1}^{u} u_i(u_i - 1)/2\right]}}$$

where t_i is the number of observations tied at a particular rank of X and u_i is the number tied at a rank of Y.

Correlation and Causality

Variables may be related with each other but this in no way implies that the change in one **causes** the change in the other. Therefore, a cause-and-effect relationship cannot be established just because a higher correlation coefficient exists between two variables.

Correlation of Nominal Variables

The Phi coefficient and Cremer's *V* statistics are used to ascertain the magnitude of the relationship between two nominal level variables. Phi coefficient describes the magnitude between two dichotomous variables. Cremer's *V* is applied on a contingency table larger than 2 × 2. Both tests are based on chi-square statistics and yield values of 0.00 to 1.00. Higher values indicate strong association between the variables.

Simple Linear Regression

Is it possible to predict the value of the dependent variable based on the value of one independent variable? Yes, simple linear regression analysis is used to predict the dependent variable (*Y*) using the independent or predictor variable (*X*). When there is only one predictor variable, the prediction method is called *simple regression.*

For example, weight can be predicted from height using simple linear regression if certain parameters of regression analysis are known.

Assumptions

Several assumptions must be satisfied if linear regression is to be used:

- Both the variables (X and Y) are measured at the interval or ratio level.
- There should be a linear relationship between the predictor and predicted variables.
- Errors in prediction of the value of Y should be normally distributed.
- Errors in prediction of the value of Y should be independent of one another.
- The distribution of the errors in the prediction of the value of the predicted variable is constant regardless of the value of the predictor variable.

The accuracy of prediction depends on the magnitude of the correlation between both the variables. The higher the correlation between the variables, the more accurate the prediction. For example, if there is perfect correlation between height and height ($r = 1$), then only one variable needs to be measured to find out the value of the other. As most variables are not perfectly correlated in the population, predictions made through regression analysis are usually imperfect.

The equation for basic linear regression is as follows:

$$Y' = a + bX$$

It is the algebraic equation for a straight line, where

Y' = predicted value of variable Y; a = intercept constant; b = slope of line (regression coefficient); X = actual value of the variable X.

Regression analysis is undertaken to compute the value of a and b so that the value of Y can be predicted for any given value of X.

The formulae for the calculation of a and b are as follows:

$$a = \overline{Y} - b\overline{X}$$

$$b = \frac{\sum xy}{\sum x^2}$$

where, x is the deviation score from the mean of the X variable, y is the deviation score from the mean of the Y variable, X is the mean of variable $\overline{X}$, $\overline{Y}$ is the mean of variable Y.

Consider the following data to understand simple linear analysis. Five observations of variable X and Y are given here:

X	2	4	5	3	6
Y	1	3	4	5	2

Steps to compute simple linear regression from the data given in the above table are explained below.

X	Y	x	x^2	y	y^2	xy	Y'	e	e^2
2	1	−2	4	−2	4	4	1.2	−0.2	0.04
4	4	0	0	1	1	0	3.0	1	1.00
5	3	1	1	0	0	0	3.9	−0.9	0.81
3	2	−1	1	−1	1	1	2.1	−0.1	0.01
6	5	2	4	2	4	4	4.8	0.2	0.04
$\sum\bar{X} = 20$	$\sum\bar{Y} = 15$		$\sum x^2 = 10$		$\sum y^2 = 10$	$\sum xy = 9$		$\sum e = 0$	$\sum e^2 = 1.9$
$X = 4$	$Y = 3$								
$r = 0.9$									

$$b = 0.9$$

$$a = 3 - (.9)(4)$$

$$= -0.6$$

$$Y' = -0.6 + 0.9X$$

The five pairs of observations of X and Y are used to calculate a and b values. Now, the value of Y can be predicted by supplying the value of a and b for a group of new people about whom information on the X variable is available. However, the predicted value (Y') is slightly different from the actual value (Y) because the correlation between X and Y is not perfect. When the correction coefficient is ±1, there will be no error in prediction ($Y' = Y$). If the value of Y is calculated from the given value of X in the above example, there is some error in the predicted value of Y as compared to the actual value. It is presented in the table under the column head e.

The data can be presented graphically, as shown in Fig. 15.9. Data is plotted across the X and Y axis and the straight line passing through it is known as the regression line.

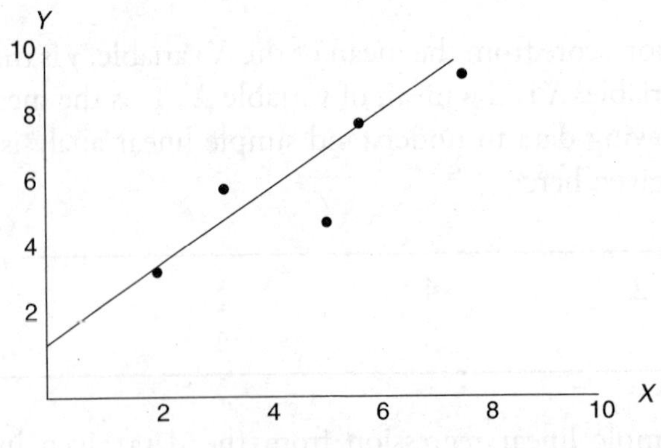

Figure 15.9 Regression line

The intercept (a) is the point at which the line crosses the Y axis. Regression coefficient (b) is the slope or angle of the line.

Simple linear regression analysis provides more insight into the relationship between two variables. In the health sciences, inferences by regression analysis are very useful to study the etiology of a disease or factors associated with a clinical condition as they put into words the impact of one variable on the other.

CHAPTER SUMMARY

- Correlation is defined as a measure that determines the type (positive or negative) and magnitude (strength) of association between two quantitatively measured variables. It is a denoted by r (correlation coefficient) and the value of r ranges from -1 to $+1$.
- Correlation data is presented on a special type of graph called a scatter plot (or scatter gram). Computation of r is logical only when the scatter diagram indicates a linear relationship.
- The plot reveals how the values on the vertical axis are scattered for a given value on the X axis and how the values on the X axis are scattered for a given value on the Y axis.
- When two variables are related positively with each other, positive correlation exists between them. Change in one variable will lead to change in the other variable in the same direction (whether positive or negative).
- When two variables are related negatively with each other, negative correlation exists between them. Change in one variable will lead to change in the other variable in the opposite direction.
- When the observations on two related variables are scattered around a central straight line on a scatter diagram, it is known as linear correlation.
- Karl Pearson's product moment method for calculation of correlation coefficient is used for variables measured on continuous or ratio level and are normally distributed in the population.
- Absence of correlation or poor correlation only means that there is no linear relation between variables; it may not mean that the two variables are unrelated.
- Spearman rho is used to compute correlation for ranked or ordinal variables. It is a non-parametric bivariate descriptive as well as inferential statistics that shows the strength and direction of the relationship between two ranked variables and confirms whether the relationship is different from zero (hypothesis testing).
- Whenever there are two identical values in the data set, it is known as a tie. In this situation, the average of the ranks that the identical values would have otherwise occupied is used for each of the tied observations.

- Kendall's tau is another test to compute the correlation coefficient between ordinal level variables.
- A concordant pair is when the rank of the second variable is greater than the rank of the first variable. A discordant pair is when the rank is equal to or less than the rank of the first variable.
- Phi coefficient and Cremer's *V* statistics are used to ascertain the magnitude of the relationship between two nominal level variables.
- Simple linear regression analysis is used to predict the dependent variable (*Y*) using the independent variable or predictor variable (*X*). When there is only one predictor variable, the prediction method is called simple regression.
- The accuracy of prediction depends on the magnitude of the correlation between both the variables X and Y. The higher the correlation between the variables, the more accurate the prediction.

EVALUATE YOURSELF

Long Answer Questions

Q1: Define correlation and explain its meaning.

Q2: What are the types of correlation? How will you interpret a correlation coefficient of +0.8 between birth weight and gestational age?

Q3: Write a short note on the scatter diagram method.

Q4: What are the assumptions of Pearson's product moment correlation? Calculate the correlation coefficient of the data given in the table below:

Maternal hemoglobin level (X)	Birth weight (g) (Y)
11	2500
14	3000
16	3800
10	2000
15	3000

Q5: What is simple linear regression analysis and prediction? What are the assumptions of simple linear analysis?

Q6: Consider the of height and weight of 10 students

Height (in cm) X	Weight (in kg) Y
150	45
160	60
165	65
175	70
180	80
175	80
155	60

What will be the predicted weight of a student with a height of 160 cm?

Short Answer Questions

Q1: Write a short note on causal relationship and correlation.

Q2: Write a short note on Pearson product moment correlation

Multiple Choice Questions

Q1: Spearman rho is used to compute the correlation for
(a) Nominal variables (b) Ordinal variables
(c) Ratio variables (d) Continuous variables

Q2: Pearson product moment correlation is used to compute the correlation for
(a) Continuous variables (b) Ratio variables
(c) Both a and b (d) Nominal variables

Q3: Cremer's *V* is a correlation statistic used for:
(a) Nominal variables (b) Ratio variables
(c) Continuous variable (d) All of the above

Q4: Pearson's correlation is what type of statistics?
(a) Descriptive (b) Inferential
(c) Both a and b (d) Non-parametric

Q5: The value of *r* ranges from:
(a) −1 to +1 (b) +1 to 0
(c) −1 to 0 (d) 0 to infinite

Answers

1. b **2.** c **3.** a **4.** c **5.** a

FURTHER READING

Agresti A. 2010. *Analysis of Ordinal Categorical Data, 2nd ed.* John Wiley & Sons, New York.

Fieller EC, Hartley HO, Pearson ES. 1957. Tests for rank correlation coefficients. I. *Biometrika* 44: 470–481.

Hollander M, Wolfe DA. 1973. *Nonparametric statistical methods*. Wiley, New York.

Kendall M. 1938. A New Measure of Rank Correlation. *Biometrica* 30 (1–2): 81–89.

Kendall MG. 1970. *Rank correlation methods, 4th ed.* Griffin, London.

Lehman A. 2005. *JMP for Basic Univariate and Multivariate Statistics: A Step-by-step Guide*. SAS Press, Cary, NC.

Mosteller F, Tukey JW. 1977. *Data Analysis and Regression,* Addison-Wesley, p. 588.

Page EB. 1963. Ordered hypotheses for multiple treatments: A significance test for linear ranks. *Journal of the American Statistical Association* 58 (301): 216–230.

Spearman C. 1904. The proof and measurement of association between two things. *Amer. J. Psychol.* 15: 72–101.

16 Parametric and Non-parametric Tests

Chapter overview

- Introduction to parametric and non-parametric tests
- Parametric tests—t- test, z-test, ANOVA, ANCOVA, MANOVA
- Non-parametric tests—chi-square test, sign test, Wilcoxon signed rank sum test, median test, Mann–Whitney test, McNemar's test, Kruskal–Wallis test, Fisher's exact test

INTRODUCTION TO PARAMETRIC AND NON-PARAMETRIC TESTS

As described in Chapter 12, there are two classes of inferential statistics: parametric and non-parametric. Parametric statistics deals with analysis and interpretation of interval or ratio level data, whereas non-parametric statistics is meant for ordinal or nominal level data. Inferential statistics is aimed at hypothesis testing with the use of parametric and non-parametric tests. This chapter describes the statistical procedure for analysing quantitative data.

PARAMETRIC TESTS

Parametric statistics is more powerful than non-parametric statistics as it estimates the parameters of a normally distributed population based on the sample statistics. This approach to data analysis emerged from the work of Fisher, and requires the following three assumptions:

- The population distribution should be normal or approximately normal.
- The data should be of at least interval level. Ordinal data with approximately normal distribution can also be analysed with parametric tests.
- The sample should be randomly drawn from the population.

Common parametric tests include Pearson's r, the t-test, the z-test and ANOVA.

t-Test

This was designed by WS Gossell, whose pen name was Student; so the test is also called Student's t-test. It is used to compare two means of small samples/groups to evaluate if they are significantly different from each other. If the sample is large then the z-test is used instead of the t-test as the data follows a normal distribution. This is used when the sample is small and population standard deviation is not known. 't' is the ratio of the observed difference between two means of small samples to the standard error of difference in the same. It follows a different distribution, known as 't' distribution, that corresponds to z in a large sample.

Criteria for using the t-test

- The sample should be randomly selected and homogeneous.
- Data should be a continuous level measure.
- Variability in data should be normally distributed.
- Sample size should be less than 30. For sample size more than 30, the z-test is more appropriate.

Types of t-test

Unpaired t-test This is also known as the independent t-test and it is used when measures from the two independent samples are compared. It is applied on the means of two independent groups of subjects (for example, control group and experimental group) and evaluates whether the difference in the means is by chance or if the treatment conditions caused this change.

Steps in the application of unpaired t-test

1. Calculate the standard error using the following formula

$$\frac{SD_1}{\sqrt{n_1}} + \frac{SD_2}{\sqrt{n_2}}$$

   where SD_1 is the standard deviation of the first sample; SD_2 is the standard deviation of the second sample; n_1 is the number of subjects in the first sample; and n_2 is the number of subjects in the second sample.
2. Calculate the observed difference between the two means.
3. Calculate t-value using the following formula
   Observed difference in mean/Standard error
4. Compute the degree of freedom: $df = n_1 + n_2 - 2$

For example: Fictitious data of 15 male and 15 female students' scores in the final BSc nursing examination is given in the table below. We need to find out whether the group difference in scores is significant or if it is only by chance.

Male (X_1)	Female (X_2)
65	63
60	85
95	90
82	98
43	90
90	92
99	98
97	93
83	97
75	98
90	87
95	76
89	72
65	47
84	89

Mean ± SD of $X_1 = 80.8 \pm 16.13$

Mean ± SD of $X_2 = 85.0 \pm 14.67$

Calculate standard error by entering values in the formula

$$SE = 4.17 + 3.79 = 7.96$$

Compute the observed difference in the means of both the groups

$$= 4.2$$

Compute the value of t

$$= \frac{4.2}{7.96} = 0.53$$

Compute the degree of freedom

$$= 15 + 15 - 2 = 28$$

The table value of t at 28 degrees of freedom and 0.05 level of significance is 2.05 (*See Annexure IV*). As the calculated value of t is less than the tabulated value, the null hypothesis is accepted. The observed difference between the mean scores of the male and female students is statistically insignificant.

Paired t-test/Dependent t-test Dependent t-test is applied to paired data of independent observations made on the same sample before and after an intervention. To evaluate the statistical significance of difference in 30 or fewer paired observations of continuous level data, the paired t-test may be used. It is the most commonly used statistical test in nursing research studies. Some common situations where paired t-test can be used for data analysis are:

- One group pretest post-study to evaluate continuous level data.
- To compare the efficacy of two treatment conditions given to the same group of individuals.
- To compare the two instruments used in nursing sciences. For example, for thermometers (mercury vs digital), we can check the accuracy of the digital thermometer by comparing the data of both the instruments.
- To compare observations made on different sites on the same individual. For example, comparing pulse rate at the radial and femoral arteries; comparing blood pressure at the upper and lower extremities.

Steps in the application of paired t-test

1. Calculate the difference in each set of paired observations.
2. Compute the mean of the difference in paired observations.
3. Calculate standard deviation of the differences.
4. Compute standard error of mean by substituting values in the formula

$$\frac{SD}{\sqrt{n}}$$

5. Determine the t-value using the formula given below

$$t = \frac{\text{Mean of differences}}{\text{Standard error of mean}}$$

6. Obtain the degree of freedom: df = $n - 1$
7. Refer the t table and check whether the calculated value of t is more or less than the tabulated value for the given degree of freedom and level of significance.
8. If the calculated value of t is more than the tabulated value, it is considered significant and the difference in the before and after mean scores is statistically significant. Hence, the null hypothesis is rejected and the alternative hypothesis is accepted.

For example: Weight of 10 obese people before aerobic exercises and at the end of two months is given in the table below.

Subject No.	Before aerobic exercises	At two months	Difference in weight	$x - \bar{x}$ Mean $\bar{x} = 4$	$(x - \bar{x})^2$
1	80	75	-5	-1	1
2	85	78	-7	-2	4
3	90	82	-8	5	25
4	95	82	-13	7	49
5	75	70	-2	0	0
6	70	58	-12	-3	9
7	85	70	-15	-1	1
8	80	70	-10	-1	1
9	90	75	-15	-3	9
10	95	80	-15	-1	1
Total			-102		100

1. Compute mean of the observed differences

$$\frac{102}{10} = -10.2 \text{ (sign can be ignored for calculation of t-value)}$$

2. Compute standard deviation of the observed differences

$$SD = 4.59$$

3. Compute standard error of observed difference

$$SE = SD\sqrt{n}$$

$$= 459\sqrt{10} = 1.45$$

4. Compute the value of t

$$t = \frac{\text{Mean observed difference}}{\text{SE of difference}}$$

$$= \frac{10.2}{1.45} = 7.03$$

5. Degree of freedom; $n - 1 = 9$

6. Referring to table values of t at 9 degrees of freedom and 0.05 level of significance, it is found to be 2.26, which is less than the computed value of t; hence the null hypothesis is rejected and the alternative hypothesis is accepted. It can be concluded that aerobic exercises caused significant reduction in weight among obese people.

z-Test

This was developed by RA Fisher. It is based on normal distribution and is widely used for testing the significance of several statistics such as measures of central tendency, coefficient of correlation and others.

Criteria for using the z-test

- The study sample must be selected through a random procedure.
- The study should involve the collection of data at continuous level of measurement.
- The variable is assumed to follow a normal distribution in the population.
- The sample size must be larger than 30.

z-test may be of one-tailed or two-tailed based on the nature of the treatment condition in the study.

Steps in the application of z-test

1. Calculate the difference in mean.
2. Find out the standard deviation of data in both groups.
3. Calculate standard error using the following formula

$$\sqrt{\frac{(SD_1)^2}{n_1} + \frac{(SD_2)^2}{n_2}}$$

4. Find the value of z

$$z = \frac{\bar{X}_1 - \bar{X}_2}{\text{SE}}$$

5. If the population variance is known then the formula used to compute standard error is

$$\sigma\sqrt{\frac{1}{n_1} + \frac{1}{n_2}}$$

Refer the z-value to find the probability of the observed difference occurring by chance. The tabled value of z at 5% of significance is 1.96. If the calculated value of z is less than the tabled value, the null hypothesis is accepted. Hence, it can be concluded that the mean of the population is equal, otherwise H_0 is rejected.

For example: In a study, 49 children were given a normal diet and iron supplements. After six months, the average hemoglobin was 12 with *SD* of 1 while the average hemoglobin of a second comparable group of 49 children who took only the normal diet was 10 with *SD* of 1.5 kg. Can the increased hemoglobin level be attributed to the iron supplements?

1. Calculate the difference between the two means

$$12 - 10 = 2$$

2. Calculate standard error of difference between two means (*SE*).

$$\sqrt{\frac{(1)^2}{49} + \frac{(1.5)^2}{49}}$$

$$SE = 0.692$$

3. Find the value of z

$$z = \frac{\bar{X}_1 - \bar{X}_2}{S}$$

$$= \frac{2}{0.692} = 2.89$$

4. As the calculated value of z is greater than the tabled value (1.96), the null hypothesis is rejected. Hence it can be concluded that iron supplements played a role in the hemoglobin increase.

Analysis of Variance (ANOVA)

ANOVA is a parametric procedure used to test mean group differences of three or more groups. The equality of two or more population (or treatment) means is judged by examining the variances of study groups/samples. It enables the researcher to determine whether the differences between the samples are simply due to random error (sampling errors) or whether there are systematic effects of treatment conditions that cause the mean in one group to differ from the mean in another. It takes into account the variations between and within the groups. ANOVA divides the variability in the dependent variable into two groups: variability caused by the independent variable and variability caused by all other factors, such as individual and environmental factors; when variability between the groups is large compared to that within the group, it may be attributed to the intervention. The statistics computed in ANOVA is the F ratio which is the ratio of *mean sum of squares between the groups* to *mean sum of squares within the groups.*

ANOVA is often used to compare three or more means; however, when the means from two samples are compared using ANOVA, it is equivalent to using an independent t-test.

Assumptions

- Samples are recruited from normally distributed populations.
- All populations have the same variance (or standard deviation).
- Samples are randomly selected and independent of one another.
- The dependent variable should be a continuous measure (interval or ratio level).
- The independent variable should consist of two or more factors/categories.
- The observation should be independent; that is, there is no relationship between the observations within each group or between the groups themselves.
- The dependent variable should be normally distributed for each level/category of the independent variable.

Types of ANOVA

- **One-way:** This is applicable when there is one continuous response variable (test score) that is compared with at least three or more levels of a factor variable (for example, occupation).
- **Two-way:** This is used when there is one continuous response variable which is compared with two or more factorial variables (occupation, marital status).
- **Factorial:** This is used for the analysis of data in factorial design, to evaluate interaction effects among the treatment conditions.
- **Repeated measures:** This is used for the analysis of data in cross-over research designs, where the same group of subjects is used for each treatment condition.
- **Multivariate analysis of variance (MANOVA):** This is a type of ANOVA used for two or more continuous level response variables. It is further divided into one-way and two-way MANOVA. In one-way MANOVA, two or more continuous response variables are compared with a single factorial variable. Two-way ANOVA is used to compare two or more continuous response variables with two or more factorial variables.

It is beyond the scope of this book to explain the computation of each type of ANOVA. However, the steps for the computation of one-way ANOVA are given here.

Steps in the application of ANOVA

1. State the null hypothesis. H_0: Means of all the groups are comparable.
2. Calculate the grand mean of all the values in all the groups by combining the data.

3. Calculate the mean of each group.
4. Calculate the sum of squares between the groups. It is the sum of squared deviation of individual group mean to grand mean.
5. Calculate the sum of squares within the groups. It is the sum of squared deviation of individual scores in the group from its own group mean.
6. Calculate between the groups and within the group degree of freedom.
   a. Between the groups degree of freedom = Number of groups – 1
   b. Within the group degree of freedom = Number of observations – Number of groups
7. Compute mean sum of squares between and within the groups.
8. Place the values in the table given below and compute the F ratio.

Source of variation 1	Degree of freedom 2	Sum of squares 3	Mean sum of squares (MSS) 4 = 3/2	F ratio = MSS1/MSS2 5
Between the groups				
Within the groups				
Total				

9. Compare the calculated F ratio with that given in the F-table at the calculated degree of freedom between the classes and at degree of freedom within the classes at 5% level of significance. If the calculated value is greater than the tabled value, H_0 is rejected and the alternative hypothesis (significant difference between the means) is accepted. If the F ratio value is smaller than the tabled value, H_0 is accepted.

For example: To know whether nicotine patch or nicotine chewing gum is effective for quitting smoking. The dependent variable is the weekly consumption of cigarettes after four weeks of intervention. About 30 smokers were randomised into three groups: nicotine patch group, nicotine chewing gum group and no intervention group. The fictitious data is presented in the table below.

Nicotine patch	Nicotine chewing gum	No intervention
50	40	90
55	35	85
60	30	80
40	25	80
35	20	85
45	20	90
50	35	95

(continued)

Continued

Nicotine patch	Nicotine chewing gum	No intervention
55	30	75
60	25	70
40	15	70
Mean = 49	Mean = 27.5	Mean = 82
Grand Mean = 52.83		

1. Calculate the sum of squares between the groups

$$(52.83 - 49)^2 + (52.83 - 27.5)^2 + (52.83 - 82)^2$$

$$= 14.67 + 641.61 + 850.89 = 1507.17$$

2. Calculate the sum of squares within the groups as follows:

Nicotine patch	Mean deviation	Nicotine chewing gum	Mean deviation	No intervention	Mean deviation
50	–1	40	–12.5	90	–8
55	–6	35	–7.5	85	–3
60	–11	30	–2.5	80	2
40	9	25	2.5	80	2
35	14	20	7.5	85	–3
45	4	20	7.5	90	–8
50	–1	35	–7.5	95	–13
55	–6	30	–2.5	75	7
60	–11	25	2.5	70	12
40	9	15	12.5	70	12
Mean = 49		Mean = 27.5		Mean = 82	

$$= 690 + 562.5 + 660 = 1912.5$$

3. Calculate the mean sum of squares between the groups

$$\frac{1507.15}{2} = 753.58$$

4. Calculate mean sum of squares within the group

$$\frac{1912.5}{27} = 70.83$$

5. Calculate the F ratio

$$f = \frac{753.58}{70.83} = 10.64$$

6. Compare the calculated value of F with the tabulated value at 0.05 level of significance, two-tailed, within the group df = 27 and between the group df = 2. The tabulated value is found to be 3.35 (*See Annexure V*).
7. As the calculated value is more than the tabled value, the null hypothesis is rejected. However, from the above result, it cannot be declared whether nicotine patch or nicotine chewing gum was more effective for cessation of smoking. To determine this, multiple comparison procedures, also known as post hoc tests, are required. These tests segregate the differences in group means which leads to rejection of the ANOVA null hypothesis. It noteworthy that the series of t-tests (nicotine patch group vs nicotine chewing gum group; nicotine patch group vs no intervention group; nicotine chewing gum vs no intervention group) will not be appropriate in place of post hoc tests as it will increase the likelihood of type I errors.

ANCOVA

Analysis of covariance (ANCOVA) is a combination of multiple regression and ANOVA. It permits control of extraneous variables/covariates and is therefore also known as method of control (statistical control). The goal of ANCOVA is to control group differences on the covariate while examining the mean difference on the response.

ANCOVA in experimental research (in which random assignment is used) provides a more precise estimation of group difference on the response variable. In quasi-experiments (non-equivalent control group design) where pre-existing group differences are found because of lack of homogeneity in the non-equivalent groups, ANCOVA provides a statistical control which takes into account these pre-existing group differences and eliminates its effect on the dependent variable. A covariate is a source of variation that affects the response variable, but which was not controlled during the study design. It cannot be related to any categorical factor being tested.

Regression is used as the first step of ANCOVA to adjust scores on the dependent variable by removing the effect of covariates. Once the covariates are controlled, it removes variability in the dependent measures that can be explained by the covariate.

ANOVA in the second step is applied to test the significance of the difference between the groups means.

For example, to test the effectiveness of guided imagery on cardiac patients' anxiety. An experimental group in one hospital is exposed to treatment, and a comparison group in another hospital is not. The patients' anxiety level is measured both before and after the intervention. As both groups are in different environments, there will be a pretest difference in anxiety levels, which needs to be controlled. In this situation, pretest anxiety scores (a covariate) can be statistically controlled through ANCOVA. A pretest measure is an excellent choice for a covariate; it can be continuous variables or dichotomous variables. However, the independent variable is always a nominal level variable (Fig. 16.1).

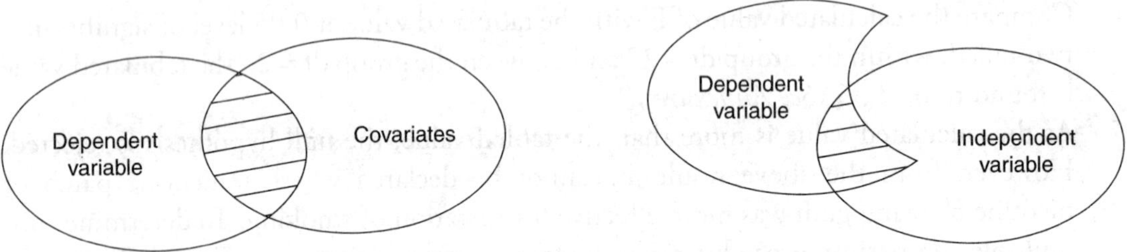

Figure 16.1 Concepts in ANCOVA

NON-PARAMETRIC TESTS

Non-parametric tests are also called distribution-free statistics, as these tests require no assumptions about the form of the population data distribution. They provide a good alternative to parametric statistics when the assumptions of parametric tests cannot be met or when the sample size is small. These tests do not involve the use of any population parameters, i.e., μ and σ are not required, and the underlying distribution does not need to be normal. Chi-square test, sign test, McNemar's test, Wilcoxon signed rank sum test, Mann–Witney U test, median test, Kruskal–Wallis one-way analysis of variance by ranks, Friedman's two-way analysis of variance by ranks, Spearman's rank correlation coefficient and Fisher's exact test are some of the important non-parametric tests used by nurse researchers.

At least one non-parametric equivalent exists for each type of parametric statistical test. Table 16.1 shows the non-parametric analogue to parametric statistical tests.

Table 16.1 Non-parametric analogue to parametric statistical tests

Analysis purpose	Parametric tests	Non-parametric analogues
To compare means between two independent groups	Two-sample/Independent t-test, z-test	Wilcoxon rank sum test, Mann–Whitney U test
To compare two quantitative measurements taken from the same individual	Dependent/Paired t-test	Wilcoxon signed rank test

(*continued*)

Continued

Analysis purpose	Parametric tests	Non-parametric analogues
To compare means between three or more independent groups	Analysis of variance (ANOVA)	Kruskal–Wallis test, median test
To estimate the association between two quantitative variables	Pearson's coefficient of correlation	Spearman's rank correlation, chi-square test, phi coefficient of concordance

Chi-square Test

The chi-square test introduced by Karl Pearson is a non-parametric test of proportions, association and goodness of fit. The test involves the calculation of a quantity, called chi-square (χ^2). As discussed earlier, non-parametric tests are not based on any assumption and do not follow any distribution of variable. This test uses chi-square distribution and is an important test in nursing research. As a test of proportion, it can evaluate the significance of the difference between two or more proportions. Another application is as a test of association to identify the significance of association between two events. In other words, using this test, the researcher can identify the probability of association of two discreet variables such as obesity and coronary artery disease, smoking and lung cancer, attention deficit hyperactivity disorder and work status of the mother. Each discreet variable may have two or more categories and accordingly 2 × 2 or 2 × 3 or 3 × 3 contingency tables are constructed for the calculation of the chi-square value. For example, to evaluate the association of obstructed sleep apnea with gender, a 2 × 3 contingency table can be constructed as follows:

Gender	Obstructed sleep apnea		
	Yes f	No f	Total
Male	17	12	29
Female	22	18	40
Transgender	06	05	11
Total	45	35	80

In the chi-square test, the observed frequency in each cell of the contingency table is compared with the expected frequency according to a specific hypothesis. For example, if according to existing prevalence of lung cancer, the researcher expected 10 of 20 smokers to have lung cancer and the actual observed number was 8, then she might want to know about the goodness of fit between the observed and expected frequency—whether the differences between observed and expected are the result of chance or due to other factors. How much deviation is probable before the researcher can conclude that something other than chance is causing the observed to differ from the expected frequency? Chi-square statistics are used to test the null hypothesis, which states that there is no significant difference between the expected and observed result.

The formula used to compute the chi-square value is:

$$\chi^2 = \frac{(O - E)^2}{E}$$

where O is the observed frequency and E is the expected frequency in each cell of the contingency table. Chi-square values are calculated for each cell and are summed to obtain the final chi-square value of the table.

Expected frequency can be calculated for each cell using the formula given below:

$$E = \frac{\text{Column total} \times \text{Row total}}{\text{Sample total}}$$

Steps to compute Chi-square statistics

1. Create 2 × 2 or 2 × 3 contingency tables as per the category system of two or more discreet variables.
2. Enter the actual observed frequency (not the percentage) in each cell of the contingency table.
3. Determine the expected frequency (E) for each cell of the contingency table using the formula given above.
4. Find the difference between the observed and expected frequencies in each cell (O – E).
5. Calculate the chi-square value for each cell using the formula given above.
6. Sum the χ^2 values of all the cells to obtain the total chi-square value.
   Calculate the degree of freedom from the number of categories in each event. Degree of freedom (df) = (C – 1) × (R – 1); where C is the number of vertical columns and R is the number of horizontal rows. Degree of freedom is placed at the foot of the chi-square symbol (χ^2_{df}) which indicates the total of χ^2 values at a particular degree of freedom.
7. Refer the χ^2 table to compare the calculated and tabulated χ^2 values at the computed degree of freedom and specific level of significance, such as .05, .02, .01, .001. If the tabulated χ^2 value is more than the calculated chi-square value, the null hypothesis is accepted; otherwise, it is rejected.

For example: To discover the effect of 24-hour fluid balance on bowel movements in post-surgical patients (Table 16.2).

Table 16.2 Effect of 24-hour fluid balance on bowel movements among post-surgical patients

Bowel movements	24-hour fluid balance		Total	Chi-square statistics
	Positive	Negative		
Present	25	30	55	$\chi^2 = 0.0166$
Absent	28	32	60	df = 1
Total	53	62	115	p = 0.8964

Steps to calculate the chi-square value for the data given in the above table.

1. This is a 2 × 2 contingency table in which the observed data for each category (fluid balance and bowel movement) is already placed.
2. Calculate the expected frequency for each cell.

$$53 \times \frac{55}{115} = 25.34$$

3. Entering values in the formula for chi-square calculation

$$\frac{(25 - 25.34)^2}{25.34} = 0.0046$$

The value of chi-square is 0.0046 for this cell.

4. Now, calculate the chi-square value of column 2 row 1 using the steps given above for column 1 row 1. The value of the chi-square is 0.0041 for this cell. Similarly, it is 0.0044 and 0.0035, for column 1 row 2 and column 2 row 2, respectively.
5. By summing all the chi-square values, the final value of chi-square for the data given in the table will be 0.0046 + 0.0041 + 0.0044 + 0.0035 = 0.0166.
6. Calculate the degree of freedom. (C – 1) × (R – 1) = (2 – 1) × (2 – 1) = 1
7. Now, compare the chi-square value of 0.0166 for df = 1 from the tabulated value.
8. When the calculated value of the chi-square is compared with the tabulated value for df = 1 at level of significance 0.05, it is found that the calculated value is lower than the tabulated value of 3.84 (*See Annexure VIII*).
9. Hence, the null hypothesis that 24-hours' fluid balance is not significantly associated with bowel movement among post-surgical patients can be accepted.

Salient features

- The chi-square test is used for nominal or ratio level data.
- The observation should be independent.

- The sample size required for a chi-square test is 50 or more.
- The expected frequency of any cell should not be less than 5 in a 2 × 2 contingency table. If it is less than 5, frequencies from the preceding or succeeding cells can be pooled together in order to make it 5 or more. Alternatively, Yate's correction can be applied to avoid misleading results. It involves reduction of 0.5 from the absolute value of O – E while calculating the expected frequency. However, this alternative is not applicable for tables larger than 2 × 2.
- If any expected frequency is well below 5, some other appropriate test should be applied.
- It does not measure the strength of association between variables. It only provides information about whether variables are associated with each other. However, it does not indicate the strength or extent of association.
- The association between variables should not be interpreted as a cause and effect relationship.
- Chi-square requires the use of numerical values, not percentages or ratios.

Sign Test

This is a non-parametric test used to test the null hypothesis in place of a one-sample t-test, paired t-test or for ordinal scaled data or categorical data where it is possible to rank the observations. Dependency of the two sample data is considered by taking the differences of paired values. The signs (positive or negative) of the individual differences are taken for the test. The null hypothesis is that the number of positive differences should approximately equal the number of negative differences. Zero differences are not considered in the test. This is a simple binomial test with probability $p = 0.5$ for a sign to be positive and probability $q = 0.5$ for a sign to be negative.

For example: To evaluate the effect of BLS training, 15 staff nurses are tested before and after the training for competence in chest compression on a seven-point scale. The researcher wants to know whether chest compression competence is enhanced by the training. Raw data is presented in the following table.

Subject	Before training	After training	Difference (after – before)	Sign of the difference
1	5	6	1	+
2	3	2	–1	–
3	4	4	0	No sign for zero difference
4	2	4	2	+
5	1	3	2	+
6	6	6	0	No sign for zero difference

(continued)

Continued

Subject	Before training	After training	Difference (after – before)	Sign of the difference
7	7	7	0	No sign for zero difference
8	3	5	2	+
9	2	3	1	+
10	3	5	2	+
11	5	5	0	No sign for zero difference
12	1	3	2	+
13	4	4	0	No sign for zero difference
14	4	5	1	+
15	3	2	–1	–

Of the 15 subjects, eight showed a positive change, two negative and five no change at all. Zero differences are not counted. The analysis is done only with the eight positive and two negative changes. The binomial test tests the probability of $k \geq 8$ positive changes, whereas the probability of a positive change is $p = 0.5$ and the probability of a negative change is $q = 0.5$.

Hypothesis testing

The null hypothesis states that there are less or equal positive and negative changes ($p \leq 0.5$) and the alternative hypothesis is that there are more positive than negative changes ($p > 0.5$). Here, $n = 10$ (number of positive changes + number of negative changes). The probability for event k equal or greater than 8 is given using the binominal formula:

$$\sum_{i=k}^{n} \binom{n}{i} p^{i} q^{n-1}$$

$$\binom{10}{8} \times 0.5^{8} \times 0.5^{2} + \binom{10}{9} \times 0.5^{9} \times 0.5^{1} + \binom{10}{10} \times 0.5^{10} \times 0.5^{0}$$

$$= 0.044 + 0.0097 + 0.00097$$

$$= 0.05467$$

Now, check the one-sided distribution. The probability of 8 or more positive changes is 0.0547 which is greater than the 5% significance level. Therefore, the alternative hypothesis is rejected and it is concluded that BLS training does not show any improvement in the competence of chest compression.

Only the one-sided test was conducted because the training was expected to produce a positive change. The probability of 8 or more positive changes is 0.0547.

For example: The table below shows the hours of relief provided by two analgesic drugs in 12 patients suffering from arthritis. Is there any evidence that one drug provides longer relief than the other?

Case	Drug A	Drug B	Case	Drug A	Drug B
1	2.0	3.5	7	14.9	16.7
2	3.6	5.7	8	6.6	6.0
3	2.6	2.9	9	2.3	3.8
4	2.6	2.4	10	2.0	4.0
5	7.3	9.9	11	6.8	9.1
6	3.4	3.3	12	8.5	20.9

In this case, the null hypothesis is that median difference is zero. The actual differences (Drug B – Drug A) are: +1.5, +2.1, +0.3, –0.2, +2.6, –0.1, +1.8, –0.6, +1.5, +2.0, +2.3, +12.4

The actual median difference is 1.65 hours. We have r+ = 9, r– = 3, n = 12, r = Max (r–, r+) = 9. Therefore, the two-sided *p* value (from binomial tables) is 0.146.

It can be concluded that there is no evidence for a difference between the two treatments.

Note that the Wilcoxon signed rank sum test would also be appropriate in this case and is a more powerful test because it takes into account the magnitude of the differences as well as the sign.

Wilcoxon Signed Rank Test

This is a non-parametric test equivalent to the parametric dependent t-test and is used to test hypothesis for median. The Wilcoxon signed rank test is different from the Wilcoxon rank sum test as it takes into consideration the sign (+, –) assigned to ranks. It compares two sets of scores (paired) generated from the same participants from one time point to another, or when participants are subjected to more than one treatment condition. Data collected in repeated measures design, matched pairs, or before and after measures can be analysed through this non-parametric statistic. Like other non-parametric tests, it also does not require any assumptions about the shape of the distribution. Therefore, it can be used as an alternative to the t-test whenever the population cannot be assumed to be normally distributed. The data should be of at least ordinal level for the application of this test.

For example, to study whether there is a difference in smokers' weekly cigarette consumption before and after six weeks of counselling. Here, the dependent variable is 'weekly cigarette consumption' and the effectiveness of counselling can be evaluated by comparing the before and after data of the same individuals.

Assumptions

- The dependent variable should be an ordinal or continuous level measure (cannot be nominal).
- The independent variable should consist of two categorical related groups or matched pairs (same subjects are present in both groups as they have been measured on two occasions on the same dependent variable).
- The distribution of differences between the scores of both groups needs to be symmetrical in shape.

Hypothesis

For paired observations: H_0: Median difference between the pairs is zero.
For a single set of observations: H_0: The median value is equal to some value M.

Steps

1. Calculate the absolute difference for each pair. For the single observation data set, calculate the difference between each observation and the hypothesised median.
2. Omit from consideration those cases where the absolute difference for the pair is zero.
3. Rank the difference, ignoring the signs (assign rank 1 to the smallest rank, 2 to the next, and so on).
4. Rank the difference, ignoring the signs (assign rank 1 to the smallest rank, 2 to the next, and so on) using tied ranks where appropriate. Average the ranks across the tied observations and reduce the variance by $t^3-t/48$ for each group of t tied ranks.
5. Assign to each rank a + sign when the difference is more than zero and a – sign when the difference is less than zero.
6. Compute the value of W for the Wilcoxon test, which is equal to the sum of the signed ranks.

$$W = \left|\sum_{i=1}^{N_r}[\operatorname{sgn}(x_{2,i} - x_{1,i}) \cdot R_i]\right|$$

7. The number of signed ranks, here designated as ns/r, is equal to the number of pairs with some differences minus the number of pairs for which the difference is zero.
8. When ns/r is ≥ 10, the sampling distribution of W is in close approximation to the normal distribution. Therefore, the z-ratio along with the associated one-tailed and two-tailed probabilities can be computed.
9. Z score can be calculated as

$$z = \frac{W - \mu_w}{\sigma_w},\ \sigma_w = \sqrt{\frac{N_r(N_r+1)(2N_r+1)}{6}}$$

$$\mu_w = \frac{n_r(n_r + 1)}{4}$$

10. If $Z > Z_{\text{Critical}}$ then reject H_0.
11. For smaller sample sizes ($n_{s/r}$ = 5 to 9), the obtained value of W can be referred to the separate table of critical values of $\pm W$. If $W > W_{\text{Critical, }Nr}$ then reject the null hypothesis.

For example: The table below shows the hours of relief provided by two analgesic drugs in nine patients suffering from arthritis of the knee joint. Is there any evidence that one drug provides longer relief than the other?

Case	Drug 1 Hours of relief	Drug 2 Hours of relief
1	2.4	3.6
2	5.5	10.5
3	8.6	5.3
4	4.1	10.7
5	8.6	4.3
6	7.2	5.1
7	6.8	5.2
8	3.2	10.9
9	9.2	7.4

1. State the null hypothesis: Median difference is zero.
2. Calculate the actual difference (Drug 2 – Drug 1)

   +1.2, +5, −3.3, +6.6, −4.3, −2.1, −1.6, +7.7, −1.8

3. Rank the differences and affix a sign to each rank.

Difference	1.2	1.6	1.8	2.1	3.3	3.6	4.3	5	6.6
Rank	1	2	3	4	5	6	7	8	9
Sign	+	–	–	–	–	+	–	+	+

   $N_{s/r}$ is 9, which is less than 10; therefore approximation to normal distribution is discarded.

4. Compute *W*.

   $$+1+6+8+9-2-3-4-5-7=3$$

5. Compare the value of W with the tabulated value, $W < W_{0.05,\ 9}$ (*See Annexure XI*). Hence the null hypothesis is accepted. There is no difference in both the drugs in terms of hours of pain relief from arthritis.

Mood's Median Test

This is a non-parametric test analogue to the parametric t-test to evaluate whether two independent samples belong to the population with the same median or not. The null hypothesis is stated as follows: the medians of the populations from which two or more independent random samples are drawn are the same. The alternative hypothesis is that the medians of the populations from which two or more independent random samples are drawn are different. It only considers the position of each observation relative to the overall median of the combined data. It has good relative power for heavy-tailed (outlier-rich) distributions; however, the power is poor for normally distributed and short-tailed data.

Assumptions

- The samples should be selected randomly from their respective populations.
- The populations from which the two independent samples are recruited should be of the same form, differing only in location.
- The variable of interest for analysis should be on continuous level of measurement.
- The two independent samples need not be of equal size.

Steps to compute the median test

1. Pool the data of both the samples.
2. Determine the median from the combined data of the two samples.
3. Determine the number of observations above and below the median in both the samples separately.
4. Tabulate the two sample observations in the form of a 2 × 2 contingency table with respect to the median, as follows:

	Observation	
	Below median	**Above median**
Sample I	A	B
Sample II	C	D

5. Execute chi-square statistics on the 2 × 2 contingency table to test the hypothesis H_0: Both the groups/samples have the same median.

$$\chi^2 = \frac{N(AD - BC)^2}{(A+B)(C+D)(A+C)(A+D)}$$

If the calculated value of chi is less than the tabled value at 5% level of significance and 1 degree of freedom, the null hypothesis is accepted and it can be concluded that there is no difference in the median of both the samples.

McNemar's Test

Quinn McNemar introduced this test in 1947. It is a non-parametric analogue to the paired t-test (within the group) in parametric statistics. McNemar's test is suitable for comparing paired nominal/dichotomous data in one group before and after or pre and post test research design or case control study. It is a useful test when the dependent variable is measured on the nominal or ordinal scale. For example, to investigate the impact of 30 minutes of daily aerobic exercises on obesity. In this study, 60 participants (30 obese and 30 non-obese) were recruited. All participants attended 30 minutes of aerobics exercises daily for four weeks. Four weeks after this intervention, the participants were assessed about whether they remained obese or non-obese. In this study, participants were categorised as being obese and non-obese before the intervention and then re-assessed as either obese or non-obese after the intervention. Therefore, this study has paired samples and a dependent variable that is dichotomous with two mutually exclusive categories (i.e., obese and non-obese). In this situation, McNemar's test is the appropriate choice to analyse the data.

Assumptions

- The dependent variable should be of categorical type with two categories.
- The two groups of dependent variables must be mutually exclusive. In other words, a participant can only be part of only one of the two groups.
- The sample should be drawn randomly from the population of interest.

Steps in the application of McNemar's test

1. Arrange the raw data in two columns, before and after the intervention.
2. Identify changes in the dependent variable after the intervention (positive or negative).
3. Tabulate the data in the form of a 2 × 2 contingency table, as follows:

Before	After	
	+	–
–	a	b
+	c	d

The cell frequencies should be the number of pairs and not the number of individuals (for case control paired data, before and after paired data). Cells b and c arc called discordant cells as they represent pairs with a difference. Cells a and d are called concordant. However, the rule of thumb is that $b + c \geq 20$.

4. Apply McNemar's test statistics

$$\chi^2 = \frac{(b-c)^2}{b+c}$$

This follows a χ^2 distribution with 1 degree of freedom. If the calculated value is less than the tabled value at 5% level of significance, the null hypothesis is accepted; otherwise it is rejected.

For example: In a case control study, the presence of stroke risk factor in 200 subjects (100 pairs) is described in a 2×2 table:

Case	Control	
	Present	Absent
Present	25	25
Absent	35	15 (d)

$$\chi^2 = \frac{(25-35)^2}{25+35} = \frac{100}{50} = 2$$

Degree of freedom = 1

From the chi-square distribution table, the value of χ^2 for 1 degree of freedom is 3.84. The calculated value of the chi-square is 2.0 which is less than the tabled value, indicating that the null hypothesis should be accepted. Therefore, it can be concluded that there is no difference in risk factor in the two groups.

Mann–Whitney U Test

The Mann–Whitney test is also called the rank sum test, Mann–Whitney–Wilcoxon test, Wilcoxon rank sum test and Wilcoxon–Mann–Whitney test. It is applied to compare two unpaired groups. It is a non-parametric test corresponding to the t-test for comparing central tendencies of two independent groups. The test requirement is that the dependent variable must be at least ordinal scaled (rank order scaled). It has greater efficiency than the t-test when the data is not normally distributed. The independent samples should be drawn randomly from the population. The null hypothesis in the Mann–Whitney test states that the distributions of both groups are identical. There is a 50% probability that an observation value randomly selected from one population exceeds an observation selected randomly from the other population.

Steps in the application of the Mann–Whitney U test

1. Pool the data of both groups and rank all the values from low to high, paying no attention to which group each value belongs to. The smallest observation is assigned a rank of 1, whereas the largest value gets a rank of N, that is, the total number of values in both the groups. If two observations are the same, they both get the average of the two ranks for which they tie.
2. Compute the sum of ranks for each group separately.
3. Calculate the Mann–Whitney U statistics for both the groups using the formula given below:

$$U_1 = n_1 n_2 + \frac{n_1(n_1+1) - R_1}{2}$$

$$U_2 = n_1 n_2 + \frac{n_1(n_1+1) - R_2}{2}$$

   where R_1 and R_2 are the sum of ranks for group 1 and group 2, respectively.
4. Determine the Mann–Whitney U test statistic value (U). It is the minimum of U_1 and U_2.
5. If the calculated value of U is more than the tabled value of U at n_1, n_2 degree of freedom, the null hypothesis is rejected (*See Annexure XIII*).

For example: Compute the Mann–Whitney U statistics for the data of two independent groups, as given below:

Group A	Group B
53	44
38	40
69	61
57	52
46	32
39	44
73	70
48	41
73	67
74	72
60	53
78	72

After pooling the data of both groups, it is arranged in ascending order and ranks are assigned to each observation as follows:

Pooled data arranged in ascending order	Rank	Group to whom the observation belongs
32	1	B
38	2	A
39	3	A
40	4	B
41	5	B
44	6.5	B
44	6.5	B
46	8	A
48	9	A
52	10	B
53	11.5	B
53	11.5	A
57	13	A
60	14	A
61	15	B
67	16	B
69	17	A
70	18	B
72	19.5	B
72	19.5	B
73	21.5	A
73	21.5	A
74	23	A
78	24	A

From the above, the sum of ranks assigned to group A items or R_1 can be found

$$R_1 = 2 + 3 + 8 + 9 + 11.5 + 13 + 14 + 17 + 21.5 + 21.5 + 23 + 24 = 167.5$$

Similarly, the sum of ranks assigned to group B or R_2 can be found

$$R_2 = 1 + 4 + 5 + 6.5 + 6.5 + 10 + 11.5 + 15 + 16 + 18 + 19.5 + 19.5 = 132.5$$

$n_1 = 12; n_2 = 12$

$$U_1 = (12)(12) + \frac{12(12+1) - 167.5}{2}$$

$$= 54.5$$

$$U_2 = (12)(12) + \frac{12(12+1) - 132.5}{2}$$

$$= 89.5$$

As $U_1 < U_2$; $U = U_1$
Compute the z score for the given value of U

$$Z = U_1 = \frac{N_1 \times N_2}{\sqrt{\frac{N_1 N_2 (N_1 + N_2 + 1)}{N_2}}}$$

$$= 54.5 - \frac{(12)(12)}{\sqrt{\frac{(12)(12)(12+12+1)}{12}}}$$

$$= 54.5 - \frac{144}{\sqrt{\frac{144(25)}{12}}}$$

$$= 54.5 - 8.31$$

$$= 46.19$$

The calculated value of *z* is more than the tabulated value (5% CI, two-tailed). Thus H_0 is rejected.

Fisher's Exact Test

This is an alternative to the chi-square test when the sample size is very small (less than 20) in two independent groups or the expected frequencies are less than 5 and each variable is with two levels. It is a type of exact test, so called because it allows the researcher to calculate exactly the significance of the deviation from a null hypothesis, rather than relying on an approximation. A contingency table (2 × 2) is constructed and the factorial method is used to compute the probability of observed cell frequencies. Factorial is notated by '!' which means multiply the number by all integers smaller than the number (example: 4! = 4 × 3 × 2 × 1 = 24). The formula used to compute chi-square in Fisher's exact test is as follows:

$$\chi^2 \text{ Fisher's or P} = \frac{r_1!r_2!c_1!c_2}{n!F_{11}!F_{12}!F_{21}!F_{22}!}$$

where, r_1 and r_2 are row totals; c_1 and c_2 are column totals; F_{11} is the observed frequency across column 1 and row 1 in a 2 × 2 contingency table; F_{12} is the observed frequency across column 1 and row 2 in a 2 × 2 contingency table; F_{21} is the observed frequency across column 2 and row 1 in a 2 × 2 contingency table; F_{22} is the observed frequency across column 2 and row 2 in a 2 × 2 contingency table.

For example: A researcher is interested in assessing the efficacy of a newly invented drug (Drug A) over an existing one (Drug B) in the cure of a rare disease. Two groups are exposed to different treatment conditions (drugs A and B) and the outcome is assessed in terms of cured and not cured.

	Cured	Not cured	Total
Drug A	5	2	7
Drug B	3	4	7
Total	8	6	14

$$P = \frac{8!6!7!7!}{14!5!3!2!4!}$$

$$P = \frac{(8\times7\times6\times5\times4\times3\times2\times1)(6\times5\times4\times3\times2\times1)(7\times6\times5\times4\times3\times2\times1)(7\times6\times5\times4\times3\times2\times1)}{14!5!3!2!4!}$$

$$P = \frac{40320\times720\times5040\times5040}{87178291200\times120\times6\times2\times24}$$

$$= \frac{737418060864000}{3012881743872000}$$

$$= 0.0245$$

As $p < 0.05$, the null hypothesis is rejected and it is concluded that Drug A is more efficacious than Drug B in the cure of a rare disease.

Kruskal–Wallis Test

This test was developed by Kruskal and Wallis (1952) and is named after them. It is a non-parametric analogue to analysis of variance (ANOVA) in parametric statistics and extends the Mann–Whitney U test to more than two groups. It is used to compare values from more than two groups based on their ranks. Like all non-parametric tests, it is not as powerful as ANOVA. The Kruskal–Wallis Test can be used:

- When the researcher wants to compare three or more treatment conditions and each treatment condition is performed by an individual group.
- When the data is not normally distributed or variances for different treatment conditions are markedly different.
- When the data is measured on at least the ordinal scale. If continuous level data of three independent groups is not normally distributed, then also it is used to analyse data instead of the parametric ANOVA test.
- When parametric test conditions are not met by the data.

For example: An experimental study to assess the effect of yoga exercises on stress levels among employees of a selected multinational company in Pune. The researcher wants to know whether yoga exercises alleviate stress. What should be the time period for yoga exercises to reduce stress effectively?

Employees who are stressed are allocated randomly to one of three treatment conditions: no exercise; 30 minutes of yoga exercises per day; 60 minutes of yoga exercises per day. At the end of a month, the researcher must ask each participant to rate how stressed they now feel, on a five-point Likert scale. The score on the Likert scale ranges 10–50, where 10 indicates 'not stressed' and 50 indicates 'highly stressed'. The raw data collected from three groups on the stress scale is presented here. The Kruskal–Wallis test is used to evaluate whether the differences among the groups have occurred by chance.

Group A (No intervention)	Group B (30 minutes of yoga exercises)	Group C (60 minutes of yoga exercises)
45	20	15
43	22	17
44	18	19
39	25	13
37	24	16
35	23	14
33	21	11
41	27	12

1. Pool the data and rank all of the scores, ignoring which group they belong to.

Group A (No intervention)		Group B (30 minutes of yoga exercises)		Group C (60 minutes of yoga exercises)	
Score	Rank	Score	Rank	Score	Rank
45	*24*	20	*10*	15	*5*
43	*22*	22	*12*	17	*7*
44	*23*	18	*8*	19	*9*
39	*20*	25	*15*	13	*3*
37	*19*	24	*14*	16	*6*
35	*18*	23	*13*	14	*4*
33	*17*	21	*11*	11	*1*
41	*21*	27	*16*		*2*

2. Calculate mean and standard deviation of ranks assigned to data group-wise:

   Group A: Mean ± SD = 20.5 ± 2.45

   Group B: Mean ± SD = 12.38 ± 2.67

   Group C: Mean ± SD = 4.63 ± 2.67

3. Compute the sum of ranks (Tc) for each group separately

   Group A: = 168

   Group B: = 99

   Group C: = 37

4. Using the following formula, find the value of H.

$$H = \frac{12}{N(N+1)} \sum \frac{Tc^2}{nc} - 3(N+1)$$

where H = Kruskal–Wallis test statistic; N = Total number of participants in all the groups = 24; nc = Number of participants in each group = 8.
(*Note:* This is not the original formula for the calculation of H. However, this formula is easier for computation of H value and yields exactly the same results as the original formula.)

$$\sum \frac{Tc^2}{nc} = \frac{168^2}{8} + \frac{99^2}{8} + \frac{37^2}{8}$$

$$= 3528 + 1225.12 + 171.12$$

$$= 4924.24$$

$$H = \frac{12}{24(24+1)} \times 4924.24 - 3(24+1)$$

$$= \frac{12}{600} \times 4924.24 - 75$$

$$= 23.49$$

5. Compute the degree of freedom (Number of groups – 1).

$$= 2$$

6. Comparing the value of H at 2 degrees of freedom and 0.05 level of confidence in a chi-square table revealed that it is higher than the tabulated value. Hence, the null hypothesis can be rejected and it can be concluded that group difference is not by chance; rather it is attributed to the interventions. Yoga exercises of 60 minutes are most effective in reducing stress among employees of a selected multinational company.

Advantages of Non-parametric Tests

- Non-parametric tests do not require any assumption about population data distribution (normal or any other distribution).
- It is applicable for quantitative as well as qualitative data.
- Computation of non-parametric statistics is easy and it is simple to understand.
- Many non-parametric tests are applicable to small sample size data. Therefore, they are useful for analysing pilot study data and for when researchers work with a rare disease.
- It allows for hypothesis testing.

Disadvantages of Non-parametric Tests

- It is useful for testing hypothesis but not for estimation of population parameters.
- Most non-parametric techniques are less powerful statistically than their parametric counterparts. Therefore, they are less able to detect differences and there is greater risk of committing type II error in hypothesis testing, if the data meets the assumptions of parametric statistics. As the non-parametric tests are performed on ranks of original data, they inevitably lose accuracy.

CHAPTER SUMMARY

- Parametric statistics is more powerful than non-parametric statistics as it estimates the parameters of a normally distributed population based on the sample statistics.
- Student's t-test is used to compare two means of small samples/groups to evaluate if they are significantly different from each other. If the sample is large then z-test is used instead of t-test as the data follows a normal distribution.
- Unpaired t-test is also known as independent t-test and is used when measures from the two independent samples are compared.
- Dependent t-test is applied to paired data of independent observations made on the same sample before and after the intervention.
- z-test is used for larger samples (more than 30) in place of the t-test.
- ANOVA is a parametric procedure used to test mean group differences of three or more groups. The equality of two or more population (or treatment) means is judged by examining the variance of the study groups/samples.
- The statistics computed in ANOVA is the F ratio which is the ratio of mean sum of squares between the groups to mean sum of squares within the group.
- Factorial ANOVA is used for analysis of data in factorial design to evaluate interaction effects among the treatment conditions.
- Repeated measures ANOVA is used for analysis of data in cross-over research designs where the same group of subjects is used for each treatment condition.
- Multivariate analysis of variance is an ANOVA used for two or more continuous level response variables.
- Analysis of covariance (ANCOVA) is a combination of multiple regression and ANOVA. It permits control of extraneous variables/covariates and is also known as method of control (statistical control).
- Non-parametric tests are also called distribution-free statistics as these tests require no assumptions about the form of the population data distribution. It provides a good alternative to parametric statistics when the assumptions of parametric tests cannot be met, or when the sample size is small.
- At least one non-parametric equivalent exists for each type of parametric statistical test.
- The chi-square test introduced by Karl Pearson is a non-parametric test of proportions, association and goodness of fit. The test involves the calculation of a quantity called chi-square (χ^2).
- The sign test is a non-parametric test used to test the null hypothesis in place of a one-sample t-test, paired t-test or for ordinal scaled data or categorical data where it is possible to rank the observations.
- Wilcoxon signed rank test is a non-parametric test equivalent to the parametric dependent t-test and is used to test hypothesis for median. It compares two sets of scores (paired) generated from the same participants from one time point to another.

- The median test is a non-parametric test analogue to the parametric t-test to evaluate whether two independent samples belong to the population with the same median or not.
- McNemar's test is a non-parametric analogue to the paired t-test (within the group) in parametric statistics. It is suitable for comparing paired nominal/dichotomous data in one group before and after or pre and post test research design or case control study.
- The Mann–Whitney test, also called the rank sum test, is applied to compare two unpaired groups. It is a non-parametric test corresponding to the t-test for comparing central tendencies of two independent groups. The test requirement is that the dependent variable must be at least ordinal scaled.
- Fisher's exact test is an alternative to the chi-square test when the sample size is very small (less than 20) in two independent groups or expected frequencies are less than 5 and each variable is with two levels.
- Kruskal–Wallis test is a non-parametric analogue to analysis of variance (ANOVA) in parametric statistics and extends the Mann–Whitney U test to more than two groups. It is used to compare more than two group values based on their ranks.
- The main advantage of non-parametric tests is that they do not require any assumption about population data distribution (normal or any other distribution).
- The disadvantage of non-parametric tests is that they are not useful for estimation of population parameters.

EVALUATE YOURSELF

Long Answer Questions

Q1: Differentiate between parametric and non-parametric tests. What are the assumptions of the chi-square test?

Q2: List the parametric tests. Explain the underlying assumptions for the use of t-test.

Q3: What are ANOVA and ANCOVA? Explain the different types of ANOVA test with relevant examples.

Q4: Fisher's exact test is a type of exact test—elaborate this statement.

Q5: Compute the chi-square value of the given 2 × 2 contingency table. Interpret the results.

Obesity	Obstructed sleep apnea	
	Yes	No
Yes	25	30
No	35	20

Q6: An experimental study to assess the effectiveness of a workshop on infection control practices among staff nurses. In this study the researcher recruited 30 staff nurses randomised into the control and experimental groups. Data was collected before and after the workshop through a checklist (mininmum score 0, maximum score 20). Answer the following questions:

- Which statistical test will be appropriate to assess the effectiveness of the workshop?
- What is your rationale for selecting that test?
- Calculate the test statistics from the data given below and interpret the results.

Scores on checklist in experimental vs control groups

N = 30

Experimental group n = 15	Control group n = 15
10	9
15	5
13	8
14	4
17	8
18	2
17	5
20	6
19	4
13	5
11	6
10	9
15	7
17	5
16	2

Q7: An experimental study to evaluate the effectiveness of Basic Life Support training on the knowledge and skills of Class 9 students. The sample of 30 randomly selected students was randomised into the control and experiment groups. The researcher wanted to know whether the students acquired relevant BLS knowledge and skills after the workshop and were able to retain the same over a period of three months. Pretest data was collected before the training and post-test data was collected on Day 7 and Day 90 of the workshop. Answer the following questions:

- Which test would you apply to ascertain the acquisition of relevant knowledge and skills? State the rationale for the selection of the test.
- Which test would you apply to evaluate the retention of knowledge and skills? Explain the assumptions on which the selected test is based.
- Compute and interpret the selected test statistics from the data given below:

Subject No.	Control group knowledge score			Experimental group knowledge score			Control group skill scores			Control group skill scores		
	Pretest	7th day	90th day	Pretest	7th day	90th day	Pretest	7th day	90th day	Pretest	7th day	90th day
1	8	9	8	9	18	19	2	1	2	2	6	5
2	9	10	9	10	20	21	1	2	2	2	8	7
3	7	8	9	3	22	20	1	2	2	1	9	10
4	10	8	7	6	24	22	2	3	2	3	6	8
5	11	10	12	8	25	24	1	1	3	1	7	8
6	13	14	11	5	28	27	2	2	1	2	8	7
7	6	8	7	9	23	23	3	2	1	3	7	5
8	8	7	8	7	21	24	2	3	2	4	7	6
9	9	10	9	6	20	22	3	2	1	2	8	7
10	10	9	9	10	20	24	1	1	2	1	6	6
11	11	10	11	10	22	23	2	1	3	2	8	6
12	10	8	8	8	23	21	2	1	1	2	9	8
13	9	7	9	9	24	26	2	4	3	3	10	9
14	9	8	9	5	27	25	3	2	1	1	9	10
15	8	7	8	7	28	27	4	5	3	2	8	10

Short Answer Questions

Write short notes on

Q1: Parametric tests

Q2: ANOVA

Q3: t-test

Q4: Kruskal–Wallis test

Q5: Fisher's exact test

Multiple Choice Questions

Q1: Population parameters can be estimated by:
(a) t-test
(b) Chi-square test
(c) Mann–Whitney U test
(d) All of the above

Q2: Which of the following statistical tests is used to compare means of three or more groups?
(a) z-test
(b) ANOVA
(c) Chi-square test
(d) McNemar's test

Q3: When the calculated value of t is more than the tabled value in t distribution, you
(a) Accept the null hypothesis
(b) Accept the alternative hypothesis
(c) Reject the null hypothesis
(d) Both b and c

Q4: The non-parametric analogue of ANOVA is:
(a) Kruskal–Wallis test
(b) Chi-square test
(c) Mann–Whitney U test
(d) McNemar's test

Q5: Which of the following is distribution-free statistics?
(a) ANOVA
(b) t-test
(c) z-test
(d) Mann–Whitney U test

Q6: Which of the following types of ANOVA test is used to analyse interaction effect between treatment conditions?
(a) Repeated measure ANOVA
(b) One-way ANOVA
(c) ANCOVA
(d) Factorial ANOVA

Q7: t-test is used in place of z-test when:
(a) Sample size is equal to or less than 30
(b) Sample is equal to or more than 50
(c) Sample is equal to or more than 40
(d) Sample is equal to or more than 100

Q8: Yate's correction in the chi-square test is only applicable on a:
(a) 2 × 2 contingency table
(b) 3 × 3 contingency table
(c) 4 × 4 contingency table
(d) All of the above

Q9: Which of the following is a method of statistical control?
(a) ANOVA
(b) ANCOVA
(c) McNemar's test
(d) Wilcoxon signed rank test

Q10: Fisher's exact test is used in place of the chi-square test when:
(a) Sample size is very small (less than 20)
(b) Expected frequencies are less than 5
(c) Both a and b
(d) None of the above

Answers

1. a **2.** b **3.** d **4.** a **5.** d
6. d **7.** a **8.** a **9.** b **10.** c

FURTHER READING

Armitage P, Berry G, Mathews JNS. 2008. *Statistical methods in medical research, 4th ed.* John Wiley and Sons.

Corder GW, Foreman DI. 2014. *Non-parametric statistics: A step-by-step approach.* Wiley.

Hollander M, Wolfe DA. 1999. *Non-parametric statistical method, 2nd ed.* Willey, New York.

Jackson SL. 2012. *Research method and statistics: A critical thinking approach, 4th ed.* Wadsworth Cengage Learning, Belmont, CA.

JD Gibbons. 1993. *Non-parametric statistics: An introduction.* Sage, Newbury Park, CA.

Mahajan BK. 2002. *Methods in statistics: For medical students and research workers, 6th ed.* Jaypee Brothers Medical Publishers (P) Ltd, New Delhi.

Munro BH. 2005. *Statistical methods for healthcare research, 5th ed.* Lippincott Williams & Wilkins, Philadelphia.

Negi KS. 2010. *Biostatistics, 2nd ed.* AITBS Publishers, New Delhi.

Parbhakaran GN. 2006. *Biostatistics.* Jaypee Publishers, New Delhi.

Pett MA. 1997. *Non-parametric statistics in healthcare research: Statistics for small samples and unusual distributions.* Sage Publications, California.

Plichta SB, Garzon LS. 2009. *Statistics for nursing and allied health.* Wolters Kluwer/ Lippincott Williams & Wilkins Health, Philadelphia.

Polit DF, Beck CT. 2008. *Nursing research: Generating and assessing evidence for nursing practice, 8th ed.* Lippincott William & Wilkins, New Delhi.

Polit DF, Hungler BP. 2001. *Nursing Research: Methods, Appraisal and Utilization, 5th ed.* Lippincott William and William, Philadelphia.

Rubin A. 2010. *Statistics for evidence-based practice and evaluation, 2nd ed.* Wadsworth Cengage Learning, Belmont, CA.

Siegel S, Castellan NJ, Jr. 1988. *Non-parametric statistics for the behavioral sciences, 2nd ed.* McGraw–Hill, New York.

Vickers AJ. 2005. Parametric versus non-parametric statistics in the analysis of randomized trials with non-normally distributed data. *BMC Medical Research Methodology* 5(35).

Vickers AJ. 2005. The use of percentage change from baseline as an outcome in a controlled trial is statistically inefficient: A simulation study. *BMC Medical Research Methodology* 1(6).

17 Use of Computers for Data Analysis

Chapter overview

- Introduction to computers
- Use of computers in statistics
- Statistical packages for quantitative research: SPSS, STATA, Microsoft Office Excel
- Statistical packages for qualitative research
- Advantages and disadvantages of statistical packages

INTRODUCTION TO COMPUTERS

The computer is an electronic device that operates under the control of instructions stored in its own memory. It processes raw data into organised, meaningful and useful information and stores the results. Computers have revolutionised our lives by offering quick and easy ways of performing various tasks which are considered tedious and lengthy if done manually. It has changed the work flow in hospitals and the face of healthcare service delivery to patients in the 21st century. In hospitals, computers are used for OPD registration, administration, patient management, monitoring of care, patient records management and discharge. Hospital informatics is a robust network of computers used for the overall management of modern hi-tech hospitals in patient assessment, diagnostic services, drug management, monitoring in critical care, documentation and electronic medical records systems. Computers have replaced paper-based systems and eliminated the problems of illegible handwriting leading to medication errors; they also help prevent patient information from going missing.

Computers have not only changed the system of healthcare but have also changed the ways of conducting research in the health sciences. Literature review, which was once considered a very difficult task, has become easy with the advent of computerised databases which facilitate rapid search and retrieval of abstracts of nursing literature. Furthermore, computer-assisted interviewing allows the researcher to capture data immediately in a usable format. Preparation, revision and formatting of research proposals/documents/theses have become less time-consuming and more convenient with computers. Research data management and analysis was very tedious as it required manual computation of statistical tests before the advent of computers, but today, with the use of statistical packages, one click generates the results of research projects.

Use of computers in statistics

The second half of the 20th century has witnessed a rapid and sustained increased in computing power which has revolutionised the practice of statistical science. Advances in computer technology have paved the way for innovative techniques for use in statistics. It has implications for the future of statistics, with new emphasis on experimental and empirical statistics. Nowadays, a researcher has a broad range of choice of general and specific purpose statistical software which facilitate the management and analysis of large volumes of data. Computation of descriptive and inferential statistics has never been as easy as it is now, with the use of computers.

Statistical Packages for Quantitative Research

It is the speed, reliability, accuracy and storage that make computers a powerful tool for statistical analysis. Statistical packages are specialised software that incorporate specific features and syntax commands to assist in data analysis. It allows for more efficient and effective processing of research data. The use of statistical packages is invaluable in handling, arranging and storing large amounts of data efficiently. Quantitative research has been revolutionised by the ability of computers to make repetitive calculations rapidly and accurately. Many statistical packages can assist with quantitative analysis. Spreadsheets such as SPSS, STATA and Microsoft Excel are some of the statistical packages that can be used in data entry, analysis and interpretation. These packages are robust and provide the most detailed and versatile results of research data analysis.

SPSS (Statistical Product and Services Solutions)

Previously known as Statistical Package for Social Sciences, SPSS was developed at Stanford University in 1960 to help statistical analysis in social sciences research. It is capable of running on all operating platforms like Windows, Macintosh and the UNIX system.

Currently in version 22.0, it has been one of the most comprehensive and flexible statistical analysis and data management solutions. It can import data from almost any type of file and conduct complex statistical analysis (both descriptive as well inferential statistics) to generate tabulated results, and graphs/chart of distributions and trends. It includes features on ad hoc analysis, hypothesis testing and predictive analytics.

The latest version of IBM SPSS statistics is loaded with some unique features:

- Its output can be deployed on multiple smart devices simultaneously
- Specialised techniques are used to improve overall performance

STATA

This is another statistical package compatible with Windows, Macintosh and Unix/Linux. Currently in version 14.0, it is a complete statistical software package that provides almost everything needed for research data management, analysis and graphics. It is fast, accurate and easy to use, with a point and click interface and powerful command syntax.

Features of STATA It is fully loaded with a range of features required for complete analysis of quantitative data.

- **Data management features:** It includes features on data transformation, import/export of data, variable labels, value labels (e.g., male and female for 0 and 1), ascending or descending sorting of data.
- Power and sample size estimation
- **Graphic features:** It includes line, bar charts, scatter plot, pie chart, hi-lo, and so on. The quality of graphs is high and they are distinctly styled with facilities to edit.
- **Basic statistical tests:** Pearson/Spearman correlation, z- and t-test, tests of proportions, ANOVA, Cronbach's alpha, test of normality, stepwise regression and random number.
- Linear models include regression, censored outcomes, quantile regression, bootstrap MANOVA, factorial ANOVA and repeated measure ANOVA
- Poisson regression, binominal tests, Fisher's exact test
- Bayesian analysis
- **Survival analysis:** Kaplan–Meier and Nelson–Aalen estimators
- Multivariate methods
- Non-parametric methods
- Epidemiological tests, ROC analysis

Microsoft Office Excel

This is a utility of Microsoft Office which provides statistical solutions for quantitative data. It allows for import of data from other sources/web/from text, direct data entry in spreadsheets, data sorting in order, checking for errors in data entry, removal of duplicates and validation of data. It can be used for a range of descriptive statistical operations like average, mean, percentage and standard deviation. Inferential statistical tests like t-test, chi-square test, Pearson product moment, F statistics and Fisher's exact test can also be executed. Graphical features enable the researcher to produce high-quality bar graphs, pie graphs, trends, line graphs and various other types. The Help menu provides useful information about the execution of various commands. Figs 17.1 to 17.9 help you understand the various features of Microsoft Office Excel.

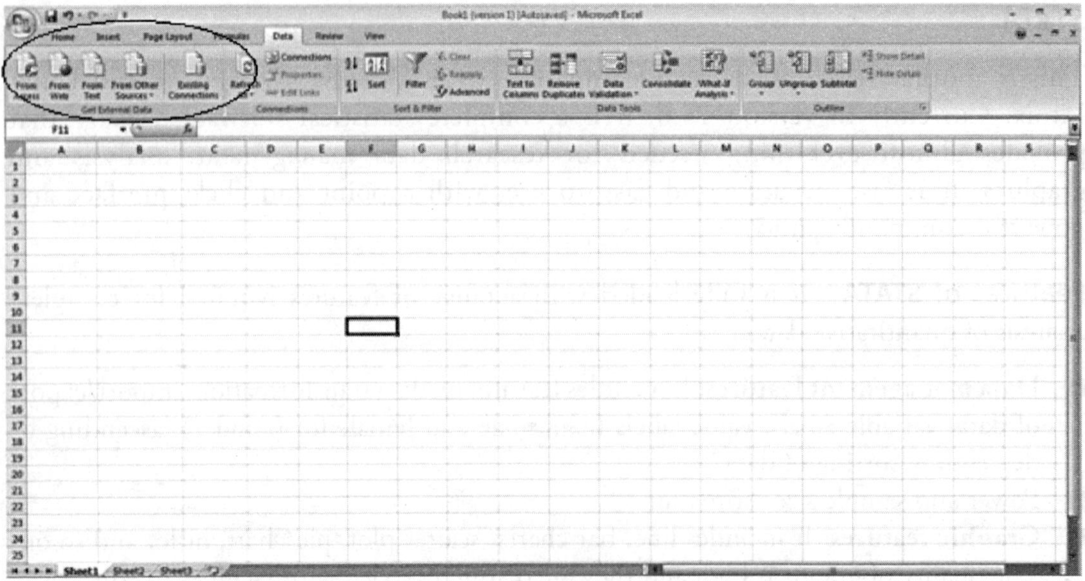

Figure 17.1 Blank Excel spreadsheet for data entry

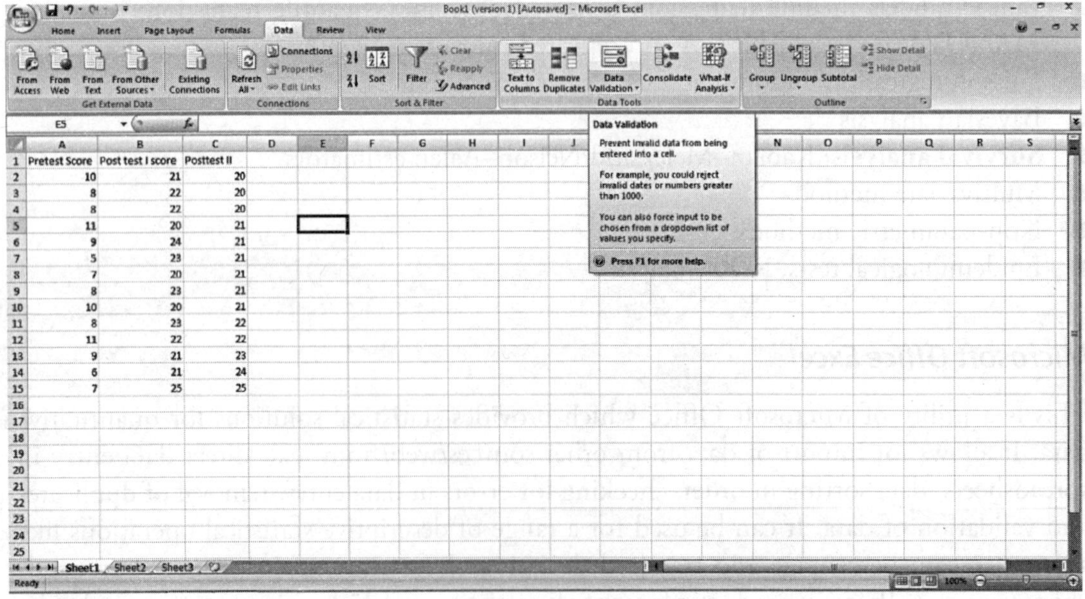

Pretest Score	Post test I score	Posttest II
10	21	20
8	22	20
8	22	20
11	20	21
9	24	21
5	23	21
7	20	21
8	23	21
10	20	21
8	23	22
11	22	22
9	21	23
6	21	24
7	25	25

Figure 17.2 Data validation tool in Excel

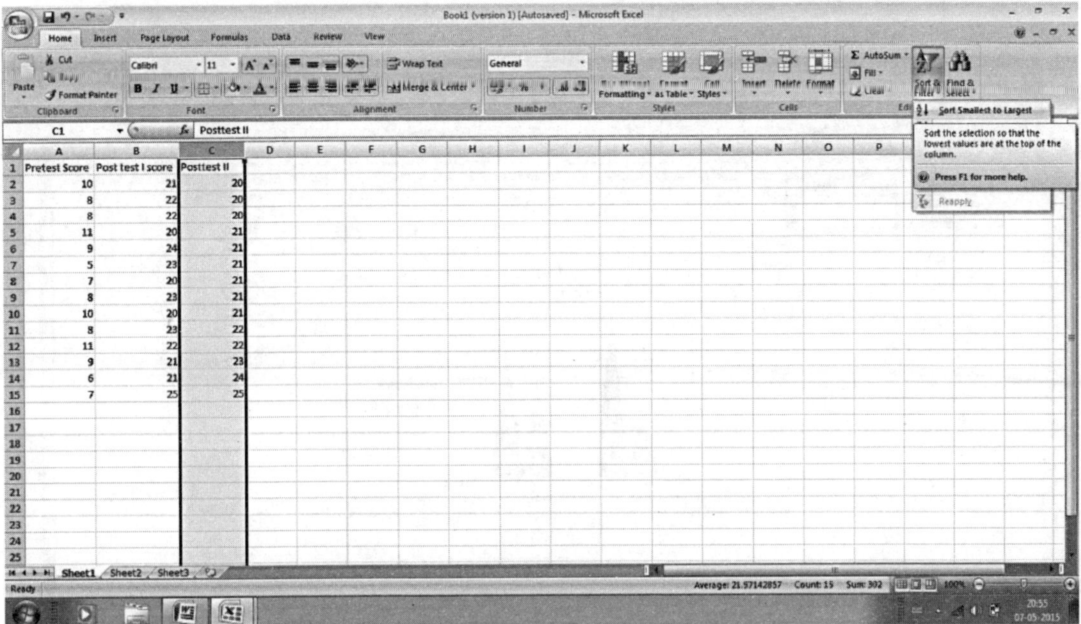

Figure 17.3 Sorting and filtering data function in Excel

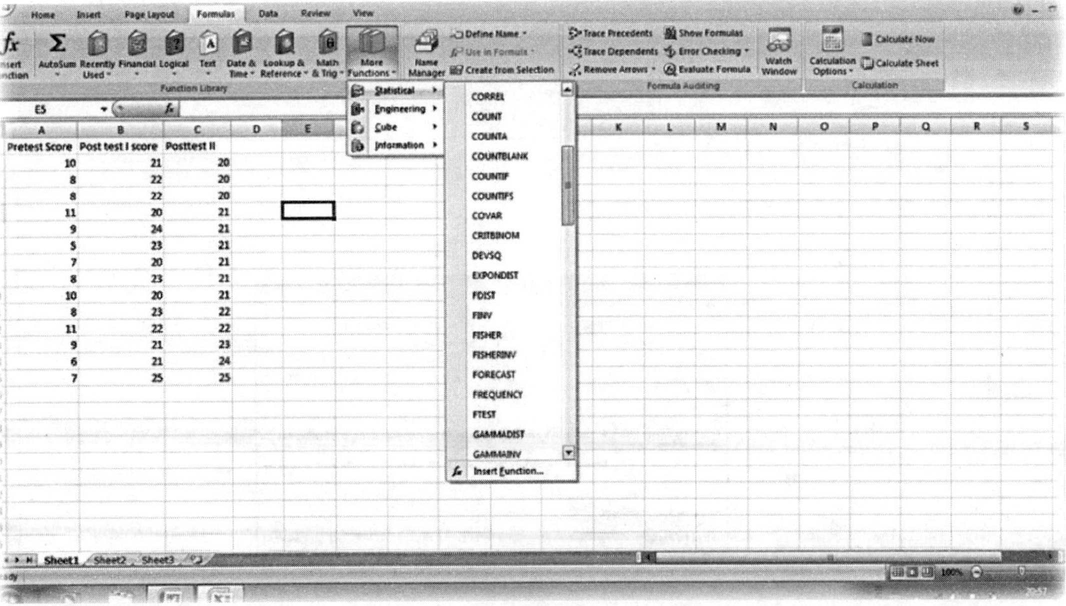

Figure 17.4 Different types of statistical tests available under the More Functions tab

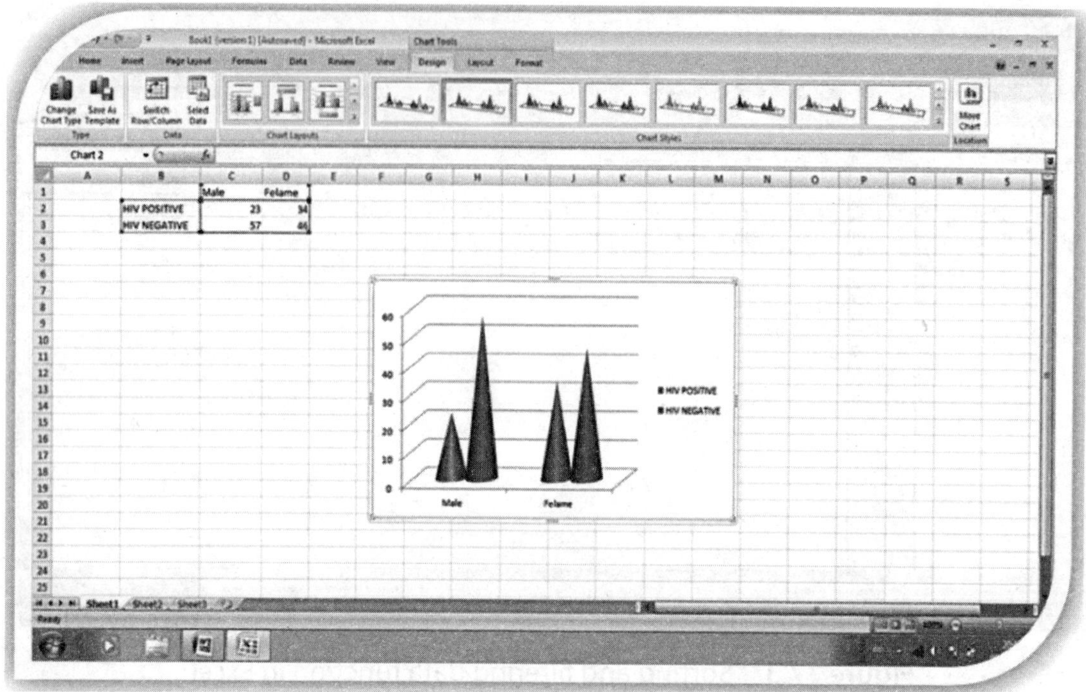

Figure 17.5 Graphical interface in Excel

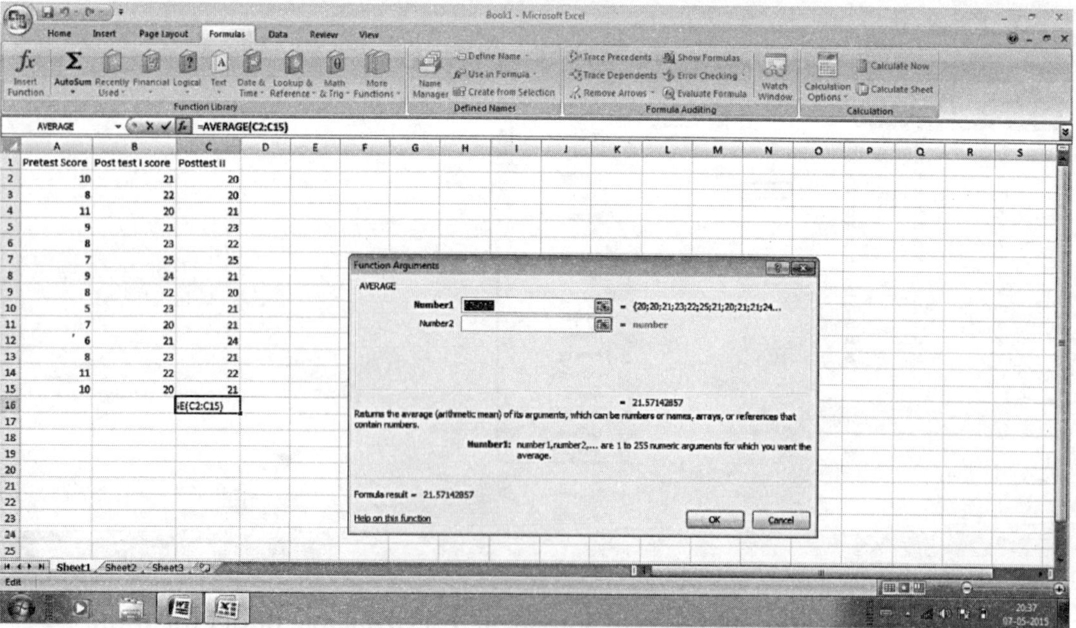

Figure 17.6 Computation of mean in Excel

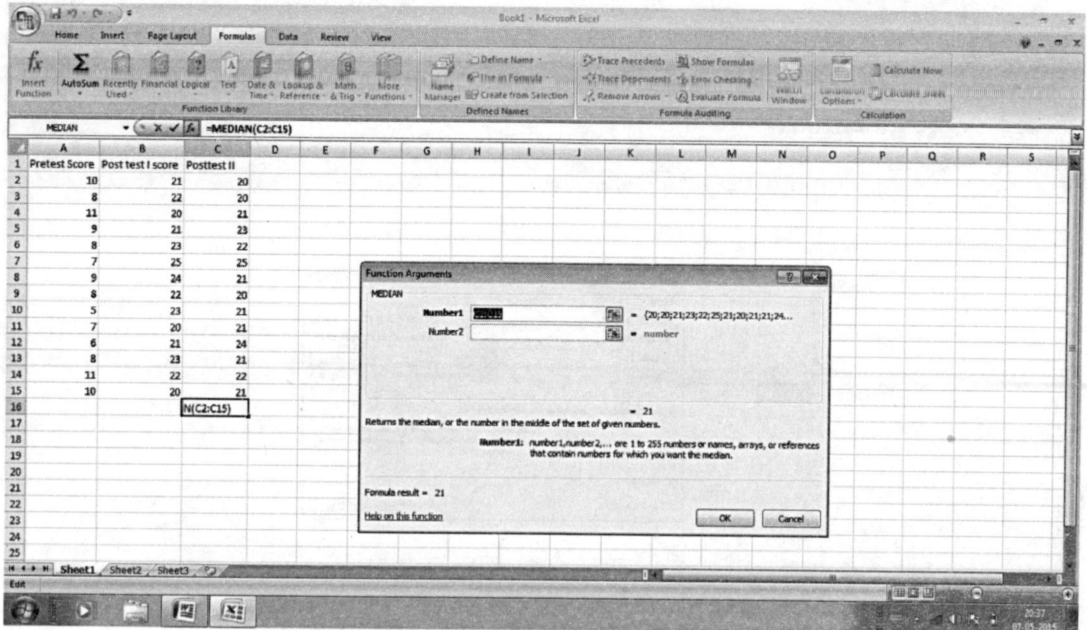

Figure 17.7 Computation of median in Excel

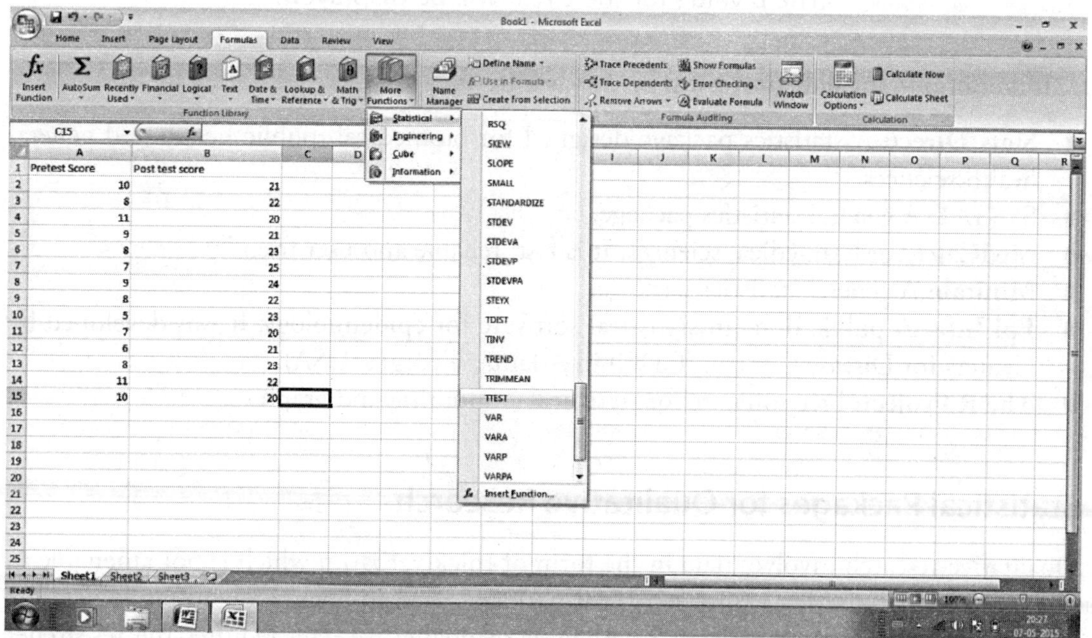

Figure 17.8 Computation of t-test in Excel

1. Enter data for two independent groups. 2. Click on the Formulas tab. Click on More Functions and select TTEST from the drop-down menu.

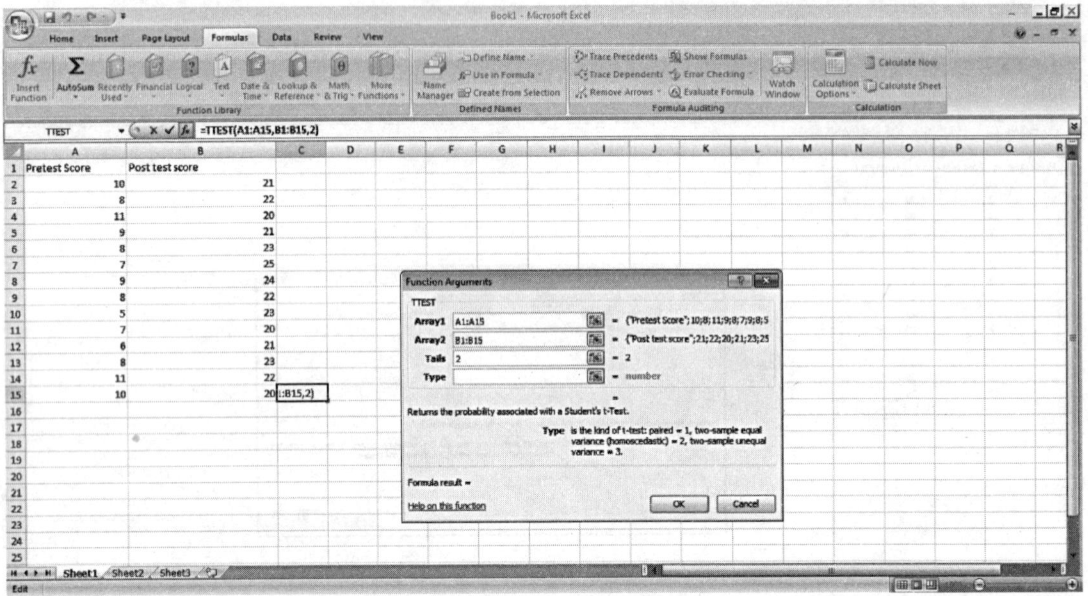

Figure 17.9 Execution of t-test in Excel

3. The Function Arguments window is displayed. Enter the column and row details of both the groups data in Array 1 and Array 2. 4. Enter the tails (one-tailed or two-tailed test) and the type of the test (independent or dependent). 5. Click OK. The *p* value for the t-test will be displayed.

Other important statistical packages are as follows:

- **Stats Direct:** A statistics package designed for biomedical, public health and general health sciences.
- **SYSTAT:** A general statistics package.
- **MedCalc:** For biomedical sciences. It is fast, reliable and user friendly.
- **Minitab:** A general statistics package.
- **Epi Info:** A public domain statistical software for epidemiology. It was developed by Centers for Disease Control (CDC) in Atlanta, Georgia (USA).
- **The R Project:** Free software for statistical computing and graphics.

Statistical Packages for Qualitative Research

Qualitative research involves data in the form of thick verbatim which is not amenable to quantitative analysis. Therefore, statistical packages used to analyse quantitative data are not useful for qualitative researchers. Analysis of qualitative data requires the researcher to immerse herself in the data to identify the relevant themes and categories leading to a theory. It is more difficult to execute manually as compared to quantitative data analysis. Therefore, attempts were made in the mid-1980s by several qualitative researchers with expertise in computer technology to develop statistical packages for qualitative data analysis. Software programs like Ethnograph, TAP and Qualpro started a chain of statistical package developments in the field of qualitative research. Initial developments were not user-friendly; later they were improved by the inclusion of many features. Today, there are more than 25 packages which are user-friendly and easy to use for qualitative data analysis (Fig. 17.10). NVivo, HyperRESEARCH, Hypersoft and Ethnograph are some of the widely used software packages among qualitative researchers. However, unlike quantitative

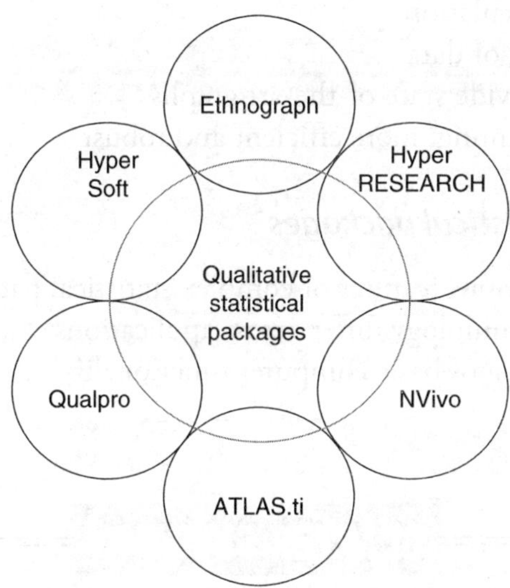

Figure 17.10 Qualitative statistical packages

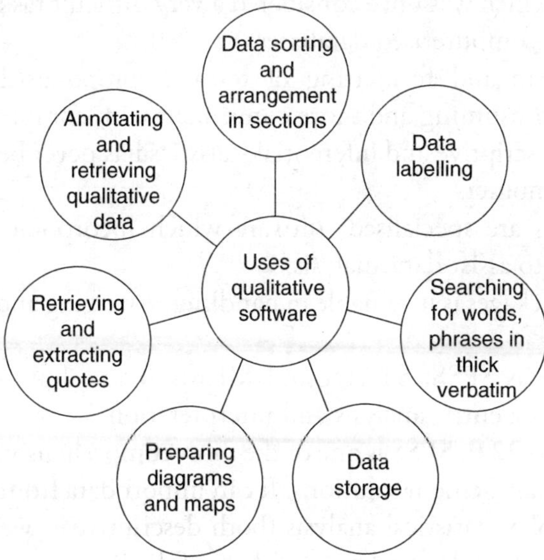

Figure 17.11 Use of qualitative software

statistical packages, qualitative packages cannot be considered as a single method that can be applied in a step-by-step manner. There is a considerable range of features in qualitative programmes: some can analyse textual information while others can handle images, sound and video captured by qualitative researchers.

These statistical packages are useful for undertaking the tasks depicted in Fig. 17.11.

Advantages of statistical packages

- Provides error-free calculation
- Efficient management of data
- Graphical utilities provide state-of-the-art graphs
- Faster, less time-consuming, more efficient and robust

Disadvantages of statistical packages

- Understanding the various features of complex statistical packages may be difficult
- Menu, syntax and terminology differ across applications
- Requires understanding of basic computer functionality

CHAPTER SUMMARY

- The computer processes raw data into organised, meaningful and useful information and stores the results.
- Literature review, which was once considered a very difficult task, has become very easy with the advent of computerised databases.
- Preparation, revision and formatting of research proposals/documents/theses have become less time-consuming and more convenient with computers.
- Computation of descriptive and inferential statistics has never been as easy as it is today with the use of computers.
- Statistical packages are specialised software which incorporate specific features and syntax commands to assist data analysis.
- Use of statistical packages is invaluable in handling, arranging and storing large amounts of data efficiently.
- Spreadsheets, such as SPSS, STATA and Microsoft Excel are some of the statistical packages used in data entry, analysis and interpretation.
- Currently in version 22.0, SPSS is one of the most comprehensive and flexible statistical analysis and data management solutions. It can import data from almost any type of file and conduct complex statistical analysis (both descriptive as well inferential statistics) to generate tabulated results, and graphs/chart of distributions and trends.

- Currently in version 14.0, STATA is a complete statistical software package that provides almost everything needed for research data management, analysis and graphics.
- Microsoft Office Excel can be used for a range of descriptive statistical operations like average, mean, percentage and standard deviation. Inferential statistical tests like t-test, chi-square test, Pearson product moment, F statistics and Fisher's exact test can also be executed in Excel.
- Stats Direct, SYSTAT, MedCalc, Minitab, R and Epi Info are some of the widely used statistical packages for data analysis in quantitative research.
- Software programs like Ethnograph, TAP and Qualpro started a chain of statistical package development in the field of qualitative research.
- NVivo, HyperRESEARCH, Hypersoft and Ethnograph are some of the widely used software among qualitative researchers.
- There is a considerable range of features in qualitative programmes: some can analyse textual information, while others can handle images, sound and video captured by qualitative researchers.
- The advantages of statistical packages include error-free calculation, less-time consuming and efficient data management solutions.
- The disadvantage of statistical packages is that understanding of various features of complex statistical packages may be difficult.

EVALUATE YOURSELF

Long Answer Questions

Q1: Describe the use of computers in the health sciences.

Q2: Define statistical packages. Explain any one commonly used comprehensive statistical package for analysis of quantitative data.

Q3: What is the role of statistical packages in the analysis of qualitative research data?

Short Answer Questions

Write short notes on

Q1: Quantitative statistical packages

Q2: Qualitative statistical packages

Q3: Use of computers in data analysis

Multiple Choice Questions

Q1: Which of following is a software package for qualitative data analysis?
(a) HyperRESEARCH (b) STATA
(c) SPSS (d) SAS

Q2: Which of the following packages is used for quantitative data analysis?
(a) HyperRESEARCH (b) Ethnograph
(c) Qualpro (d) MATLAB

Answers

1. a **2.** d

FURTHER READING

IBM SPSS Statistics. (http://spss.co.in/spssstatistics.aspx)

Kelle U (ed). 1995. *Computer-aided qualitative data analysis. Theory, methods and practice.* Sage, London.

Seidel J, Kelle U. 1995. Different functions of coding in the analysis of textual data. In: *Computer-aided qualitative data analysis. Theory, methods and practice.* U Kelle (ed). Sage, London.

STATA. Data Analysis and Statistical Software. (http://www.stata.com/)

Weitzman E, Miles MB. 1995. *Computer programs for qualitative data analysis.* Sage, Thousand Oaks, CA.

Annexure

STANDARD NORMAL DISTRIBUTION

Table values represent area to the *left* of the *Z* score (cumulative probabilities for positive *z*-values)

Z	0	0.01	0.02	0.03	0.04	0.05	0.06	0.07	0.08	0.09
0.0	0.5000	0.5040	0.5080	0.5120	0.5159	0.5199	0.5239	0.5279	0.5319	0.5359
0.1	0.5398	0.5438	0.5478	0.5517	0.5557	0.5596	0.5636	0.5675	0.5714	0.5753
0.2	0.5793	0.5832	0.5871	0.5909	0.5948	0.5987	0.6026	0.6064	0.6103	0.6141
0.3	0.6179	0.6217	0.6255	0.6293	0.6331	0.6368	0.6406	0.6443	0.6480	0.6517
0.4	0.6554	0.6591	0.6628	0.6664	0.6700	0.6736	0.6772	0.6808	0.6844	0.6879
0.5	0.6915	0.6950	0.6985	0.7019	0.7054	0.7088	0.7123	0.7157	0.7190	0.7224
0.6	0.7257	0.7291	0.7324	0.7356	0.7389	0.7421	0.7454	0.7486	0.7517	0.7549
0.7	0.7580	0.7611	0.7642	0.7673	0.7703	0.7734	0.7764	0.7793	0.7823	0.7852
0.8	0.7881	0.7910	0.7939	0.7967	0.7995	0.8023	0.8051	0.8078	0.8106	0.8133
0.9	0.8159	0.8186	0.8212	0.8238	0.8264	0.8289	0.8315	0.8340	0.8365	0.8389
1.0	0.8413	0.8437	0.8461	0.8485	0.8508	0.8531	0.8554	0.8577	0.8599	0.8621
1.1	0.8643	0.8665	0.8686	0.8708	0.8729	0.8749	0.8770	0.8790	0.8810	0.8829
1.2	0.8849	0.8869	0.8888	0.8906	0.8925	0.8943	0.8962	0.8980	0.8997	0.9015
1.3	0.9032	0.9049	0.9066	0.9082	0.9099	0.9115	0.9131	0.9147	0.9162	0.9177
1.4	0.9192	0.9207	0.9222	0.9236	0.9251	0.9265	0.9278	0.9292	0.9306	0.9319
1.5	0.9332	0.9345	0.9357	0.9370	0.9382	0.9394	0.9406	0.9418	0.9429	0.9441
1.6	0.9452	0.9463	0.9474	0.9484	0.9495	0.9505	0.9515	0.9525	0.9535	0.9545
1.7	0.9554	0.9564	0.9573	0.9582	0.9591	0.9599	0.9608	0.9616	0.9625	0.9633
1.8	0.9641	0.9648	0.9656	0.9664	0.9671	0.9678	0.9686	0.9693	0.9699	0.9706
1.9	0.9713	0.9719	0.9726	0.9732	0.9738	0.9744	0.9750	0.9756	0.9761	0.9767
2.0	0.9773	0.9778	0.9783	0.9788	0.9793	0.9798	0.9803	0.9808	0.9812	0.9817

(*Continued*)

Continued

Z	0	0.01	0.02	0.03	0.04	0.05	0.06	0.07	0.08	0.09
2.1	0.9821	0.9826	0.9830	0.9834	0.9838	0.9842	0.9846	0.9850	0.9854	0.9857
2.2	0.9861	0.9864	0.9868	0.9871	0.9874	0.9878	0.9881	0.9884	0.9887	0.9890
2.3	0.9893	0.9896	0.9898	0.9901	0.9904	0.9906	0.9909	0.9911	0.9913	0.9916
2.4	0.9918	0.9920	0.9922	0.9924	0.9927	0.9929	0.9930	0.9932	0.9934	0.9936
2.5	0.9938	0.9940	0.9941	0.9943	0.9945	0.9946	0.9948	0.9949	0.9951	0.9952
2.6	0.9953	0.9955	0.9956	0.9957	0.9958	0.9960	0.9961	0.9962	0.9963	0.9964
2.7	0.9965	0.9966	0.9967	0.9968	0.9969	0.9970	0.9971	0.9972	0.9973	0.9974
2.8	0.9974	0.9975	0.9976	0.9977	0.9977	0.9978	0.9979	0.9979	0.9980	0.9981
2.9	0.9981	0.9982	0.9983	0.9983	0.9984	0.9984	0.9985	0.9985	0.9986	0.9986
3.0	0.9986	0.9987	0.9987	0.9988	0.9988	0.9989	0.9989	0.9989	0.9989	0.9990

Annexure

STANDARD NORMAL DISTRIBUTION

Table values represent area to the *right* of the *Z* score (cumulative probabilities for negative *z*-values)

z	0.00	0.01	0.02	0.03	0.04	0.05	0.06	0.07	0.08	0.09
−3.0	0.0013	0.0013	0.0013	0.0012	0.0012	0.0011	0.0011	0.0011	0.001	0.001
−2.9	0.0019	0.0018	0.0018	0.0017	0.0016	0.0016	0.0015	0.0015	0.0014	0.0014
−2.8	0.0026	0.0025	0.0024	0.0023	0.0023	0.0022	0.0021	0.0021	0.002	0.0019
−2.7	0.0035	0.0034	0.0033	0.0032	0.0031	0.003	0.0029	0.0028	0.0027	0.0026
−2.6	0.0047	0.0045	0.0044	0.0043	0.0041	0.004	0.0039	0.0038	0.0037	0.0036
−2.5	0.0062	0.006	0.0059	0.0057	0.0055	0.0054	0.0052	0.0051	0.0049	0.0048
−2.4	0.0082	0.008	0.0078	0.0075	0.0073	0.0071	0.0069	0.0068	0.0066	0.0064
−2.3	0.0107	0.0104	0.0102	0.0099	0.0096	0.0094	0.0091	0.0089	0.0087	0.0084
−2.2	0.0139	0.0136	0.0132	0.0129	0.0125	0.0122	0.0119	0.0116	0.0113	0.011
−2.1	0.0179	0.0174	0.017	0.0166	0.0162	0.0158	0.0154	0.015	0.0146	0.0143
−2.0	0.0228	0.0222	0.0217	0.0212	0.0207	0.0202	0.0197	0.0192	0.0188	0.0183
−1.9	0.0287	0.0281	0.0274	0.0268	0.0262	0.0256	0.025	0.0244	0.0239	0.0233
−1.8	0.0359	0.0351	0.0344	0.0336	0.0329	0.0322	0.0314	0.0307	0.0301	0.0294
−1.7	0.0446	0.0436	0.0427	0.0418	0.0409	0.0401	0.0392	0.0384	0.0375	0.0367
−1.6	0.0548	0.0537	0.0526	0.0516	0.0505	0.0495	0.0485	0.0475	0.0465	0.0455
−1.5	0.0668	0.0655	0.0643	0.063	0.0618	0.0606	0.0594	0.0582	0.0571	0.0559
−1.4	0.0808	0.0793	0.0778	0.0764	0.0749	0.0735	0.0721	0.0708	0.0694	0.0681
−1.3	0.0968	0.0951	0.0934	0.0918	0.0901	0.0885	0.0869	0.0853	0.0838	0.0823
−1.2	0.1151	0.1131	0.1112	0.1093	0.1075	0.1056	0.1038	0.102	0.1003	0.0985
−1.1	0.1357	0.1335	0.1314	0.1292	0.1271	0.1251	0.123	0.121	0.119	0.117
−1.0	0.1587	0.1562	0.1539	0.1515	0.1492	0.1469	0.1446	0.1423	0.1401	0.1379

(*Continued*)

Continued

z	0.00	0.01	0.02	0.03	0.04	0.05	0.06	0.07	0.08	0.09
–0.9	0.1841	0.1814	0.1788	0.1762	0.1736	0.1711	0.1685	0.166	0.1635	0.1611
–0.8	0.2119	0.209	0.2061	0.2033	0.2005	0.1977	0.1949	0.1922	0.1894	0.1867
–0.7	0.242	0.2389	0.2358	0.2327	0.2296	0.2266	0.2236	0.2206	0.2177	0.2148
–0.6	0.2743	0.2709	0.2676	0.2643	0.2611	0.2578	0.2546	0.2514	0.2483	0.2451
–0.5	0.3085	0.305	0.3015	0.2981	0.2946	0.2912	0.2877	0.2843	0.281	0.2776
–0.4	0.3446	0.3409	0.3372	0.3336	0.33	0.3264	0.3228	0.3192	0.3156	0.3121
–0.3	0.3821	0.3783	0.3745	0.3707	0.3669	0.3632	0.3594	0.3557	0.352	0.3483
–0.2	0.4207	0.4168	0.4129	0.409	0.4052	0.4013	0.3974	0.3936	0.3897	0.3859
–0.1	0.4602	0.4562	0.4522	0.4483	0.4443	0.4404	0.4364	0.4325	0.4286	0.4247
0.0	0.5	0.496	0.492	0.488	0.484	0.4801	0.4761	0.4721	0.4681	0.4641

Annexure

DISTRIBUTION OF *T* PROBABILITY (ONE-TAILED TEST)

Degree of freedom	α = 0.10	α = 0.05	α = .025	α = .01	α = .005	α = .0005
1	3.078	6.314	12.706	31.821	63.657	636.619
2	1.886	2.920	4.303	6.965	9.925	31.598
3	1.638	2.353	3.182	4.541	5.841	12.941
4	1.533	2.132	2.776	3.747	4.604	8.610
5	1.476	2.015	2.571	3.376	4.032	6.859
6	1.440	1.953	2.447	3.143	3.707	5.959
7	1.415	1.895	2.365	2.998	3.449	5.405
8	1.397	1.860	2.306	2.896	3.355	5.041
9	1.383	1.833	2.262	2.821	3.250	4.781
10	1.372	1.812	2.228	2.765	3.169	4.587
11	1.363	1.796	2.201	2.718	3.106	4.437
12	1.356	1.782	2.179	2.681	3.055	4.318
13	1.350	1.771	2.160	2.650	3.012	4.221
14	1.345	1.761	2.145	2.624	2.977	4.140
15	1.341	1.753	2.131	2.602	2.947	4.073
16	1.337	1.746	2.120	2.583	2.921	4.015
17	1.333	1.740	2.110	2.567	2.898	3.965
18	1.330	1.734	2.101	2.552	2.878	3.922
19	1.328	1.729	2.093	2.539	2.861	3.883
20	1.325	1.725	2.086	2.528	2.845	3.850
21	1.323	1.721	2.080	2.518	2.831	3.819
22	1.321	1.717	2.074	2.508	2.819	3.792
23	1.319	1.714	2.069	2.500	2.807	3.767
24	1.318	1.711	2.064	2.492	2.797	3.745
25	1.316	1.708	2.060	2.485	2.787	3.725

(*Continued*)

Continued

Degree of freedom	α = 0.10	α = 0.05	α = .025	α = .01	α = .005	α = .0005
26	1.315	1.706	2.056	2.479	2.779	3.707
27	1.314	1.703	2.052	2.473	2.771	3.690
28	1.313	1.701	2.048	2.467	2.763	3.674
29	1.311	1.699	2.045	2.462	2.756	3.659
30	1.310	1.697	2.042	2.457	2.750	3.646
40	1.303	1.684	2.021	2.423	2.704	3.551
60	1.296	1.671	2.000	2.390	2.660	3.460
120	1.289	1.658	1.980	2.358	2.617	3.373
∞	1.282	1.645	1.960	2.326	2.576	3.291

Annexure

DISTRIBUTION OF *T* PROBABILITY (TWO-TAILED TEST)

Degree of freedom	$\alpha = 0.20$	$\alpha = .10$	$\alpha = .05$	$\alpha = .02$	$\alpha = .01$	$\alpha = .001$
1	3.078	6.314	12.706	31.821	63.657	636.619
2	1.886	2.920	4.303	6.965	9.925	31.598
3	1.638	2.353	3.182	4.541	5.841	12.941
4	1.533	2.132	2.776	3.747	4.604	8.610
5	1.476	2.015	2.571	3.376	4.032	6.859
6	1.440	1.953	2.447	3.143	3.707	5.959
7	1.415	1.895	2.365	2.998	3.449	5.405
8	1.397	1.860	2.306	2.896	3.355	5.041
9	1.383	1.833	2.262	2.821	3.250	4.781
10	1.372	1.812	2.228	2.765	3.169	4.587
11	1.363	1.796	2.201	2.718	3.106	4.437
12	1.356	1.782	2.179	2.681	3.055	4.318
13	1.350	1.771	2.160	2.650	3.012	4.221
14	1.345	1.761	2.145	2.624	2.977	4.140
15	1.341	1.753	2.131	2.602	2.947	4.073
16	1.337	1.746	2.120	2.583	2.921	4.015
17	1.333	1.740	2.110	2.567	2.898	3.965
18	1.330	1.734	2.101	2.552	2.878	3.922
19	1.328	1.729	2.093	2.539	2.861	3.883
20	1.325	1.725	2.086	2.528	2.845	3.850
21	1.323	1.721	2.080	2.518	2.831	3.819
22	1.321	1.717	2.074	2.508	2.819	3.792
23	1.319	1.714	2.069	2.500	2.807	3.767
24	1.318	1.711	2.064	2.492	2.797	3.745
25	1.316	1.708	2.060	2.485	2.787	3.725

(*Continued*)

Continued

Degree of freedom	α = 0.20	α = .10	α = .05	α = .02	α = .01	α = .001
26	1.315	1.706	2.056	2.479	2.779	3.707
27	1.314	1.703	2.052	2.473	2.771	3.690
28	1.313	1.701	2.048	2.467	2.763	3.674
29	1.311	1.699	2.045	2.462	2.756	3.659
30	1.310	1.697	2.042	2.457	2.750	3.646
40	1.303	1.684	2.021	2.423	2.704	3.551
60	1.296	1.671	2.000	2.390	2.660	3.460
120	1.289	1.658	1.980	2.358	2.617	3.373
∞	1.282	1.645	1.960	2.326	2.576	3.291

Annexure

F VALUES FOR α = 0.05 (TWO-TAILED TEST) AND α = 0.025 (ONE-TAILED TEST)

df_B / df_W	1	2	3	4	5	6	8	10	12	20	30	∞
1	161.4	199.5	215.7	224.6	230.2	234	238.9	241.9	243.9	248.0	250.1	254.3
2	18.51	19.00	19.16	19.25	19.30	19.33	19.37	19.39	19.41	19.44	19.46	19.50
3	10.13	9.55	9.28	9.12	9.01	8.94	8.85	8.79	8.75	8.66	8.62	8.53
4	7.71	6.94	6.59	6.39	6.26	6.16	6.04	5.96	5.91	5.80	5.75	5.63
5	6.61	5.79	5.41	5.19	5.05	4.95	4.82	4.74	4.68	4.56	4.50	4.36
6	5.99	5.14	4.76	4.53	4.39	4.28	4.15	4.06	4.00	3.87	3.81	3.67
7	5.59	4.74	4.35	4.12	3.97	3.87	3.73	3.64	3.58	3.44	3.38	3.23
8	5.32	4.46	4.07	3.84	3.69	3.58	3.44	3.35	3.28	3.15	3.08	2.93
9	5.12	4.26	3.86	3.63	3.48	3.37	3.23	3.14	3.07	2.94	2.86	2.71
10	4.96	4.10	3.71	3.48	3.33	3.22	3.07	2.98	2.91	2.77	2.70	2.54
11	4.84	3.98	3.59	3.36	3.20	3.09	2.95	2.85	2.79	2.65	2.57	2.40
12	4.75	3.89	3.49	3.26	3.11	3.00	2.85	2.75	2.69	2.54	2.47	2.30
13	4.67	3.81	3.41	3.18	3.03	2.92	2.77	2.67	2.60	2.46	2.38	2.21
14	4.60	3.74	3.34	3.11	2.96	2.85	2.70	2.60	2.53	2.39	2.31	2.13
15	4.54	3.68	3.29	3.06	2.90	2.79	2.64	2.54	2.48	2.33	2.25	2.07
16	4.49	3.63	3.24	3.01	2.85	2.74	2.59	2.49	2.43	2.28	2.19	2.01
17	4.45	3.59	3.20	2.97	2.81	2.70	2.55	2.45	2.38	2.23	2.15	1.96
18	4.41	3.55	3.16	2.93	2.77	2.66	2.51	2.41	2.34	2.19	2.11	1.92
19	4.38	3.52	3.13	2.90	2.74	2.63	2.48	2.38	2.31	2.15	2.07	1.88
20	4.35	3.49	3.10	2.87	2.71	2.60	2.45	2.35	2.28	2.12	2.04	1.84
21	4.32	3.47	3.07	2.84	2.69	2.57	2.42	2.32	2.25	2.10	2.01	1.81
22	4.30	3.44	3.05	2.82	2.66	2.55	2.40	2.30	2.23	2.07	1.98	1.78
23	4.28	3.42	3.03	2.80	2.64	2.53	2.38	2.28	2.20	2.05	1.96	1.76

(*Continued*)

Continued

df_B / df_w	1	2	3	4	5	6	8	10	12	20	30	∞
24	4.26	3.40	3.01	2.78	2.62	2.51	2.36	2.26	2.18	2.03	1.94	1.73
25	4.24	3.39	2.99	2.76	2.60	2.49	2.34	2.24	2.17	2.01	1.92	1.71
26	4.22	3.37	2.98	2.74	2.59	2.47	2.32	2.22	2.15	1.99	1.90	1.69
27	4.21	3.35	2.96	2.73	2.57	2.46	2.31	2.20	2.13	1.97	1.88	1.67
28	4.20	3.34	2.95	2.71	2.56	2.45	2.29	2.19	2.12	1.96	1.87	1.65
29	4.18	3.33	2.93	2.70	2.55	2.43	2.28	2.18	2.10	1.94	1.85	1.64
30	4.17	3.32	2.92	2.69	2.53	2.42	2.27	2.17	2.09	1.93	1.84	1.62
40	4.08	3.23	2.84	2.61	2.45	2.34	2.18	2.08	2.00	1.84	1.74	1.51
60	4.00	3.15	2.76	2.53	2.37	2.25	2.10	1.99	1.92	1.75	1.65	1.39
120	3.92	3.07	2.68	2.45	2.29	2.18	2.02	1.91	1.83	1.66	1.55	1.25
∞	3.84	3.00	2.60	2.37	2.21	2.10	1.94	1.83	1.75	1.57	1.46	1.00

Annexure

F VALUES FOR α = 0.01 (TWO-TAILED TEST) AND α = 0.005 (ONE-TAILED TEST)

df_B / df_w	1	2	3	4	5	6	8	10	12	20	30	∞
1	4052	4999	5403	5624	5763	5858	5981	6055	6106	6208	6260	6365
2	98.50	99	99.17	99.25	99.30	99.33	99.37	99.40	99.42	99.45	99.47	99.5
3	34.12	30.82	29.46	28.71	28.24	27.91	27.49	27.23	27.05	26.69	26.50	26.12
4	21.20	18.00	16.69	15.98	15.52	15.21	14.80	14.55	14.37	14.02	13.84	13.46
5	16.26	13.27	12.06	11.39	10.97	10.67	10.29	10.05	9.89	9.55	9.38	9.02
6	13.74	10.92	9.78	9.15	8.75	8.47	8.10	7.87	7.72	7.40	7.23	6.88
7	12.25	9.55	8.45	7.85	7.46	7.19	6.84	6.62	6.47	6.16	5.99	5.65
8	11.26	8.65	7.59	7.01	6.63	6.37	6.03	5.81	5.67	5.36	5.20	4.86
9	10.56	8.02	6.99	6.42	6.06	5.80	5.47	5.26	5.11	4.81	4.65	4.31
10	10.04	7.56	6.55	5.99	5.64	5.39	5.06	4.85	4.71	4.40	4.25	3.91
11	9.65	7.20	6.22	5.67	5.32	5.07	4.74	4.54	4.40	4.10	3.94	3.60
12	9.33	6.93	5.95	5.41	5.06	4.82	4.50	4.30	4.15	3.86	3.70	3.36
13	9.07	6.70	5.74	5.20	4.86	4.62	4.30	4.10	3.96	3.66	3.51	3.16
14	8.86	6.51	5.56	5.03	4.69	4.46	4.14	3.94	3.80	3.50	3.35	3.00
15	8.68	6.36	5.42	4.89	4.56	4.32	4.00	3.81	3.67	3.37	3.21	2.87
16	8.53	6.23	5.29	4.77	4.44	4.20	3.89	3.69	3.55	3.26	3.10	2.75
17	8.40	6.11	5.18	4.67	4.34	4.10	3.79	3.59	3.45	3.16	3.00	2.65
18	8.28	6.01	5.09	4.58	4.25	4.01	3.70	3.51	3.37	3.08	2.92	2.57
19	8.18	5.93	5.01	4.50	4.17	3.94	3.63	3.43	3.30	3.00	2.84	2.49
20	8.10	5.85	4.94	4.43	4.10	3.87	3.56	3.37	3.23	2.94	2.78	2.42
21	8.02	5.78	4.87	4.37	4.04	3.81	3.51	3.31	3.17	2.88	2.72	2.36
22	7.94	5.72	4.82	4.31	3.99	3.76	3.45	3.26	3.12	2.83	2.67	2.30
23	7.88	5.66	4.76	4.26	3.94	3.71	3.41	3.21	3.07	2.78	2.62	2.26

(*Continued*)

Continued

df_B / df_w	1	2	3	4	5	6	8	10	12	20	30	∞
24	7.82	5.61	4.72	4.22	3.89	3.67	3.36	3.17	3.03	2.74	2.58	2.21
25	7.77	5.57	4.67	4.18	3.85	3.63	3.32	3.13	2.99	2.70	2.54	2.17
26	7.72	5.53	4.64	4.14	3.82	3.59	3.29	3.09	2.96	2.66	2.50	2.13
27	7.68	5.49	4.60	4.11	3.78	3.56	3.26	3.06	2.93	2.63	2.47	2.10
28	7.64	5.45	4.57	4.07	3.75	3.53	3.23	3.03	2.90	2.60	2.44	2.06
29	7.60	5.42	4.54	4.04	3.72	3.50	3.20	3.00	2.87	2.57	2.41	2.03
30	7.56	5.39	4.51	4.02	3.70	3.47	3.17	2.98	2.84	2.55	2.39	2.01
40	7.31	5.18	4.31	3.83	3.51	3.29	2.99	2.80	2.67	2.37	2.20	1.80
60	7.08	4.98	4.13	3.65	3.34	3.12	2.82	2.63	2.50	2.20	2.03	1.60
120	6.85	4.79	3.95	3.48	3.17	2.96	2.66	2.47	2.34	2.03	1.86	1.38
∞	6.63	4.60	3.78	3.32	3.02	2.80	2.51	2.32	2.19	1.88	1.70	1.00

Annexure

F VALUES FOR $\alpha = 0.001$ (TWO-TAILED TEST) AND $\alpha = 0.0005$ (ONE-TAILED TEST)

df_B / df_w	1	2	3	4	5	6	8	12	24	∞
1	405284	500000	540379	562500	576405	585937	598144	610667	623497	636619
2	998.5	999	999.2	999.2	999.3	999.3	999.4	999.4	999.5	999.5
3	167.5	148.5	141.1	137.1	134.6	132.8	130.6	128.3	125.9	123.5
4	74.14	61.25	56.18	53.44	51.71	50.53	49	47.41	45.77	44.05
5	47.04	36.61	33.2	31.09	29.75	28.84	27.64	26.42	25.14	23.78
6	35.51	27	23.7	21.9	20.81	20.03	19.03	17.99	16.89	15.75
7	29.22	21.69	18.77	17.19	16.21	15.52	14.63	13.71	12.73	11.69
8	25.42	18.49	15.83	14.39	13.49	12.86	17.04	11.19	10.3	9.34
9	22.86	16.39	13.9	12.56	11.71	11.13	10.37	9.57	8.72	7.81
10	21.04	14.91	12.55	11.28	10.48	9.92	9.2	8.45	7.64	6.76
11	19.69	13.81	11.56	10.35	9.58	9.05	8.35	7.63	6.85	6
12	18.64	12.97	10.8	9.63	8.89	8.38	7.71	7	6.25	5.42
13	17.81	12.31	10.21	9.07	8.35	7.86	7.21	6.52	5.78	4.97
14	17.14	11.78	9.73	8.62	7.92	7.43	6.8	6.13	5.41	4.6
15	16.59	11.34	9.34	8.25	7.57	7.09	6.47	5.81	5.1	4.31
16	16.12	10.97	9	7.94	7.27	6.81	6.19	5.55	4.85	4.06
17	15.72	10.66	8.73	7.68	7.02	6.56	5.96	5.32	4.63	3.85
18	15.38	10.39	8.49	7.46	6.81	6.35	5.76	5.13	4.45	3.67
19	15.08	10.16	8.28	7.26	6.61	6.18	5.59	4.97	4.29	3.52
20	14.82	9.95	8.1	7.10	6.46	6.02	5.44	4.82	4.15	3.38
21	14.59	9.77	7.94	6.95	6.32	5.88	5.31	4.7	4.03	3.26
22	14.38	9.61	7.8	6.81	6.19	5.76	5.19	4.58	3.92	3.15
23	14.19	9.47	7.67	6.69	6.08	5.65	5.09	4.48	3.82	3.05

(*Continued*)

Continued

df_B / df_w	1	2	3	4	5	6	8	12	24	∞
24	14.03	9.34	7.55	6.59	5.98	5.55	4.99	4.39	3.74	2.97
25	13.88	9.22	7.45	6.49	5.88	5.46	4.91	4.31	3.66	2.89
26	13.74	9.12	7.36	6.41	5.8	5.38	4.83	4.24	3.59	2.82
27	13.61	9.02	7.27	6.33	5.73	5.31	4.76	4.17	3.52	2.75
28	13.50	8.93	7.19	6.25	5.66	5.24	4.69	4.11	3.46	2.7
29	13.39	8.85	7.12	6.19	5.59	5.18	4.64	4.05	3.41	2.64
30	13.29	8.77	7.05	6.12	5.53	5.12	4.58	4	3.36	2.59
40	12.61	8.25	6.6	5.7	5.13	4.73	4.21	3.64	3.01	2.23
60	11.97	7.76	6.17	5.31	4.76	4.37	3.87	3.31	2.69	1.9
120	11.38	7.31	5.79	4.95	4.42	4.04	3.55	3.02	2.4	1.56
∞	10.83	6.91	5.42	4.62	4.1	3.74	3.27	2.74	2.13	1.00

Annexure

DISTRIBUTION OF CHI SQUARE PROBABILITY

df	Level of significance					
	.10	.05	.02	.01	.005	.001
1	2.706	3.841	5.41	6.635	7.879	10.83
2	4.605	5.991	7.82	9.210	10.597	13.82
3	6.251	7.815	9.84	11.345	12.838	16.27
4	7.779	9.488	11.67	13.277	14.860	18.46
5	9.236	11.070	13.39	15.086	16.750	20.52
6	10.645	12.592	15.03	16.812	18.548	22.46
7	12.017	14.067	16.62	18.475	20.278	24.32
8	13.362	15.507	18.17	20.090	21.955	26.12
9	14.684	16.919	19.68	21.666	23.589	27.88
10	15.987	18.307	21.16	23.209	25.188	29.59
11	17.275	19.675	22.62	24.725	26.757	31.26
12	18.549	21.026	24.05	26.217	28.300	32.91
13	19.812	22.362	25.47	27.688	29.819	34.53
14	21.064	23.685	26.87	29.141	31.319	36.12
15	22.307	24.996	28.26	30.578	32.801	37.7
16	23.542	26.296	29.63	32.000	34.267	39.25
17	24.769	27.587	31	33.409	35.718	40.79
18	25.989	28.869	32.35	34.805	37.156	42.31
19	27.204	30.144	33.69	36.191	38.582	43.82
20	28.412	31.410	35.02	37.566	39.997	45.32
21	29.615	32.671	36.34	38.932	41.401	46.80
22	30.813	33.924	37.66	40.289	42.796	48.27
23	32.007	35.172	38.97	41.638	44.181	49.73
24	33.196	36.415	40.27	42.980	45.559	51.18
25	34.382	37.652	41.57	44.314	46.928	52.62
26	35.563	38.885	42.86	45.642	48.290	54.05
27	36.741	40.113	44.14	46.963	49.645	55.48
28	37.916	41.337	45.42	48.278	50.993	56.89
29	39.087	42.557	46.69	49.588	52.336	58.30
30	40.256	43.773	47.96	50.892	53.672	59.7

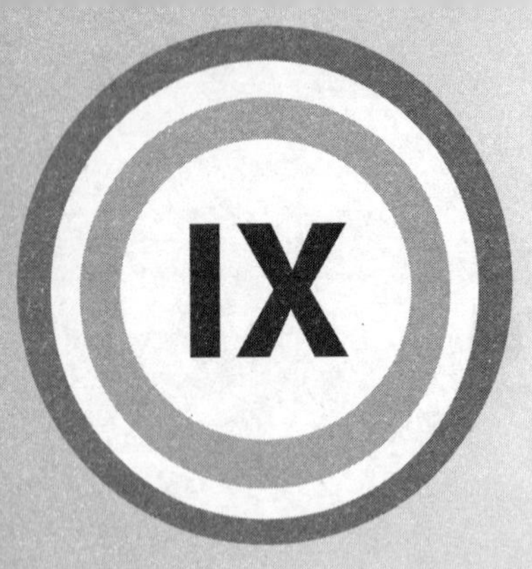

Annexure

SIGNIFICANT VALUES OF THE CORRELATION COEFFICIENT

df	Level of significance (one tailed/two tailed)				
	.05/.10	.025/.05	.01/.02	.005/.01	.0005/.001
1	.988	.997	.9995	.9999	0.9999
2	.900	.950	.980	.990	0.999
3	.805	.878	.934	.959	0.991
4	.729	.811	.882	.917	0.974
5	.669	.754	.833	.874	0.951
6	.622	.707	.789	.834	0.925
7	.582	.666	.750	.798	0.898
8	.549	.632	.716	.765	0.872
9	.521	.602	.685	.735	0.847
10	.497	.576	.658	.708	0.823
11	.476	.553	.634	.684	0.801
12	.458	.532	.612	.661	0.780
13	.441	.514	.592	.641	0.760
14	.426	.497	.574	.623	0.742
15	.412	.482	.558	.606	0.725
16	.400	.468	.542	.590	0.708
17	.389	.456	.528	.575	0.693
18	.378	.444	.516	.561	0.679
19	.369	.433	.503	.549	0.665
20	.360	.423	.492	.537	0.652
21	.352	.413	.482	.526	0.640
22	.344	.404	.472	.515	0.629
23	.337	.396	.462	.505	0.618
24	.330	.388	.453	.496	0.607
25	.323	.381	.445	.487	0.597

(*Continued*)

Continued

df	Level of significance (one tailed/two tailed)				
	.05/.10	.025/.05	.01/.02	.005/.01	.0005/.001
26	.317	.374	.437	.479	0.588
27	.311	.367	.430	.471	0.579
28	.306	.361	.423	.463	0.570
29	.301	.355	.416	.456	0.562
30	.296	.349	.409	.449	0.554
35	.275	.325	.381	.418	0.519
40	.257	.304	.358	.393	0.490
45	.243	.288	.338	.372	0.465
50	.231	.273	.322	.354	0.443
60	.211	.250	.295	.325	0.408
70	.195	.232	.274	.303	0.380
80	.183	.217	.256	.283	0.357
90	.173	.205	.242	.267	0.338
100	.164	.195	.230	.254	0.321

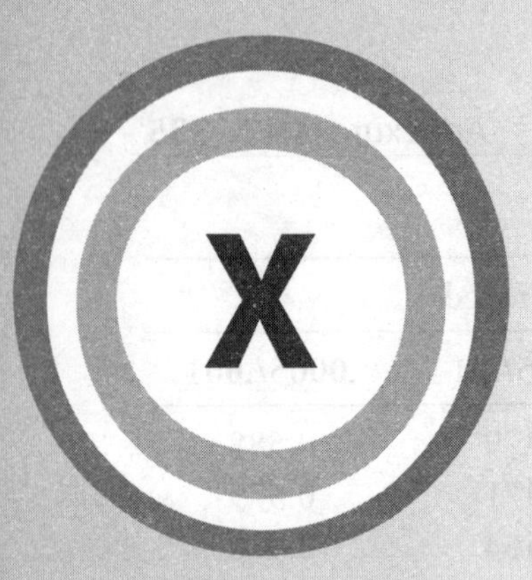

Annexure

SPEARMAN'S RANK CORRELATION COEFFICIENT

N	Level of significance (one tailed/two tailed)		
	0.05/0.10	0.025/0.05	0.005/0.01
5	.900	1.00	–
6	.829	.886	1.00
7	.714	.786	.929
8	.643	.738	.881
9	.600	.700	.833
10	.564	.648	.794
11	.536	.618	.755
12	.503	.587	.727
13	.484	.560	.703
14	.464	.538	.679
15	.446	.521	.654
16	.429	.503	.635
17	.414	.488	.618
18	.401	.472	.600
19	.391	.460	.584
20	.380	.447	.570
21	.370	.436	.556
22	.361	.425	.544
23	.353	.416	.532
24	.344	.407	.521
25	.337	.398	.511
26	.331	.390	.501
27	.324	.383	.492
28	.318	.375	.483
29	.312	.368	.475
30	.306	.362	.467
35	.283	.335	.433
40	.264	.313	.405
45	.248	.294	.382
50	.235	.279	.363

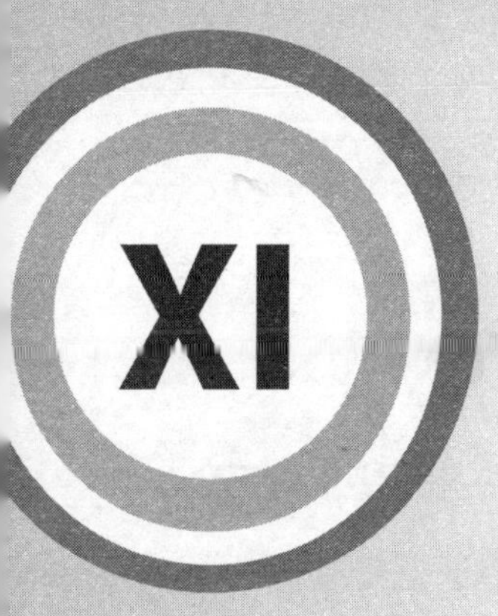

Annexure

WILCOXON SIGNED RANK TEST

N	Level of significance (one tailed/two tailed)	
	0.025/0.05	0.005/0.01
6	0	–
7	2	–
8	3	0
9	5	1
10	8	3
11	10	5
12	13	7
13	17	9
14	21	12
15	25	15
16	29	19
17	34	23
18	40	27
19	46	32
20	52	37
21	58	42
22	65	48
23	73	54
24	81	61
25	89	68

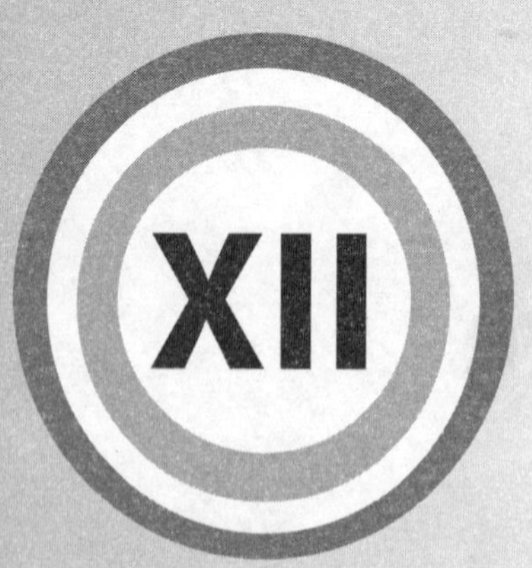

Annexure

SIGN TEST

N	Level of significance (one tailed/two tailed)		
	0.05/0.10	0.025/0.05	0.01/0.02
5	0	–	–
6	0	0	–
7	0	0	0
8	1	0	0
9	1	1	0
10	1	1	0
11	2	1	1
12	2	2	1
13	3	2	1
14	3	2	2
15	3	3	2
16	4	3	2
17	4	4	3
18	5	4	3
19	5	4	4
20	5	5	4
21	6	5	4
22	6	5	5
23	7	6	5
24	7	6	5
25	7	7	6

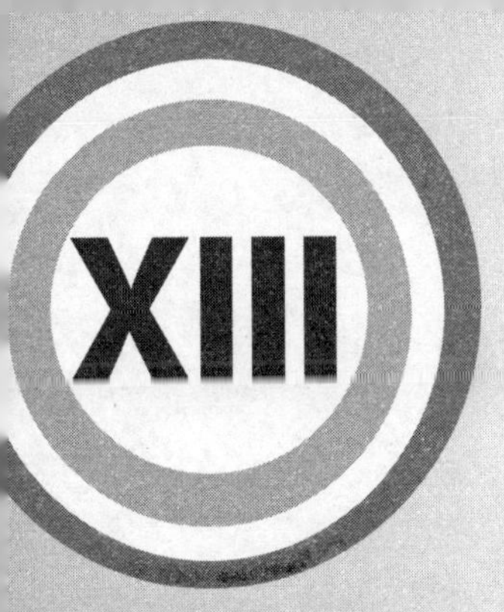

Annexure

MANN–WHITNEY U TEST

$\alpha = 0.05$ (two-tailed); 0.025 (one-tailed)

		N2															
		5	6	7	8	9	10	11	12	13	14	15	16	17	18	19	20
	5	2	3	5	6	7	8	9	11	12	13	14	15	17	18	19	20
	6		5	6	8	10	11	13	14	16	17	19	21	22	24	25	27
	7			8	10	12	14	16	18	20	22	24	26	28	30	32	34
	8				13	15	17	19	22	24	26	29	31	34	36	38	41
	9					17	20	23	26	28	31	34	37	39	42	45	48
	10						23	26	29	33	36	39	42	45	48	52	55
	11							30	33	37	40	44	47	51	55	58	62
N1	12								37	41	45	49	53	57	61	65	69
	13									45	50	54	59	63	67	72	76
	14										55	59	64	69	74	78	83
	15											64	70	75	80	85	90
	16												75	81	86	92	98
	17													87	93	99	105
	18														99	106	112
	19															113	119
	20																127

Annexure

MANN–WHITNEY U TEST

$\alpha = 0.01$ (two-tailed); $\alpha = 0.005$ (one-tailed)

		N2															
		5	6	7	8	9	10	11	12	13	14	15	16	17	18	19	20
	5	0	1	1	2	3	4	5	6	7	7	8	9	10	11	12	13
	6		2	3	4	5	6	7	9	10	11	12	13	15	16	17	18
	7			4	6	7	9	10	12	13	15	16	18	19	21	22	24
	8				7	9	11	13	15	17	18	20	22	24	26	28	30
	9					11	13	16	18	20	22	24	27	29	31	33	36
	10						16	18	21	24	26	29	31	34	37	39	42
	11							21	24	27	30	33	36	39	42	45	48
N1	12								27	31	34	37	41	44	47	51	54
	13									34	38	42	45	49	53	57	60
	14										42	46	50	54	58	63	67
	15											51	55	60	64	69	73
	16												60	65	70	74	79
	17													70	75	81	86
	18														81	87	92
	19															93	99
	20																105

Model Question Paper I

Time: 3 hours **Max. Marks: 80**

Note: Attempt all questions.

Marks are indicated against each question.

1. Define problem statement. Enlist the criteria of good research problem. Discuss in brief the steps of research process. *(2 + 6 + 8)*
2. Differentiate between qualitative and quantitative research designs. Discuss experimental design in detail. *(8 + 8)*
3. Define population and sample. Discuss the types of sampling techniques. *(4 + 12)*
4. Write short notes on (any four) *4*
   (a) Hypothesis
   (b) Reliability
   (c) Ethics in research
   (d) Variables
   (e) Data collection procedures
   (f) Scale of measurement
5. Define statistics. Discuss in detail the graphical presentation of data. *(4 + 12)*
6. Discuss in brief:- *(8 + 8)*
   (i) Review of literature
   (ii) Utilization of research finding
7. Calculate mean, median and mode of the following data:- *(5 + 6 + 5)*

Marks	Frequency
0–20	10
20–40	24
40–60	36
60–80	20
80–100	10

Model Question Paper II

Time: 3 hours **Max. Marks: 80**

Note: Attempt any five questions.

Marks are indicated against each question.

1. Define research and nursing research. Describe the characteristics of a good research. *(3 + 3 + 10)*
2. Define sampling and discuss different types of sampling techniques. *(3 + 13)*
3. Write short notes on (any four)
   (a) Questionnaires
   (b) Pilot study
   (c) Review of literature
   (d) Variables
   (e) Hypothesis
   (f) Steps of nursing research
4. Define research design, explain about experimental research design. *(4 + 12)*
5. Explain in brief:- *(8 + 8)*
   (a) Methods of data collection
   (b) Writing a research report
6. Calculate mean, median and mode for the following data *(5 + 6 + 5)*

   X – 10, 20, 30, 40, 50
   Frequency – 4, 5, 3, 2, 5

7. Calculate mean, median and standard deviation for the following data *(5 + 5 + 6)*

   X – 2, 4, 6, 8, 10, 12, 14
   Frequency – 4, 6, 11, 12, 14, 13, 10

Model Question Paper III

Time: 3 hours (180 Min) **Maximum: 100 marks**

Answer ALL questions in the same order.
Answer Section A and Section B Separately

SECTION A
(NURSING RESEARCH)

I. Elaborate on: *(2 × 20 = 40)*

1. Explain the Purpose, Scope, Sources and the steps in Review of Literature in Detail
2. Describe Non-experimental Research Design in detail with Suitable Example.

II. Write Notes on: *(4 × 5 = 20)*

1. Need for Research In Nursing.
2. List the steps in development and refinement of Research Problem.
3. Pilot Study.
4. List the components of a Research Report.

III. Short Answers on: *(5 × 2 = 10)*

1. List the types of Qualitative Design.
2. Types of validity.
3. List the component of critiquing Published Research.
4. List 4 features influencing sampling process.
5. Define Nursing Research.

SECTION B
(STATISTICS)

I. Write Notes on: *(4 × 5 = 20)*

1. Calculate the Co-efficient of Correlation for the Data.

X	10	12	18	24	23	27
Y	13	18	12	25	30	10

2. Nine students are chosen at random from a group and their heights are found to be 63, 63, 64, 65, 69, 69, 70, 70, 71. Test whether the mean height may be taken to be 65. [t0.05 = 2.31]
3. Types of diagrams and its uses in Statistics.
4. Define.
   (a) Test of Hypothesis
   (b) Type I error and Type II error

II. Short Answers on: *(5 × 2 = 10)*

1. Write short noes on Classification of data.
2. Write 4 properties of normal distribution.
3. List the uses of Chi-square test.
4. Find the mode of the following data
   24, 28, 20, 28, 36, 37, 36, 50, 80, 28.
5. Properties of Correlation Coefficient.

Model Question Paper IV

Time: 3 hours **Maximum: 75 marks**

SECTION A
NURSING RESEARCH

I. Elaborate on: *(1 × 15 = 15)*

1. Explain the data collection tools with examples.

II. Write Notes on: *(4 × 5 = 20)*

1. Conceptual framework
2. Item analysis
3. Interview method
4. Utilization of research findings

III. Short Answer Questions: *(7 × 2 = 14)*

1. Need for nursing research
2. Randomization
3. Types of validity
4. Sampling error
5. Population
6. Case study
7. Define problem statement

SECTION B
STATISTICS

I. Elaborate on: *(1 × 15 = 15)*

1. A random sample of size 15 from a normal population yields a mean value of 2.23 and a variance of 7.33. Does this support the hypothesis that the population mean is '0'? (Table value: 2.145).

II. Write Notes on: *(1 × 5 = 5)*

1. Define type-I and type-II error

III. Short Answer Questions: *(3 × 2 = 6)*

1. Explain Bar chart.
2. Explain measures of Dispersion.
3. Which test is used for samples of two different times, namely pre and post?

Model Question Paper V

Time: 3 hours **Max Marks: 75**

Note: Attempt all questions. Use of calculators or any electronic device is not allowed.

(Nursing Research) *(50)*

1. Define the following Terms:
   (a) Research Hypothesis (b) Research Population
   (c) Research Variable (d) Quantitative Research
   (e) Sample and sampling *(2 × 5 = 10)*
2. Differenciate the following:
   (a) Probability and Non Probability sampling
   (b) Experimental and Non Experimental research.
   (c) Dependent and Independent variables.
   (d) Validity and Reliability of a research tool.
   (e) Self Report and observation method. *(3 × 5 = 15)*
3. (a) Define Research & Nursing Research
   (b) Discuss in brief Need & significance of Nursing Research.
   (c) Describe in brief steps of research process. *(2 + 6 + 7 = 15)*
4. Write short notes on any five of the following.
   (a) Pilot Study (b) Sources of literatures Review
   (c) Characteristics of a good research (d) Communication of research finding
   (e) Historical survey (f) Methods of data collection *(2 × 5 = 10)*

(Statistics) *(25)*

1. Define the following terms.
   (a) Statistics (b) Data & Datum
   (c) Standard Deviation (d) Normal distribution
   (e) Measures of variability *(2 × 5 = 10)*
2. Describe Frequency distribution and Graphical presentation of data. *(10)*
3. Calculate Arithmetic mean of the following data.
   23, 22, 20, 24, 16, 17, 18, 19, 21 *(5)*

Model Question Paper VI

Time: 3 Hrs **Max. Marks: 75**

- Answer all questions
- Use Only Ordinary Calculator

Essay *(15)*

1. Define sampling. Discuss the types of sampling and the factors influencing the sampling process. *(2 + 8 + 5 = 15)*

Short Notes *(5 × 5 = 25)*

2. Criteria of good research problem.
3. Types of research instruments.
4. Human rights in nursing research
5. Experimental designs.
6. Pilot study

Answer the following *(5 × 5 = 25)*

7. Birth weights of 10 newborns are 3.3 kg, 6.1 kg, 5.8 kg, 3.8 kg, 2.7 kg, 4.1 kg, 3.9 kg, 5.1 kg, 3.0 kg and 3.8 kg. Find out the mean value and median value.
8. The blood sugar of the patients attending diabetes clinic is as follows draw a histogram using this data.

Blood sugar (mg/DI)	No. of patients
70–80	5
80–90	10
90–100	20
100–110	30
110–120	25

9. Utilization of research findings
10. Inferential statistics
11. Purpose of literature review.

Differentiate between *(5 × 2 = 10)*

12. Hypothesis and Assumption
13. Dependent and Extraneous variables
14. Phenomenology and Historical research.
15. CINHAL and COCHRANE
16. Manipulation and Control in true experimental study.

Index

A

analysis of variance (ANOVA) 327
  assumptions 328
  steps in 328
  types 328
assent 17

B

Betty Neuman's healthcare systems model 114, 126
bio-physiological methods 177
  advantages 179
  disadvantages 179
  in vitro 178
  in vivo 178
biostatistics 262–263
bivariate statistics 265

C

causality 314
chi-square test 333
  salient features 335
  steps in 334
class interval width 195
communication and utilisation of research **212–234**
  abstract 222
  disseminating results at conferences 214
    oral presentation 214
    poster presentation 215
  how to communicate findings 213
  introduction to communication of findings 212
  publishing a journal article 216
    preparing the article 217
  preparing theses and dissertations 218
    characteristics 218
    outline 219
    writing 218
  research utilisation 227
    barriers to 227
    bridging the research and practice gap 229
    CURN project 229
    facilitators of 228
    innovation diffusion model 229
    Stetler model 230
  Vancouver reference style 225
confidence interval 264
construct 114
correlation coefficient 181
critical region 264
critiquing research articles/reports **235–246**
  introduction to 235
  definitions of 235
  example 240
  steps in qualitative research critiquing 243
  steps in quantitative research critiquing 236
Cronbach's alpha 182
crude
  birth rate 268
  death rate 269
CURN project 229

D

data analysis 104, **192–211**
  analysis and interpretation 205

classification 192
chronological 193
geographical 192
qualitative 193
quantitative 193
graphical presentation 198
constructing a graph 199
types 199
introduction to 192
organisation 193
frequency distribution 194
tabulation 196
classification 198
constructing a table 196
data collection tools and techniques **156–191**, 254
developing the plan 157
bio-physiological methods 177
interviews 160
observations 164
projective techniques 176
Q sorts 177
questionnaires 157
vignettes 175
data collection procedure 184
introduction to 156
pilot study 184
reliability of instrument 180
validity of instrument 179
definition
literature review 60
research and nursing research 3
research approach/design 74
research critiquing 235
research problem/question 32
sampling techniques 133
theoretical/conceptual framework 114
degree of freedom 265
demography 270

E

ethics in nursing research 14
informed consent 16
format 17
principle of beneficence 15
principle of justice 16
principle of respect for human dignity 16
evidence-based nursing practice
barriers to implement 13
importance 13
steps involved 14
evolution of nursing research
in India10
in the West 9

F

factor analysis 265
factorial 85
feasibility 39
FINER criteria 41

G

general fertility rate (GFR) 268
graphs, types
frequency polygon 201
histogram 200
multiple bar chart 200
simple bar chart 200
subdivided bar chart 200
Ogive 202
pictogram 205
pie diagram 202

H

how to rank data 310–312
hypothesis 33, 48, 339
characteristics of 49
testing 52, 337–338
types of 49
hypothesis, testing
errors in 53
steps in 52
hypothesis testing, errors
alpha 53
beta 53
effect size 54
p value 54
type I 53

type II 53
hypothesis, types
alternative 50
one-tailed 51
two-tailed 51
complex 51
directional 52
non-directional 52
null 49
research 50
simple 51
statistical 49

I

Imogene King
systems interaction model 126
theory of goal attainment 115
incidence rate 268–269
index of equivalence 183
infant mortality rate 270
interviews
advantages 163
conducting 163
disadvantages 164
instructions to conduct 162
types of 161
semi-structured 161
structured 161
unstructured 161
vs questionnaires 164
introduction to statistics **262–274**
applications and scope in health 266
anatomy 267
microbiology 267
nursing 266
pathology 267
pharmacology 267
physiology 267
public health 267
basic terminology 263
biostatistics 262
types and levels of data 270
interval scale 270
nominal scale 270
ordinal scale 270
ratio scale 271
types of methods 265
descriptive 265
inferential 265
vital health statistics 267
relating to fertility 268
relating to morbidity 268
relating to mortality 269

L

level of significance 263–264
Ludwig von Bertalanffy's systems theory 125

M

manipulation 79
marriage rate 268
maternal mortality rate 269
McNemar's test 342
assumptions 342
steps in 342
measures of central tendency **275–288**
introduction to 275
mean 276
advantages 280
calculation for class interval data 278
calculation for grouped data 277
calculation for ungrouped data 276
characteristics 276
limitations 280
median 280
advantages 281
calculation 280
limitations 281
mode 282
advantages 283
calculation 282
limitations 284
position of measures 284
skewed distribution 284
negative skewness 285
selecting the measure 284
measures of relationship **302–320**
correlation, meaning and need 302

correlation statistics 306
Karl Pearson's product moment method 306
Kendall's tau 312
nominal variables 314
simple linear regression 314
Spearman rho 309
scatter diagram method 303
types of correlation 303
linear 305
multiple 304
negative 304
no correlation 305
non-linear 305
positive 303
simple 304
measures of variability **289–301**
choosing the measure 298
interquartile range 290
advantages 293
disadvantages 293
introduction 289
range 289
advantages 290
disadvantages 290
standard deviation 295
in normal distribution data set 297
shortcut method 296
using Microsoft Excel 296
variance 293
methods of acquiring knowledge 4
problem-solving 4
scientific method 6
modified Berlin questionnaire 183
Mood's median test 341
assumptions 341
steps in 341

N

non-experimental design, research objectives dimension
descriptive 93
exploratory 94
non-experimental design, time dimension
cross-sectional 92
longitudinal 92
prospective 92
retrospective 92
non-probability sampling techniques
consecutive sampling 144
advantage 144
disadvantage 144
convenience sampling 144
advantages 144
disadvantages 144
judgmental/purposive sampling 145
advantages 146
disadvantages 146
quota sampling 144
advantages 145
disadvantages 145
non-proportional 145
proportional 145
sample size determination 148
sequential sampling 148
advantages 148
disadvantages 148
snowball/network sampling 146
advantages 146
disadvantages 147
types 146
use of 148
nursing research during
Nightingale's era 11
twentieth century 11
twenty-first century 12

O

observations
advantages 165
checklist/structured 168
advantages 168
disadvantages 168
disadvantages 166
Guttman scale 173
Likert scale 171
constructing items for 172
guidelines 172
how to improve 172
reliability of 173

Osgood's semantic differential scale
participation 166
planning for 165
rating scale 169
types 169
visual analog scale 174
advantages 174
disadvantages 174
outliers 264

P

P value 54
parametric and non-parametric tests **321–356**
introduction 321
non-parametric tests 332
advantages 350
chi-square 333
disadvantages 350
Fisher's exact 346
Kruskal–Wallis 348
Mann–Whitney U 343
McNemar's 342
Mood's median 341
sign 336
Wilcoxon signed rank test 338
parametric tests 321
analysis of covariance (ANCOVA) 331
analysis of variance (ANOVA) 327
t-test 322
z-test 326
PICOT format 41
point estimation 263
population 34, 133
power of study 264
pre-experimental design
one-shot case study 90
static group comparison 90
pregnancy rate 268
prevalence rate 269
probability sampling techniques
cluster random sampling 141
advantages 141
disadvantages 141
simple random sampling 137
advantages 138
disadvantages 139
steps in 137
stratified random sampling 139
advantages 140
disadvantages 141
disproportionate 140
need for 140
proportionate 139
systematic random sampling 142
advantages 143
disadvantages 143
steps in 142
problem statement, characteristics of 38
format of research problem title 38
problem-solving method 4
steps in 5
projective techniques 176
design 176
structure 176
proposition 115

Q

Q sorts 177
definition of concourse 177
development of Q-set 177
selection of P-set 177
sorting 177
qualitative research designs 96
ethnography 101
data collection techniques 101
finding research sites 101
gaining access to the site 102
keeping field notes and journals 102
writing a report 102
grounded theory 98
methodological characteristics 99
types 99
historical research 96
aims of 97
methodology 97
phenomenology 103
data collection/analysis 104
types 103
qualitative research process 25
analytic phase 27

conceptual phase 25
design 26
dissemination phase 27
quantitative research designs 78
experimental 79
pre- 90
quasi- 88
true 79
non-experimental 91
essential criteria for cause and effect relationship 91
research objectives dimension 91
time dimension 91
validity of 94
external 96
internal 95
quantitative research process 19
analytic phase 24
conceptual phase 20
designing and planning the methodology 20
dissemination phase 25
empirical phase 24
quasi-experimental design 88
advantages 90
disadvantages 90
non-equivalent control group 88
time series 89
questionnaires
advantages 160
characteristics of 158
disadvantages 160
guidelines for constructing and administering 158
methods of administration 159
mail 159
self-administered 160
web-based 159

R

reliability of instrument 180
index of equivalence 183
internal consistency 181
inter-rater 183
modified Berlin questionnaire 183
Spearman–Brown prophecy formula 182
specificity 184
test–retest 180
RRFNS approach 39
feasibility 39
relevance 39
researchability 39
significance 39
research and research process **1–31**
characteristics of good research 8
definitions 3
ethics 14
evidence-based nursing practice 12
evolution of nursing research, India 10
evolution of nursing research, West 9
introduction to nursing research 1
methods of acquiring knowledge 4
need for nursing research 2
qualitative research 25
quantitative research 19
research approaches/designs 26, **74–112**, 104, 252
definition of 74
factors influencing selection of 75
introduction to 74
mixed methods/pragmatic 77
others 104
case study 104
evaluation research 106
focus group interviews 107
meta-analysis 106
secondary data analysis 105
participatory/action 78
qualitative 76, 96
quantitative 76, 78
research objectives, 32, 42
characteristics of 43
research problem/question **32–59**
assumptions 46
characteristics of a good problem statement 38
definitions 32
delimitations 47
evaluation of 38

hypothesis 48
identification of 35
introduction to 34
limitations 47
research objectives 42
research question 40
research variables 43
sources of 36
research proposals **247–261**
introduction to 247
reasons for rejection 257
types of 248
continuation 248
pre-proposals 248
solicited 248
unsolicited 248
writing 248
research question 33, 40
characteristics of 40
FINER criteria 41
types of 41
PICOT format 41
research question, types
causal 42
descriptive 42
relational 42
research variables 43, 45
categorical 44
continuous 44
dependent 44
independent 44
operational definition 45
others 45
review of literature **60–73**
definition of 60
examples 70
format 69
introduction to 60
process 66
purpose of 61
sources of 62
electronic 62
print 66
Roy's adaptation model 114, 116

S

sampling techniques **132–155**, 253
characteristics of good sample 132
definitions 133
factors influencing sampling process 134
need for sample 132
sampling process 135
sampling errors 151
sampling distribution of mean 151
standard error of mean 152
types of 136
non-probability 143
probability 137
scientific method 6
advantages 7
characteristics 6
limitations 8
steps of 7
secondary data analysis 105
secondary sources 62
sensitivity 183
sex ratio 270
sign test 336
hypothesis testing 337
significance of theory 116
significance 39
specific death rate 269
statistical methods, inferential
non-parametric 266
parametric 266
statistically significant result
Stetler model of research utilisation 230

T

t-test
criteria for using 322
types 322
paired/dependent 324
unpaired 322
theoretical/conceptual framework **113–131**, 237–238
characteristics of theory 115
classification of theories 120
grand 120

meta 120
middle-range 120
nursing practice 120
common concepts in nursing theory 116
conceptual model/framework/scheme 121
criteria for evaluating 123
criticism of 127
definition of 114
introduction to 113
selection of 122
significance of theory 116
systems theory 124
theory, research and practice relationship 117
total fertility rate 268
true experiment design 79
control 79
limitations 88
manipulation 79
randomisation 80
strengths 87
types 81
true experiment design, types
cross-over 85
factorial 85
post-test only 81
pretest–post-test 81
randomised block 87
Solomon four-group 82
treatment sequence 86

U

use of computers for data analysis **357–368**
advantages 366
disadvantages 366
introduction 357
use in statistics 358
statistical packages for qualitative research 364
statistical packages for quantitative research 358
Microsoft Office Excel 359
SPSS 358
STATA 359

V

validity of instrument 179
construct 179
content 180
criterion-related 180
face 179
multi-trait multi-method matrix (MTMM) 179
vignettes 175
designing 175
visual analog scale 174
advantages 174
disadvantages 174
vital health statistics, 267–270

W

Wilcoxon signed rank test 338
assumptions 339
hypothesis 339
steps 339

Z

z-test 326
criteria for using 326
steps in 326